The New NOTES

Editor

STAVROS N. STAVROPOULOS

GASTROINTESTINAL ENDOSCOPY
CLINICS OF NORTH AMERICA

www.giendo.theclinics.com

Consulting Editor
CHARLES J. LIGHTDALE

April 2016 • Volume 26 • Number 2

ELSEVIER

1600 John F. Kennedy Boulevard • Suite 1800 • Philadelphia, Pennsylvania, 19103-2899

http://www.theclinics.com

GASTROINTESTINAL ENDOSCOPY CLINICS OF NORTH AMERICA Volume 26, Number 2
April 2016 ISSN 1052-5157, ISBN-13: 978-0-323-41754-9

Editor: Kerry Holland
Developmental Editor: Donald Mumford

Gastrointestinal Endoscopy Clinics of North America (ISSN 1052-5157) is published quarterly by Elsevier Inc., 360 Park Avenue South, New York, NY 10010-1710. Months of issue are January, April, July, and October. Business and Editorial Offices: 1600 John F. Kennedy Blvd., Suite 1800, Philadelphia, PA, 19103-2899. Periodicals postage paid at New York, NY and additional mailing offices. Subscription prices are $335.00 per year for US individuals, $538.00 per year for US institutions, $100.00 per year for US students and residents, $370.00 per year for Canadian individuals, $637.00 per year for Canadian institutions, $465.00 per year for international individuals, $637.00 per year for international institutions, and $245.00 per year for Canadian and foreign students/residents. To receive student/resident rate, orders must be accompanied by name of affiliated institution, date of term, and the *signature* of program/residency coordinator on institution letterhead. Orders will be billed at individual rate until proof of status is received. Foreign air speed delivery is included in all *Clinics* subscription prices. All prices are subject to change without notice. **POSTMASTER:** Send address change to *Gastrointestinal Endoscopy Clinics of North America*, Elsevier Health Sciences Division, Subscription Customer Service, 3251 Riverport Lane, Maryland Heights, MO 63043. **Customer Service: 1-800-654-2452 (US). From outside the United States, call 1-314-447-8871. Fax: 1-314-447-8029. E-mail: JournalsCustomerService-usa@elsevier.com (for print support) or JournalsOnlineSupport-usa@elsevier.com (for online support).**

Reprints. For copies of 100 or more, of articles in this publication, please contact the Commercial Reprints Department, Elsevier Inc., 360 Park Avenue South, New York, NY 10010-1710. Tel. 212-633-3874; Fax: 212-633-3820; E-mail: reprints@elsevier.com.

Gastrointestinal Endoscopy Clinics of North America is covered in *Excerpta Medica*, *MEDLINE/PubMed (Index Medicus), and MEDLINE/MEDLARS.*

Contributors

CONSULTING EDITOR

CHARLES J. LIGHTDALE, MD
Professor of Medicine, Division of Digestive and Liver Diseases, Professor of Medicine, Columbia University Medical Center, New York, New York

EDITOR

STAVROS N. STAVROPOULOS, MD, FASGE
Director of Endoscopy, Director, Program in Advanced Gastrointestinal Endoscopy (P.A.G.E.), Department of Medicine, Division of Digestive and Liver Diseases, Winthrop University Hospital, Mineola, New York; Adjunct Professor of Clinical Medicine, Columbia University, New York, New York; Adjunct Clinical Professor of Medicine, Temple University, Philadelphia, Pennsylvania

AUTHORS

WOOJIN AHN, PhD
Research Assistant Professor, Department of Mechanical, Aerospace and Nuclear Engineering, Center for Modeling, Simulation and Imaging in Medicine, Rennselaer Polytechnic Institute, Troy, New York

JOSEPH RAMON ARMENGOL-MIRO, MD
Professor, World Institute for Digestive Endoscopy (WIDER); Professor, Digestive Endoscopy, Vall D'Hebron University Hospital, Barcelona, Spain

MARKUS BAUDER, MD
Department of Gastroenterology and Oncology, Klinikum Ludwigsburg, Medizinische Klinik I, Ludwigsburg, Germany

ROBERT BECHARA, MD
Assistant Professor, Queen's University Division of Gastroenterology Kingston General and Hotel Dieu Hospitals, Kingston Ontario; Digestive Diseases Centre, Showa University Koto-Toyosu Hospital, Tokyo, Japan

KAREL CACA, MD
Department of Gastroenterology and Oncology, Klinikum Ludwigsburg, Medizinische Klinik I, Ludwigsburg, Germany

MINGYAN CAI, MD
Endoscopy Center and Endoscopy Research Institute, Zhongshan Hospital, Fudan University, Shanghai, China

SUVRANU DE, ScD
J Erik Jonsson '22 Distinguished Professor of Engineering, Director, Department of Mechanical, Aerospace and Nuclear Engineering, Center for Modeling, Simulation and Imaging in Medicine, Rennselaer Polytechnic Institute, Troy, New York

CHRISTOPHER J. GOSTOUT, MD
Professor of Medicine, Division of Gastroenterology and Hepatology, Mayo Clinic, Rochester, Minnesota

OSAMU GOTO, MD, PhD
Division of Research and Development for Minimally Invasive Treatment, Cancer Center, Keio University School of Medicine, Tokyo, Japan

MARK A. GROMSKI, MD
Clinical Fellow, Division of Gastroenterology/Hepatology, Indiana University School of Medicine, Indianapolis, Indiana

ROBERT H. HAWES, MD
Florida Hospital Center for Interventional Endoscopy; Professor of Medicine, University of Central Florida College of Medicine; Medical Director, Florida Hospital Institute for Minimally Invasive Therapy, Orlando, Florida

HARUHIRO INOUE, MD, PhD
Professor and Director, Digestive Diseases Centre, Showa University Koto-Toyosu Hospital, Tokyo, Japan

SERGEY V. KANTSEVOY, MD, PhD
Professor of Medicine, University of Maryland School of Medicine; Director of Therapeutic Endoscopy, Institute for Digestive Health and Liver Diseases, Mercy Medical Center, Baltimore, Maryland; Professor, World Institute for Digestive Endoscopy (WIDER), Barcelona, Spain

MOUEN A. KHASHAB, MD
Director of Therapeutic Endoscopy, Associate Professor, Department of Medicine, Johns Hopkins Hospital; Division of Gastroenterology and Hepatology, Department of Medicine, The Johns Hopkins Medical Institutions, Baltimore, Maryland

HYUNG HUN KIM, MD
Chief Physician, Department of Gastroenterology, Endoscopy Center for Gastrointestinal Oncology, Hansol Hospital, Seoul, Korea

YUKO KITAGAWA, MD, PhD
Department of Surgery, Keio University School of Medicine, Tokyo, Japan

HIDEKI KOBARA, MD, PhD
Department of Gastroenterology and Neurology, Kagawa University, Kita, Kagawa, Japan

CARTER LEBARES, MD
Assistant Professor of Surgery, University of California San Francisco, San Francisco, California

BING-RONG LIU, MD, PhD
Department of Gastroenterology and Hepatology, The Second Affiliated Hospital of Harbin Medical University, Harbin, People's Republic of China

LUÍS CARVALHO LOURENÇO, MD
Gastroenterology Department, Hospital Professor Doutor Fernando Fonseca, Amadora, Portugal

TSUTOMU MASAKI, MD, PhD
Department of Gastroenterology and Neurology, Kagawa University, Kita, Kagawa, Japan

KAI MATTHES, MD, PhD
Department of Anesthesiology, Perioperative and Pain Medicine, Children's Hospital Boston, Harvard Medical School, Boston, Massachusetts

RANI MODAYIL, MD
Winthrop University Hospital, Mineola, New York

HIROHITO MORI, MD, PhD
Department of Gastroenterology and Neurology, Kagawa University, Kita, Kagawa, Japan; Department of Gastroenterological Surgery, Ehime Rosai Hospital, Niihama, Ehime, Japan

SAURABH S. MUKEWAR, MBBS
Fellow Gastroenterology, Division of Gastroenterology and Hepatology, Mayo Clinic, Rochester, Minnesota

PAYAL SAXENA, MBBS, FRACP
Division of Gastroenterology and Hepatology, Assistant Professor, Department of Medicine, Royal Prince Alfred Hospital, Caperdown, New South Wales, Australia; Division of Gastroenterology and Hepatology, Department of Medicine, The Johns Hopkins Medical Institutions, Baltimore, Maryland

ARTHUR SCHMIDT, MD
Department of Gastroenterology and Oncology, Klinikum Ludwigsburg, Medizinische Klinik I, Ludwigsburg, Germany

JI-TAO SONG, MD
Department of Gastroenterology and Hepatology, The Second Affiliated Hospital of Harbin Medical University, Harbin, People's Republic of China

STAVROS N. STAVROPOULOS, MD, FASGE
Director of Endoscopy, Director, Program in Advanced Gastrointestinal Endoscopy (P.A.G.E.), Department of Medicine, Division of Digestive and Liver Diseases, Winthrop University Hospital, Mineola, New York; Adjunct Professor of Clinical Medicine, Columbia University, New York, New York; Adjunct Clinical Professor of Medicine, Temple University, Philadelphia, Pennsylvania

LEE L. SWANSTROM, MD, FACS, FASGE
Institute of Image-guided Minimally Invasive Surgery, Institut Hospitalo Universitair, University of Strasbourg, Strasbourg, France

HIROYA TAKEUCHI, MD, PhD
Department of Surgery, Keio University School of Medicine, Tokyo, Japan

NORIYA UEDO, MD
Vice Director, Department of Gastrointestinal Oncology, Osaka Medical Center for Cancer and Cardiovascular Diseases, Osaka, Japan

NAOHISA YAHAGI, MD, PhD
Division of Research and Development for Minimally Invasive Treatment, Cancer Center, Keio University School of Medicine, Tokyo, Japan

DANFENG ZHANG, MD
Endoscopy Center and Endoscopy Research Institute, Zhongshan Hospital, Fudan University, Shanghai, China

PINGHONG ZHOU, MD, PhD
Endoscopy Center and Endoscopy Research Institute, Zhongshan Hospital, Fudan University, Shanghai, China

Contents

Foreword: The New NOTES Expands Interventional Endoscopy   xiii

Charles J. Lightdale

Preface: The New NOTES: More "E" and Less "S" Leads to Success!   xv

Stavros N. Stavropoulos

Lessons Learned from Traditional NOTES: A Historical Perspective   221

Robert H. Hawes

> The idea of natural orifice surgery was conceived by Kantsevoy and Kalloo in the late 1990s. A group of surgeons formed the Apollo Group in 1997. Their vision and mission were to impact the practice of therapeutic endoscopy through innovation in techniques and technologies. The concept of natural orifice surgery was introduced at the initial meeting held on Kiawah Island, South Carolina in 1998. The original concept of flexible endoscopic surgery involved per-oral passage of a flexible endoscope into the stomach followed by entrance into the peritoneal cavity via a gastrotomy.

The Evolution of "New Notes," Origins, and Future Directions   229

Saurabh S. Mukewar and Christopher J. Gostout

> The transformation of the submucosa into a working space provided a paradigm shift for endolumenal endoscopic intervention. The submucosal space can provide an undermining access to the removal of overlying mucosal disease. This space can also provide a protective mucosal barrier accommodating interventions into the deep layers of the gut wall and body cavities, such as the abdomen and mediastinum.

POEM, the Prototypical "New NOTES" Procedure and First Successful NOTES Procedure   237

Robert Bechara and Haruhiro Inoue

 Video content accompanies this article at www.giendo.theclinics.com

> Peroral endoscopic myotomy (POEM) was first performed in 2008 as a novel treatment of achalasia. It is now performed globally, demonstrating the evolution of the first successful natural orifice transluminal endoscopic surgery (NOTES) procedure. There is extensive data demonstrating the safety and efficacy of POEM, and now long-term data has emerged demonstrating that the efficacy is durable. POEM is also being used to successfully treat diffuse esophageal spasm (DES) and jackhammer esophagus. With jackhammer esophagus and DES, inclusion of the lower esophageal sphincter in the myotomy minimizes the risk of symptom development from iatrogenic ineffective esophageal motility.

Per-Oral Pyloromyotomy (POP): An Emerging Application of Submucosal Tunneling for the Treatment of Refractory Gastroparesis   257

Carter Lebares and Lee L. Swanstrom

A growing body of literature supports the use of laparoscopic pyloroplasty as a minimally invasive treatment of refractory gastroparesis that has failed conservative measures and for benign gastric outlet obstruction. Endoscopic pyloric dilation, stent placement, and Botox have been described for similar indications, but often with transient or mixed results. Per-oral pyloromyotomy has recently been proposed as an endoscopic alternative to surgical pyloroplasty or pylormyotomy because it is less invasive by its nature and potentially more durable than current endoscopic treatments.

Submucosal Tunneling Endoscopic Resection (STER) and Other Novel Applications of Submucosal Tunneling in Humans   271

Bing-Rong Liu and Ji-Tao Song

The submucosal tunneling technique was originally developed to provide safe access to the peritoneal cavity for natural orifice transluminal endoscopic surgery procedures. With this technique, the submucosal tunnel becomes the working space for partial myotomy and tumor resection. The submucosal space has come to represent the "third space" distinguished from gastrointestinal lumen (first space) and peritoneal cavity (second space). New applications continue to be developed and further clinical applications in the future are anticipated. This article summarizes the current applications of submucosal tunneling endoscopic resection for subepithelial tumors and describes other related uses of submucosal tunneling.

Endoscopic Full-thickness Resection (EFTR) for Gastrointestinal Subepithelial Tumors   283

Mingyan Cai, Pinghong Zhou, Luís Carvalho Lourenço, and Danfeng Zhang

 Video content accompanies this article at www.giendo.theclinics.com

There has been booming interest in the endoscopic full-thickness resection (EFTR) technique since it was first described. With the advent of improved and more secure endoscopic closure techniques and devices, such as endoscopic suturing devices, endoscopists are empowered to perform more aggressive procedures than ever. This article focuses on the procedural technique and clinical outcomes of EFTR for gastrointestinal subepithelial tumors.

Non-Exposure, Device-Assisted Endoscopic Full-thickness Resection   297

Markus Bauder, Arthur Schmidt, and Karel Caca

 Video content accompanies this article at www.giendo.theclinics.com

Recent developments have expanded the frontier of interventional endoscopy toward more extended resections following surgical principles. This article presents two new device-assisted techniques for endoscopic full-thickness resection in the upper and lower gastrointestinal tract. Both

methods are nonexposure techniques avoiding exposure of gastrointestinal contents to the peritoneal cavity by a "close first–cut later" principle. The full-thickness resection device is a novel over-the-scope device designed for clip-assisted full-thickness resection of colorectal lesions. Endoscopic full-thickness resection of gastric subepithelial tumors can be performed after placing transmural sutures underneath the tumor with a suturing device originally designed for endoscopic antireflux therapy.

Endoscopic Submucosal Dissection (ESD) and Related Techniques as Precursors of "New Notes" Resection Methods for Gastric Neoplasms   313

Osamu Goto, Hiroya Takeuchi, Yuko Kitagawa, and Naohisa Yahagi

Endoscopic full-thickness resection for subepithelial tumors is one of the more attractive proposed methods for less-invasive transluminal surgery but remains challenging in terms of safety and feasibility. Currently, laparoscopic endoscopic cooperative surgery is thought to be a more clinically acceptable approach. In targeting cancers, however, more advanced non-exposure techniques are required to avoid the risk of iatrogenic tumor seeding. By combining these techniques with possible regional lymphadenectomy using sentinel node navigation surgery, an ideal minimally invasive, function-preserving gastric resection can be achieved even in possible node-positive cancers. Further development for this type of advanced endoscopic surgery is expected.

Novel NOTES Techniques and Experimental Devices for Endoscopic Full-thickness Resection (EFTR)   323

Hirohito Mori, Hideki Kobara, and Tsutomu Masaki

Natural orifice transluminal endoscopic surgery (NOTES), in which a flexible endoscope is used to perform operations that have traditionally required laparoscopic surgery, has garnered attention as a minimally invasive surgery that does not leave a surgical wound on the body. Among the various forms of NOTES, endoscopic full-thickness resection (EFTR) is an ultraminimally invasive endoscopic surgery that allows for radical resection, which is an extension of endoscopic submucosal dissection and involves full-thickness excision of a tumor of the gastrointestinal tract wall. With further development of the equipment, including full-thickness suture instruments, nonexposed EFTR could be a feasible surgical procedure.

Hybrid NOTES: Combined Laparo-endoscopic Full-thickness Resection Techniques   335

Hyung Hun Kim and Noriya Uedo

Advances in laparoscopic surgery and therapeutic endoscopy have allowed these minimally destructive procedures to challenge conventional surgery. Because of its theoretic advantages and technical feasibility, laparoendoscopic full-thickness resection is considered to be the most appropriate option for subepithelial tumor removal. Furthermore, combination of laparoscopic and endoscopic approaches for treatment of neoplasia can be important maneuvers for gastric cancer resection without contamination of the peritoneal cavity if the sentinel lymph node concept is established. We are certain that the use of laparoendoscopic full-thickness resection will provide valuable experience that will allow operators to safely develop endoscopic full-thickness resection skills.

Endoscopic Suturing, an Essential Enabling Technology for New NOTES Interventions   375

Sergey V. Kantsevoy and Joseph Ramon Armengol-Miro

Natural orifice transluminal endoscopic surgery (NOTES) was developed as a new, minimally invasive approach for various interventions inside the peritoneal cavity. Since the first reports of NOTES animal interventions, various devices have been used for closure of the transluminal entrance site. This article reviews the most commonly used endoscopic closure devices and advantages of the latest generation of endoscopic suturing devices enabling reliable, surgical-quality closure of the full-thickness gastrointestinal wall defects.

New NOTES Clinical Training and Program Development   385

Payal Saxena and Mouen A. Khashab

Natural orifice translumenal endoscopic surgery (NOTES) is an intense area of research, and is arguably the most significant endoscopic innovation of this decade. Training for new NOTES is relatively long, encompassing advanced endoscopy training, mastery of endoscopic dexterity within the narrow submucosal or "third space" with an in-depth understanding of the tissue planes. Proficiency with new closure and hemostatic devices is also essential. Few institutions worldwide can provide all the cognitive and technical elements essential to train new NOTES trainees. Trainees may need to spend time across several institutions to ensure safe and effective practice of new NOTES.

Pre-clinical Training for New Notes Procedures: From Ex-vivo Models to Virtual Reality Simulators   401

Mark A. Gromski, Woojin Ahn, Kai Matthes, and Suvranu De

Natural orifice transluminal endoscopic surgery (NOTES) is a newer field of endoscopic surgery that allows for scarless treatment of pathologic entities, using novel transluminal approaches. There has been a shift of focus from a clinical and research standpoint from the development and dissemination of "first-generation" NOTES procedures to "new NOTES" procedures that traverse the mucosa of luminal structures, yet do not stray far into the peritoneal cavity. It has been a challenge to find appropriate and effective ways to train gastroenterologists and surgeons in these novel approaches. We review the importance of simulation in training and discuss available simulation options.

A Western Perspective on "New NOTES" from POEM to Full-thickness Resection and Beyond   413

Rani Modayil and Stavros N. Stavropoulos

Most new natural orifice translumenal endoscopic surgery procedures originated in Asia; therefore, most data come from operators and a health care environment different from those in the West. We provide a Western perspective. We discuss East–West differences; review areas in which the United States is leading the way; and discuss the vagaries of coding and reimbursement. In the United States, reimbursement remains problematic. A Current Procedural Terminology code for peroral endoscopic myotomy is inevitable given the rapidly accumulating overwhelmingly positive outcomes data. However, coordinated efforts may help accelerate the process.

GASTROINTESTINAL ENDOSCOPY CLINICS OF NORTH AMERICA

FORTHCOMING ISSUES

July 2016
Sedation and Monitoring in Gastrointestinal Endoscopy
John Vargo, *Editor*

October 2016
Endoscopy in Inflammatory Bowl Disease
Maria T. Abreu, *Editor*

January 2017
Evaluation of the Small Bowel
Laura B. Gerson, *Editor*

RECENT ISSUES

January 2016
Pediatric Endoscopy
Jenifer R. Lightdale, *Editor*

October 2015
Advances in ERCP
Adam Slivka, *Editor*

July 2015
Upper Gastrointestinal Bleeding Management
John R. Saltzman, *Editor*

April 2015
Advances in Colonoscopy
Charles J. Kahi and
Douglas K. Rex, *Editors*

Foreword

The New NOTES Expands Interventional Endoscopy

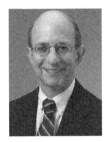

Charles J. Lightdale, MD
Consulting Editor

Natural orifice translumenal endoscopic surgery (NOTES) has been around for a dozen years or more without gaining much traction. Early pioneers had visions of incisionless removal of organs (eg, the gallbladder) using flexible endoscopes to breach an organ (eg, the stomach) to get the job done. These types of NOTES procedures were accomplished in some cases, but usually with no great benefit over standard laparoscopic technique. The New NOTES procedures emerged from Japan, where endoscopic submucosal dissection was extensively utilized mainly for en bloc removal of superficially spreading gastric cancer. This led to the development of POEM (per-oral endoscopic myotomy) for achalasia, which is finding new proponents all over the world. STER (submucosal tunneling for endoscopic resection of subepithelial tumors) and POP (per-oral pyloromyotomy) have also been introduced with seemingly great potential. Endoscopic suturing has concurrently been improved, allowing closure after EFTR (endoscopic full-thickness resection) of gastrointestinal tumors. This alphabet soup array of acronyms for New NOTES procedures may just be the beginning and promises to greatly expand the role of the interventional endoscopist.

It was almost preordained that Dr Stavros Stavropoulos would be leading the charge of the New NOTES. I have been able to watch Stavros develop as an interventionist from his days as a highly skilled Gastrointestinal Fellow (mentored by the late Dr Peter D. Stevens at Columbia-Presbyterian) to a master endoscopist in his own right, ready to explore the boundaries of flexible endoscopic surgery. He has gathered a Hall-of-Fame lineup of NOTES experts, covering all aspects of the New NOTES: the procedures, the perspectives, and the training.

If you are an interventional endoscopist in training or in practice, you should own this issue of the *Gastrointestinal Endoscopy Clinics of North America*. I believe it is a

Gastrointest Endoscopy Clin N Am 26 (2016) xiii–xiv
http://dx.doi.org/10.1016/j.giec.2016.01.002
1052-5157/16/$ – see front matter © 2016 Published by Elsevier Inc.

giendo.theclinics.com

landmark volume, setting a different direction for the New NOTES that is up and rolling. Don't miss the train.

Charles J. Lightdale, MD
Division of Digestive and Liver Diseases
Columbia University Medical Center
161 Fort Washington Avenue, Room 812
New York, NY 10032, USA

E-mail address:
CJL18@columbia.edu

Preface

The New NOTES: More "E" and Less "S" Leads to Success!

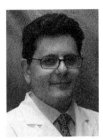

Stavros N. Stavropoulos, MD, FASGE
Editor

In this issue, renowned natural orifice translumenal endoscopic surgery (NOTES) pioneers offer several cogent reasons for the perceived demise of "traditional NOTES" procedures, such as transvaginal cholecystectomy. We would like to add to these reasons the lack of a critical mass of operators who, while skilled in endoscopic techniques such as endoscopic submucosal dissection (ESD), also had a firm grasp of surgical anatomy and principles. NOTES flourished with the advent of per-oral endoscopic myotomy (POEM) and its offshoots, precisely because, while still requiring superior flexible endoscopic resection skills, these "New NOTES" procedures eschewed the requirement for extensive surgical expertise and the formidable surgical instrumentation demands (eg, triangulation/retraction, illumination and wide-range visualization, robust hemostasis) imposed by the ambitious surgical procedures, including organ resections envisioned by "traditional NOTES." In this "post mortem" of traditional NOTES however, we should remember and appreciate that it is largely the vision and pioneering work of the luminaries of "traditional NOTES" that led to novel techniques (most prominently submucosal endoscopy) and devices (most prominently endoscopic suturing) that are fueling the "New NOTES" revolution. This issue focuses on this exciting rebirth of NOTES in the form of "short-range" endoscopic interventions that breech the gastrointestinal tract wall but stay close to it: interventions such as POEM, submucosal tunnel endoscopic resection (STER), endoscopic full-thickness resection (EFTR), and per-oral pyloromyotomy (POP). Whereas traditional NOTES, with its grand vision of deep incursions into the abdominal and chest cavities and major organ resections, failed to gain wide adoption, it planted the seeds for the "New NOTES" procedures, which are thriving and enjoying rapid growth. These "New NOTES" interventions are finally delivering on the great promise of NOTES, replacing traditional surgical procedures with minimally invasive, scarless ones. This issue brings together a "dream team" of New NOTES masters from Asia, Europe and the US. It features the "first-in-humans" pioneers of POEM, EFTR, STER, POP and device-assisted FTR and

Gastrointest Endoscopy Clin N Am 26 (2016) xv–xvi
http://dx.doi.org/10.1016/j.giec.2016.01.001
1052-5157/16/$ – see front matter © 2016 Published by Elsevier Inc.

giendo.theclinics.com

internationally recognized gurus of laparoendoscopic resection and ESD (the "parent techniques" of New NOTES) and endoscopic suturing (a critical enabling technology for New NOTES procedures). We hope that this issue will not only educate readers but also excite them about the great potential of this nimble and versatile NOTES that capitalizes on the strengths of the flexible endoscope to challenge laparoscopic surgery via a highly successful "target of opportunity" approach rather than the unsuccessful brute-force "frontal assault" attempted in the past by traditional NOTES.

Stavros N. Stavropoulos, MD, FASGE
Department of Medicine
Division of Digestive and Liver Diseases
Winthrop University Hospital
Mineola, NY, USA

222 Station Plaza North
Suite 429
Mineola, NY 11501, USA

E-mail address:
sns10md@gmail.com

Lessons Learned from Traditional NOTES
A Historical Perspective

Robert H. Hawes, MD

KEYWORDS

- Natural orifice transluminal endoscopic surgery (NOTES) • Natural orifice surgery
- White paper • Therapeutic endoscopy

KEY POINTS

- The concept of natural orifice surgery has begun with the concept of submucosal tunneling.
- It is likely that lessons learned from "new NOTES" will lead to the clinical application of traditional NOTES.
- One of the most significant outcomes from traditional and new NOTES is that it has brought therapeutic endoscopists together with minimally invasive surgeons and these relationships will be a powerful driver for innovation in minimally invasive therapies in the future.

The idea of natural orifice surgery (NOS) was conceived by Sergey Kantsevoy and Tony Kalloo in the late 1990s. A group of physicians got together to form the Apollo Group (Sydney Chung, Peter Cotton, Chris Gostout, Rob Hawes, Tony Kalloo, Sergey Kantsevoy, and Jay Pasricha) in 1997. Their vision and mission were to impact the practice of therapeutic endoscopy through innovation in techniques and technologies. The Apollo Group initially partnered with Olympus in an effort to accelerate product development. The concept of NOS was introduced at the initial meeting between the Apollo Group and Olympus held on Kiawah Island, South Carolina in 1998. Several acronyms for the procedure were initially proposed, with the first being flexible endoscopic surgery (FES). The original concept of FES presented by Kalloo and Kantsevoy involved per-oral passage of a flexible endoscope into the stomach followed by entrance into the peritoneal cavity via a gastrostomy. The rationale presented to support investment in the development of this procedure hypothesized that it would cause less postoperative pain, have improved cosmesis, avoid laparoscopic port hernias, and could potentially be performed in an environment less costly

Center for Interventional Endoscopy, Florida Hospital Orlando, 601 E. Rollins St, Orlando, Florida 32803, USA
E-mail address: robert.hawesmd@gmail.com

Gastrointest Endoscopy Clin N Am 26 (2016) 221–227
http://dx.doi.org/10.1016/j.giec.2015.12.010
1052-5157/16/$ – see front matter © 2016 Elsevier Inc. All rights reserved.

than a traditional operating room (OR). Kalloo and Kantsevoy worked diligently in the laboratory between 1998 and 2002 and settled on an approach that involved making an incision in the anterior wall of the stomach with a needle knife, augmenting the incision with balloon dilation, and then placing a double-balloon overtube to secure stable access to the peritoneal cavity and avoid leakage of gastric contents during the procedure. Their preliminary data on transgastric peritoneoscopy were presented to the Society for Surgery of the Alimentary Tract during Digestive Diseases Week (DDW) 2000.[1] Their work in the laboratory eventually culminated in the historic presentation of endoscopic gastrojejunostomy presented at DDW in 2002.[2] This work was the first demonstration that an established surgical procedure could be successfully performed entirely with a flexible endoscope through a natural orifice. The implications of FES and the potential for it to cause a significant paradigm shift in minimally invasive surgery (MIS) and therapeutic endoscopy were quickly recognized by the Society of American Gastrointestinal and Endoscopic Surgeons (SAGES) and the American Society for Gastrointestinal Endoscopy (ASGE). In an effort to guide the investigation and responsible development of this new approach to surgery, a joint committee was formed and chaired by David Rattner (representing SAGES) and the author (representing ASGE). The formal committee work was preceded by a meeting in New York of a working group consisting of equal representation from SAGES and ASGE. From this working group came 3 important items:

1. The acronym for the procedure: NOTES—Natural Orifice Transluminal Endoscopic Surgery
2. The acronym for the committee: NOSCAR—Natural Orifice Consortium for Assessment and Research
3. A White Paper—jointly published by SAGES (Surgical Endoscopy)[3] and ASGE (Gastrointestinal Endoscopy)[4]

The primary goal of the White Paper was to assure the responsible evolution of NOTES by providing a road map for its development. The White Paper was critically important because it carried enormous impact and influence by virtue of its support by the most important MIS and flexible endoscopic societies. The NOSCAR committee was equally important because its mission was to implement the principles and recommendations put forth by the White Paper.

The White Paper outlined the most significant obstacles to the clinical viability of NOTES. NOSCAR went about organizing an annual meeting to bring interested stakeholders together. Initially, there was significant corporate interest on the part of laparoscopic, flexible endoscopic, and accessory companies. The first NOSCAR meeting was held in Phoenix, Arizona in 2006 and perhaps the most important component of this first meeting was the formation of working groups. These working groups were charged with developing recommendations that would provide solutions to the list of obstacles to the clinical implementation of NOTES as outlined in the White Paper. Working group participants included both laparoscopic surgeons and therapeutic endoscopists (primarily gastroenterologists) who engaged in uninhibited discussion, often including frank disagreement, and openly expressed their thoughts and ideas. Each learned from the other, but because the opinions and recommendations were offered in a spirit of striving to achieve a common goal, progress was swift and steady. Research dollars flowed into NOSCAR; a research committee was established, and Requests for Proposal were established with priority going to those grants that had the greatest potential to solving issues raised within the working groups. The funds were administered through SAGES and ASGE, assuring that the maximal amount of money would go to the investigators. In looking back, although society involvement, the White Paper, the NOSCAR meetings, and the research generated were all of great importance, the most important force driving NOTES forward was the extraordinary group of physicians and surgeons who were brought together by the singular mission to responsibly develop NOTES. The enduring friendships and ongoing collaborations between therapeutic endoscopists and laparoscopic surgeons will be an important lasting legacy of the initial NOTES movement, and it is this group that created the foundation and brought to life the *New NOTES*.

As time progressed, many of the perceived "obstacles" to the clinical implementation of NOTES dissolved when targeted research studies were completed. Many began thinking that NOTES could become a reality. Two philosophies emerged about how the development of NOTES should proceed. Some advocated for a slow developmental course with the initial aim being to try to address unmet needs. Another camp thought that further progress in NOTES would require a "killer application." This idea caused surgeons to recall that "as goes cholecystectomy, so goes general surgery." Investigators began working on transgastric cholecystectomy, and after discovering how difficult it was with existing flexible scopes and accessories, surgeons moved to transvaginal cholecystectomy (strictly speaking "a natural orifice" but one that was already well established by our gynecologic colleagues and "naturally" excluded approximately 50% of patients). Surgeons found that transvaginal cholecystectomy could be safely accomplished if they had a good understanding of principles of safe vaginal access and closure and used long rigid laparoscopic tools. Multiple dynamics were now strongly influencing the development of NOTES, and these influences would fundamentally change the direction of development and lead to "New NOTES." These dynamics included the following:

1. It was becoming apparent that surgeons were frustrated with the limitations of the flexible endoscope as the platform for NOTES. They desired the cutting/hemostasis, suturing, and triangulation capability familiar to them with laparoscopic surgery. As a result, surgeons moved strongly toward transvaginal cholecystectomy, and this opened the door to the development of single-port surgery. Both approaches held the potential for less invasive access and improved cosmesis. The development of single-port surgery had a damaging effect on NOTES because it carried away valuable resources provided by laparoscopic companies (who saw greater potential for sales with single-port surgery), and it also further alienated gastroenterologists.

2. The movement toward use of laparoscopic instruments to accomplish a less invasive cholecystectomy had many negative ramifications for NOTES. It alienated gastroenterologists, who thought that NOTES was being high-jacked and excluded their continued participation. The move toward cholecystectomy was ill conceived because the margin to improve the procedure over standard laparoscopic cholecystectomy was so small that it would never be widely adopted.

3. With the demise of the grand dream of NOTES and the evolution toward new approaches to laparoscopic surgery, corporate money was redirected from NOSCAR to internal development and promotion of each company's vision for single-port surgery.

4. In the opinion of this author, the final "nail in the coffin" for NOTES occurred when a decision was made to increase corporate funds for a randomized trial between standard laparoscopic and NOTES cholecystectomy. Industry had become skeptical that NOTES would be widely adopted, and without the support of industry for research and device development, the evolution of NOTES could not be realized. It was thought that if it could be demonstrated that a "killer app" procedure could be

safely and effectively done with an NOTES approach, that this would reinvigorate the industry and the medical/surgical community and re-establish the NOTES movement. NOSCAR members advised that transgastric cholecystectomy could be done, and transvaginal cholecystectomy had now become reasonably well established. A multicenter, randomized, noninferiority study was designed comparing laparoscopic with transgastric and transvaginal cholecystectomy. Industry money was secured for the trial; very innovative mechanisms were developed for malpractice coverage and to cover extra costs to the institution, and the trial was begun.

The cumulative effect of these events essentially ended (for the present) the NOTES movement as it was originally conceived by Kalloo and Kantsevoy. The flexible endoscope was not embraced by surgeons, in part because of the lack of effective accessories. Most gastroenterologists (who had the greatest expertise and knowledge of therapeutic endoscopy) had become marginalized; industry money was gone. Research had come to a standstill, and the only tangible evidence of the original NOTES was the annual NOSCAR meeting, which now was run on a shoestring budget but still attracted this very special group of MIS and therapeutic endoscopists who had formed an unbreakable bond and came together with the singular purpose of moving minimally invasive therapy forward.

To understand the development of New NOTES, one has to first understand the state of the evolution of the original NOTES concept (outlined above) and then go back to the Apollo Group. It was the brilliance of Chris Gostout and his group working in the Mayo Clinic Developmental Endoscopy Unit that initiated the journey toward New NOTES. In 1998, they began working to solve the riddle of safe and easy en bloc resection. This work slowly evolved over a decade but was accelerated in 2005 when Kazuki Sumiyama, an advanced endoscopy Fellow from Jikei University in Tokyo, joined the team. Three very important concepts emerged from the work of Dr Gostout and his team: (1) the concept of tunneling to create a submucosal space; (2) the idea that the submucosa could be "opened" to create a working space (submucosal endoscopy, submucosal surgery, third-space surgery); and (3) the concept of safe closure using a mucosal flap. Their work with submucosal tunneling came about from their experience with creating a space by tunneling through the submucosa. They then went on to conceive that by making an incision through the muscularis propria and serosa at the end of the tunnel; they could accomplish safe entry into the peritoneal cavity as well as safe closure using the mucosal flap. They called this "tunneled offset viscerotomy."[5] Their work on creating a submucosal working space came about from their desire to improve the technique of en bloc resection. Their concept was called Submucosal Inside Out Project, in which they lifted a lesion, made a mucosal incision, dissected the submucosa underneath the lesion to create a working space, and then made the circumferential incision from inside the submucosal space toward the gut lumen, thus avoiding any chance of perforation.[6] Gostout's group began work on transluminal mediastinal access in parallel with their work on peritoneal access. They found that their tunneling technique had great appeal when working in the esophagus, and it was from this work that they discovered the value of the mucosal flap. They found that they could safely tunnel down the esophageal submucosal space, incise the muscle layer, enter the mediastinum, and then withdraw the scope and achieve safe and effective closure by simply clipping the small mucosal incision.[7–9]

By virtue of being a member of the Apollo Group, Jay Pasricha was aware of Dr Gostout's work in submucosal tunneling. Pasricha's innovative mind combined with his knowledge of motility disorders and therapeutic endoscopy led him to conceive of the idea of performing a submucosal tunnel to facilitate a myotomy in the treatment of achalasia. He used the tunneling and flap closure technique outlined by Gostout and Sumiyama and thought that the myotomy could be as effectively performed from within the submucosal space. Dr Pasricha did the preliminary work in pigs and published this idea in 2007.[10] The work of Drs Gostout, Sumiyama, and Pasricha was noted by Dr Haruhiro Inoue, who was working in Yokohama. In retrospect, Dr Inoue was the ideal person to further develop Dr Pasricha's idea. Dr Inoue is trained as a foregut surgeon and was, and still is, active in MIS of the esophagus, including Heller myotomy. Dr Inoue is also an internationally recognized expert in flexible endoscopy and is known for his work in endoscopic mucosal resection and endoscopic submucosal dissection (ESD). Taking the idea of Pasricha and leveraging his skill as a foregut surgeon and ESD expert, he brought Dr Pasricha's idea to clinical fruition and named the procedure per oral endoscopic myotomy (POEM). He published his first series of POEM in 2010.[11,12]

In many respects, the development of POEM was a benevolent "perfect storm" for the NOTES movement. It was a procedure that required excellent endoscopic skills and could be performed by surgeons and gastroenterologists. It represents an endoscopic procedure performed through a natural orifice that has the potential for replacing an accepted standard surgical procedure (Heller myotomy). It also fulfilled one of the promises of NOTES in that it brought the procedure from the OR to a less costly environment within the endoscopy suite. It also brought to clinical reality Gostout's original idea of third space (submucosal) surgery. The success of POEM has now provided a basis for endoscopic full-thickness resection techniques (submucosal tunneling endoscopic resection) being applied to small stromal tumors and potentially for endoscopic pyloromyotomy.[13]

In retrospect, Kalloo and Kantsevoy's vision of NOTES was perhaps too far ahead of its time. Very few surgeons had the requisite endoscopic skills; gastroenterologists were not in a position to perform traditional surgical procedures. Available endoscopic devices were in the dark ages compared with laparoscopic instruments, and industry was not prepared for a systematic, well-organized, long-term investment to allow NOTES to be responsibly developed. The obstacles to NOTES had to be systematically studied and resolved; devices had to be developed to enable safe and effective outcomes, and time was needed to allow these new techniques to be applied first in cases of unmet needs to allow refinement to optimize outcomes before competing with standard surgical procedures. Gostout's vision of creating an operating environment within the submucosa and the effectiveness of the mucosal flap closure, Pasricha's vision of NOS using the flexible endoscope for the treatment of achalasia, and Inoue's remarkable work to make POEM a standard procedure around the world have come together to create a discipline some are calling New NOTES. The development of these New NOTES procedures establishes a very important basis from which further development can proceed and serves as a bridge to true NOTES. It demonstrates to the industry the potential of the flexible endoscope through a natural orifice. Procedures can now evolve at a responsible rate, and industry can invest in new device development with a reasonable assurance that they can obtain a return on investment. As experience grows in submucosal surgery, confidence will build that mucosal flap closure is reliable. These techniques combined with new technologies may provide the segue into transesophageal mediastinal or transgastric peritoneal exploration that will ultimately lead to the clinical application of true NOTES as originally envisioned by Kalloo and Kantsevoy.

It has now been almost 20 years since the initial concept of NOTES was presented by Kalloo and Kantsevoy. Their vision has followed a somewhat traditional course that began with exuberant enthusiasm (usually too optimistic) and then morphed into tempered optimism. This phase was followed by a time of discouragement when unanticipated problems were encountered. Working through the discouraging times is dependent on the group of true believers who are invested for the long haul. In the opinion of this author, we have emerged from the discouragement phase and are now in a position to move forward toward true NOTES. In part, this is due to the bridging techniques of New NOTES but also to the work of some of the faithful. The careful and systematic investigative work of Lee Swanstom, Patricia Sylla, and Antonio Lacy on transanal colon resection is coming to fruition, and this will likely be recognized as the first NOTES procedure to cause a paradigm shift in surgery.[14-17] Optimism that true NOTES will be a broad clinical reality has now re-emerged. The course is set, and the ultimate success of NOTES will be attributed to the pioneering idea of Kalloo and Kantsevoy, the concepts of Gostout and Pasricha, the pioneering work of Inoue, but perhaps most importantly, the remarkable collaboration worldwide between minimally invasive surgeons and therapeutic endoscopists who have formed a cohesive community with a common goal of developing less invasive therapies to benefit patients.

REFERENCES

1. Kalloo AN, Singh VK, Jagannath SB, et al. Flexible transgastric peritoneoscopy: a novel approach to diagnostic and therapeutic interventions in the peritoneal cavity. Gastrointest Endosc 2004;60(1):114-7.
2. Kantsevoy SV, Jagannath SB, Niiyama H, et al. Endoscopic gastrojejunostomy with survival in a porcine model. Gastrointest Endosc 2005;62(2):287-92.
3. Rattner D, Kalloo A, ASGE/SAGES Working Group. ASGE/SAGES Working Group on natural orifice translumenal endoscopic surgery. October 2005. Surg Endosc 2006;20(2):329-33.
4. ASGE, SAGES. ASGE/SAGES Working Group on natural orifice translumenal endoscopic surgery white paper october 2005. Gastrointest Endosc 2006; 63(2):199-203.
5. Sumiyama K, Gostout CJ, Rajan E, et al. Transgastric cholecystectomy: transgastric accessibility to the gallbladder improved with the SEMF method and a novel multibending therapeutic endoscope. Gastrointest Endosc 2007;65(4):679.
6. Gostout CJ, Knipschield MA. Submucosal endoscopy with mucosal resection: a hybrid endoscopic submucosal dissection in the porcine rectum and distal colon. Gastrointest Endosc 2012;76(4):829.
7. Sumiyama K, Gostout CJ, Rajan E, et al. Submucosal endoscopy with mucosal flap safety valve. Gastrointest Endosc 2007;65(4):688.
8. Sumiyama K, Gostout CJ, Rajan E, et al. Transesophageal mediastinoscopy by submucosal endoscopy with mucosal flap safety valve technique. Gastrointest Endosc 2007;65(4):679.
9. Sumiyama K, Tajiri H, Gostout CJ. Submucosal endoscopy with mucosal flap safety valve (SEMF) technique: a safe access method into the peritoneal cavity and mediastinum. Minim Invasive Ther Allied Technol 2008;17(6):365-9.
10. Pasricha PJ, Hawari R, Ahmed I, et al. Submucosal endoscopic esophageal myotomy: a novel experimental approach for the treatment of achalasia. Endoscopy 2007;39(9):761-4.
11. Inoue H, Kudo SE. Per-oral endoscopic myotomy (POEM) for 43 consecutive cases of esophageal achalasia. Nihon Rinsho 2010;68(9):1749-52.
12. Inoue H, Minami H, Kobayashi Y, et al. Peroral endoscopic myotomy (POEM) for esophageal achalasia. Endoscopy 2010;42:265-71.

13. Khashab MA, Stein E, Clarke JO, et al. Gastric peroral endoscopic myotomy for refractory gastroparesis: first human endoscopic pyloromyotomy (with video). Gastrointest Endosc 2013;78(5):764–8.
14. Denk PM, Swanström LL, Whiteford MH. Transanal endoscopic microsurgical platform for natural orifice surgery. Gastrointest Endosc 2008;68(5):954–9.
15. Sylla P, Rattner DW, Delgado S, et al. NOTES transanal rectal cancer resection using transanal endoscopic microsurgery and laparoscopic assistance. Surg Endosc 2010;24(5):1205–10.
16. Telem DA, Han KS, Kim MC, et al. Transanal rectosigmoid resection via natural orifice translumenal endoscopic surgery (NOTES) with total mesorectal excision in a large human cadaver series. Surg Endosc 2013;27(1):74–80.
17. de Lacy AM, Rattner DW, Adelsdorfer C, et al. Transanal natural orifice transluminal endoscopic surgery (NOTES) rectal resection: "down-to-up" total mesorectal excision (TME)–short-term outcomes in the first 20 cases. Surg Endosc 2013; 27(9):3165–72.

The Evolution of "New Notes," Origins, and Future Directions

Saurabh S. Mukewar, MBBS, Christopher J. Gostout, MD*

KEYWORDS

- New NOTES • Submucosa • Endoscopic intervention • Submucosal endoscopy
- Hybrid endoscopic submucosal dissection

KEY POINTS

- The submucosa is a loosely attached gut wall layer between the mucosa and muscularis propria.
- The histologic uniqueness of the submucosa allows simple mechanical forces such as from fluid instillation or blunt balloon dissection to transform this gut wall layer into a working space.
- Submucosal endoscopy is a new concept based on using the submucosa as a working space.
- Submucosal endoscopy can be used to perform extensive mucosal excision, removal of subepithelial tumors, per-oral endoscopic myotomy, and potential new applications.

Endolumenal flexible endoscopic excision of precancerous and cancerous mucosal lesions has become an expectation. Removal of lesions up to 2 cm is possible and reliable with cap-based endoscopic mucosal resection. However, removal of larger mucosal lesions poses a challenge requiring piecemeal resection, suboptimal histologic assessment, and a likely need for multiple endoscopic sessions. In the 1990s in the Development Endoscopy Unit (DEU) of the Mayo Clinic, attempts were made to achieve complete resection of large lesions (>2 cm) with en bloc techniques. To facilitate resection of large lesions, reliable submucosal fluid cushions (SFC) were created identifying hydroxypropyl methylcellulose as a readily available, inexpensive injectate equal to hyaluronic acid.[1] Working with the SFC led to an important observation: the mucosa could easily be separated from the underlying submucosa, referred to as "delamination" (**Fig. 1**). Using a robust and diffuse SFC, wide endoscopic mucosal resection (WEMR) of the esophagus was successful with removal of large

Division of Gastroenterology & Hepatology, Mayo Clinic, 200 First Street SW, Rochester, MN 55905, USA
* Corresponding author.
E-mail address: gostout.christopher@mayo.edu

Gastrointest Endoscopy Clin N Am 26 (2016) 229–235
http://dx.doi.org/10.1016/j.giec.2015.12.004
1052-5157/16/$ – see front matter © 2016 Elsevier Inc. All rights reserved.

giendo.theclinics.com

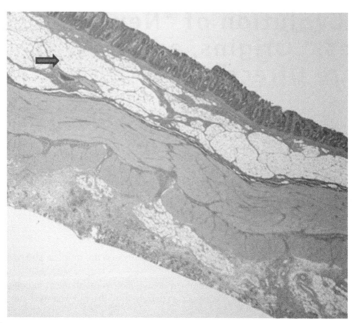

Fig. 1. The submucosa (*arrow*) is composed of loosely organized connective tissue, which can be easily disrupted, as for example, creating an SFC, separating the mucosa above from the muscle layer below.

areas greater than 5 cm in size involving up to 50% of circumference without inducing severe stricture.[2]

The experience with the development of WEMR directed attention to the submucosa. The submucosa can now be accessed and converted to a working space within which endoscopes and devices can be placed for diagnostic and therapeutic application. Initially, this was not included within the concept of natural orifice translumenal endoscopic surgery (NOTES). The vision for the submucosa is that within this space further intervention can be performed, "inside" toward the lumen or "outside" toward the deeper layers of gut and even beyond the gut wall (**Fig. 2**). For removal of mucosal lesions, going inward from submucosa toward mucosa for WEMR was theorized to be safer compared with traditionally going outward from the lumen toward the serosa, with an inherent risk of perforation and bleeding, whether using snare resection or endoscopic submucosal dissection (ESD). The submucosal space also allows access to the deeper layers of gut wall for diagnostic and therapeutic indications. For example, muscle biopsies from the muscular layers of the gut wall could thus be obtained, which previously required surgery. Offset entry through the mucosa and subsequent exit from the bowel wall at the far end of a submucosal space carries practical appeal for potential NOTES applications.[3]

TECHNIQUE FOR CREATION OF THE SUBMUCOSAL WORKING SPACE

The submucosal technique that can incorporate the above interventions is performed in a stepwise fashion with major procedural steps: isolating the submucosal layer, mucosal entry, conversion of the submucosal layer into a space, targeted interventions, and mucosal entry closure.

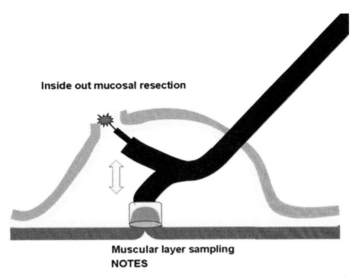

Fig. 2. Concept illustration highlighting the submucosal working space as a safe access to the deep layers of the gut wall, and an alternative safe directional means to excise overlying mucosal disease.

First, the submucosa is isolated by instilling an SFC, gaining access to submucosa. The SFC is important in order to prevent a full-thickness injury to the bowel wall. Historically, this was initially accomplished by forced gas insufflation using carbon dioxide (CO_2), but is currently accomplished more easily with liquid solutions, such as saline or hydroxypropyl methylcellulose. Studies have shown improved visualization and ease of performing excision procedures with more robust durable substances compared with saline.[4,5] Mucosal entry into the submucosa is achieved by a needle knife incision of the mucosa overlying the SFC, sufficiently large enough to accommodate the endoscope. Once submucosal access is gained, the space is created by blunt balloon dissection (**Fig. 3**). Alternatively, this can be accomplished using traditional needle knife dissection of the submucosa with continual placement of supplemental SFCs to facilitate safe needle knife dissection. In the author's experience, blunt dissection with small balloons is preferred over the needle knife for several reasons: it is quicker and easier to perform; it is protective of overlying mucosa; and given its atraumatic nature, there is reduced risk of bleeding with this technique. Blunt dissection involves advancement of deflated balloon distally, and inflating the balloon to create a space or in the esophagus, a tunnel, followed by pulling the balloon back to the scope, expanding the space. The scope is then advanced further and the cycle is repeated. Biliary stone retrieval balloons are typically used. Especially designed cylindrical balloons have been used to facilitate submucosal dissection.[6] To facilitate creating the space, a chemical substance, mesna (sodium-2-mercaptoethanesulfonate), can be used. It acts by chemically disrupting the submucosal connective tissue and has been shown to expedite mechanical dissection.[7–9] After the submucosal space is created, the endoscope itself or endoscopic tools followed by endoscope can be placed into the space. After an intended intervention that does not involve removal of overlying mucosal disease is accomplished, the endoscope is withdrawn from the space and the mucosal entry point is closed. The intact overlying mucosa serves as a protective healing tissue barrier.

A

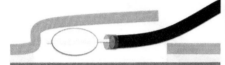

Balloon dissection of the submucosa

B

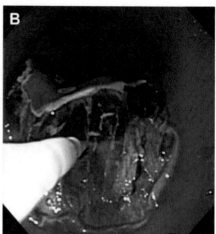

C

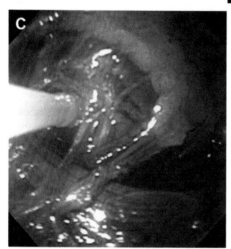

Fig. 3. (*A*) The submucosal space is conveniently and safely created by blunt balloon dissection. (*B*) A standard "blunt-tipped" endoscopic retrograde cholangiopancreatography stone extraction balloon is inserted into a robust submucosal fluid cushion in this example from a pig rectum. (*C*) Blunt balloon dissection is carried out by drawing the inflated balloon toward the endoscope. This technique of catheter insertion, balloon up, and balloon pull back, can supplement conventional ESD.

NEW NATURAL ORIFICE TRANSLUMENAL ENDOSCOPIC SURGERY PROCEDURES

What has been detailed above is now referred to as submucosal endoscopy. Submucosal endoscopy is transformative and has become the "new NOTES," gaining in popularity and with worldwide acceptance. The "new NOTES" procedures include per-oral endoscopic myotomy (POEM), STER (submucosal tunneling and endoscopic resection), and per-oral pyloromyotomy. These procedures evolved from the seminal preclinical studies conducted by the DEU beginning in 2004 with the submucosal inside out project, which transformed the submucosa into a working space. In 2007, the submucosal endoscopy with mucosal flap safety valve (SEMF) technique formed the basis of the first of the new NOTES procedures, POEM. SEMF was initially demonstrated in porcine foregut models.[10,11] In first of these 2 seminal studies, the SEMF technique permitted resection of a large full-thickness gastric muscle layer permitting access to peritoneal cavity without contamination from intragastric contents.[10] In the second study, transesophageal mediastinoscopy was performed successfully and safely in a porcine model.[11] Mediastinoscopy required a full-thickness myotomy for access, which immediately led to the consideration of converting the Heller myotomy to a submucosal endoscopic procedure. Subsequently, the author, along with the Apollo Group led by Pasricha, demonstrated that a partial esophageal myotomy of the inner circular muscle layer could be performed using SEMF technique.[12] Inoue and Kudo then went on to demonstrate the success of this technique in humans for the treatment of achalasia.[13]

EMERGING APPLICATIONS OF SUBMUCOSAL ENDOSCOPY

The ongoing resection of small localized subepithelial tumors by submucosal endoscopy is an intuitive application. Pyloromyotomy is another technically feasible extension of submucosal endoscopy. A useful clinical indication for this intervention will require careful scrutiny.[14]

The original intent for submucosal endoscopy was to provide a safer and more efficient replacement for time-consuming WEMR, which at this time is accomplished using ESD to provide en bloc resection. The Mayo DEU reported "hybrid ESD" using blunt balloon dissection in conjunction with traditional ESD to more rapidly open the submucosa and release a mucosal lesion for en bloc excision.[15] This hybrid ESD was compared directly with ESD and was found at an early stage to be at least equivalent in successfully providing complete en bloc excision.[16,17] Submucosal tunneling has also been applied experimentally to facilitate safe endoscopic full-thickness resection.[18] Endoscopic full-thickness resection has entered the clinical space and also represents the "new NOTES."

Submucosal endoscopy is being applied to enhance the diagnosis of motility disorders. Direct sampling of the muscle layer may be obtained from submucosal tunnels by full-thickness muscle layer biopsy or imaging of the neural elements in situ using confocal endoscopy with special staining of the neural elements.[19]

Transrectal SEMF for staging of gastric cancer has been studied in the porcine model. Submucosal tunneling with entry into the peritoneum has demonstrated improved visualization of the upper abdomen and highly accurate anatomic targeting for staging of foregut cancers.[20]

The protective mucosal (overlying) flap created by the SEMF technique can allow safe entry and egress for other purposes. Using this feature combined with direct access to the muscle layer, it is possible to secure lead placement for electrophysiologic monitoring and therapy. The lower esophageal sphincter (LES) can now be accessed under direct controlled visualization with renewed possibilities for the treatment of gastroesophageal reflux disease.

The submucosal space itself provides only access. It is not a functional location to deposit desirable materials for long-term intent, which is a common appealing thought. Magnets of varying sizes and shapes have been placed for potential control of reflux in studies that have been performed, only to be expelled back into the lumen in a short interval of time. Materials that can serve as repositories for drug elution to treat chronic diseases long term, such as eosinophilic esophagitis, and use of chemopreventive agents in Barrett's patients also are eventually expelled before true long-term therapeutic benefit can be seen. The muscle layer, on the other hand, offers a key to long-term applications. The ability to safely exit the intestinal wall offers access to attaching desirable therapies to the serosal or mediastinal side of the gastrointestinal tract.

Safe exit into the mediastinum via the submucosal esophageal tunnel has been shown to allow access to the heart.[21] This project was an early project that was pursued to examine the feasibility of endoscopically removing the left atrial appendage in patients with chronic atrial fibrillation, which has now been demonstrated by others.[22] These projects are some of the new horizons for submucosal endoscopy.

REFERENCES

1. Feitoza AB, Gostout CJ, Burgart LJ, et al. Hydroxypropyl methylcellulose: a better submucosal fluid cushion for endoscopic mucosal resection. Gastrointest Endosc 2003;57(1):41–7.
2. Rajan E, Gostout CJ, Feitoza AB, et al. Widespread EMR: a new technique for removal of large areas of mucosa. Gastrointest Endosc 2004;60(4):623–7.
3. Sumiyama K, Gostout CJ. Clinical applications of submucosal endoscopy. Curr Opin Gastroenterol 2011;27(5):412–7.
4. Yamamoto H, Yube T, Isoda N, et al. A novel method of endoscopic mucosal resection using sodium hyaluronate. Gastrointest Endosc 1999;50(2):251–6.
5. Conio M, Rajan E, Sorbi D, et al. Comparative performance in the porcine esophagus of different solutions used for submucosal injection. Gastrointest Endosc 2002;56(4):5.
6. Dobashi A, Sumiyama K, Gostout CJ, et al. Can mechanical balloon dissection be applied to cleave fibrotic submucosal tissues? A pilot study in a porcine model. Endoscopy 2013;45(8):661–6.
7. Sumiyama K, Gostout CJ, Rajan E, et al. Chemically assisted endoscopic mechanical submucosal dissection by using mesna. Gastrointest Endosc 2008;67(3):534–8.
8. Sumiyama K, Tajiri H, Gostout CJ, et al. Chemically assisted submucosal injection facilitates endoscopic submucosal dissection of gastric neoplasms. Endoscopy 2010;42(8):627–32.
9. Kawahara Y, Sumiyama K, Tajiri H. Chemically assisted peroral endoscopic myotomy with submucosal mesna injection in a porcine model. Minim Invasive Ther Allied Technol 2015;24(6):334–9.
10. Sumiyama K, Gostout CJ, Rajan E, et al. Submucosal endoscopy with mucosal flap safety valve. Gastrointest Endosc 2007;65(4):688–94.
11. Sumiyama K, Gostout CJ, Rajan E, et al. Transesophageal mediastinoscopy by submucosal endoscopy with mucosal flap safety valve technique. Gastrointest Endosc 2007;65(4):679–83.
12. Pasricha PJ, Hawari R, Ahmed I, et al. Submucosal endoscopic esophageal myotomy: a novel experimental approach for the treatment of achalasia. Endoscopy 2007;39(9):761–4.
13. Inoue H, Kudo SE. Per-oral endoscopic myotomy (POEM) for 43 consecutive cases of esophageal achalasia. Nihon Rinsho 2010;68(9):1749–52 [in Japanese].
14. Khashab MA, Stein E, Clarke JO, et al. Gastric peroral endoscopic myotomy for refractory gastroparesis: first human endoscopic pyloromyotomy (with video). Gastrointest Endosc 2013;78(5):764–8.
15. Gostout CJ, Knipschield MA. Submucosal endoscopy with mucosal resection: a hybrid endoscopic submucosal dissection in the porcine rectum and distal colon. Gastrointest Endosc 2012;76(4):829–34.
16. Takizawa K, Gostout CJ, Knipschield MA. Submucosal endoscopy with mucosal resection (SEMR): a new hybrid technique of endoscopic submucosal dissection. Endoscopy 2013;45(Suppl 2 UCTN):E38–9.
17. Takizawa K, Knipschield MA, Gostout CJ. Submucosal endoscopy with mucosal resection (SEMR): a new hybrid technique of endoscopic submucosal balloon dissection in the porcine rectosigmoid colon. Surg Endosc 2013;27(12):4457–62.

18. Takizawa K, Knipschield MA, Gostout CJ. Submucosal endoscopy as an aid to full-thickness resection: pilot study in the porcine stomach. Gastrointest Endosc 2015;81(2):450–4.
19. Sumiyama K, Tajiri H, Kato F, et al. Pilot study for in vivo cellular imaging of the muscularis propria and ex vivo molecular imaging of myenteric neurons (with video). Gastrointest Endosc 2009;69(6):1129–34.
20. Takizawa K, Brahmbhatt R, Knipschield MA, et al. Transcolonic peritoneoscopy by using submucosal endoscopy with mucosal flap for the detection of peritoneal bead targeting in the porcine survival model: a feasibility and effectiveness study. Gastrointest Endosc 2014;79(1):127–34.
21. Sumiyama K, Gostout CJ, Rajan E, et al. Pilot study of transesophageal endoscopic epicardial coagulation by submucosal endoscopy with the mucosal flap safety valve technique (with videos). Gastrointest Endosc 2008;67(3):497–501.
22. Moreira-Pinto J, Ferreira A, Miranda A, et al. Left atrial appendage ligation with single transthoracic port assistance: a study of survival assessment in a porcine model (with videos). Gastrointest Endosc 2012;75(5):1055–61.

POEM, the Prototypical "New NOTES" Procedure and First Successful NOTES Procedure

Robert Bechara, MD[a,b,]*, Haruhiro Inoue, MD, PhD[a]

KEYWORDS

- Peroral endoscopic myotomy (POEM)
- Natural orifice transluminal endoscopic surgery (NOTES) • Achalasia
- Diffuse esophageal spasm • Jackhammer esophagus • Hypercontractile esophagus

KEY POINTS

- Peroral endoscopic myotomy (POEM) is the first clinically successful natural orifice transluminal endoscopic surgery (NOTES) procedure that has achieved surgical efficacy with a safety profile comparable with endoscopic therapy.
- For the treatment of achalasia, there are now long-term data that demonstrate sustained clinical efficacy after POEM.
- POEM for diffuse esophageal spasm and hypercontractile esophagus should include the lower esophageal sphincter to prevent symptom development secondary to ineffective esophageal motility.
- The incidence of reflux after POEM is comparable with that after laparoscopic Heller myotomy.
- Infection-related adverse events with POEM have been rare, which should support further development of transesophageal mediastinal/peritoneal NOTES.

Disclosure Statement: The authors have nothing to disclose.
[a] Digestive Diseases Centre, Showa University Koto-Toyosu Hospital, Toyosu 5-1-38, Koto-Ku, Tokyo 135-8577, Japan; [b] Queen's University Division of Gastroenterology Kingston General and Hotel Dieu Hospitals, 166 Brock Street, Kingston, Ontario K7L 5G2, Canada
* Corresponding author. Gastrointestinal Diseases Research Unit, Hotel Dieu Hospital, Queen's University, 166 Brock Street, Kingston, Ontario K7L 5G2, Canada.
E-mail address: bechara.robert@gmail.com

Gastrointest Endoscopy Clin N Am 26 (2016) 237–255
http://dx.doi.org/10.1016/j.giec.2015.12.002
1052-5157/16/$ – see front matter © 2016 Elsevier Inc. All rights reserved.

Video content accompanies this article at www.giendo.theclinics.com

EVOLUTION OF PERORAL ENDOSCOPIC MYOTOMY

The first report of myotomy for achalasia was in Germany in 1914 by Ernest Heller. Heller performed 2 parallel myotomies along the anterior and posterior distal esophagus that extended to the gastric cardia.[1] Subsequently, in Holland in 1921, Johannes Henricus Zaaijer[2] reported performing a single anterior myotomy without compromise in efficacy. This procedure was eventually named the Heller myotomy and was performed by surgeons worldwide for achalasia. In Minnesota in 1958, Ellis and colleagues[3] reported the first successful transthoracic approach of the modified Heller myotomy. The first report of an endoscopic myotomy for achalasia was in Venezuela in 1980 by Ortega and colleagues[4] where they performed two 1-cm myotomies through the mucosa to a depth of 3 mm at the lower esophageal sphincter (LES). However, because of the limitation in myotomy length, poor efficacy, and safety concerns, the procedure was not adopted. In the 1990s, minimally invasive surgery was evolving; the laparoscopic and thoracoscopic myotomies were introduced in 1991 and 1992 by Shimi and colleagues[5] and Pellegrini and colleagues,[6] respectively. In the 2000s, advanced endoscopists became interested in using natural orifices as alternate routes for carrying out procedures in the peritoneum and mediastinum. In 2004, Kalloo and colleagues[7] performed the first transgastric peritoneoscopy in a porcine model. Subsequently in 2007, the first cases of human transluminal cholecystectomy were reported by Marescaux and colleagues[8] and Zorrón and colleagues.[9] In the same year, Pasricha and colleagues[10] described an endoscopic myotomy in a porcine model whereby a mucosal incision was made 5 cm above the gastroesophageal junction (GEJ) and a biliary dilating balloon was placed into the submucosal space to create a tunnel down to the GEJ where a selective circular muscle myotomy was performed using a needle knife. In 2008, the authors' team performed the first human peroral endoscopic myotomy (POEM); in 2010, Inoue and colleagues[11] published the first series of POEM. Since then, more than 5000 POEM procedures have been performed worldwide; it is arguably becoming the preferred treatment of achalasia. Currently, POEM and its offshoot peroral endoscopic tumorectomy remain the only thriving natural orifice transluminal endoscopic surgery (NOTES) procedures that rival or even surpass conventional surgical treatment.

ADVANTAGES OF PERORAL ENDOSCOPIC MYOTOMY

POEM offers benefits for the patients, physician, and health care system. POEM is at least as effective as laparoscopic Heller myotomy (LHM); however, it is performed endoscopically and, therefore, is associated with a shorter hospital stay, quicker recovery, and less blood loss.[12–14] From a procedural perspective, POEM provides the ability to tailor the length and position of the myotomy to patients. Procedural freedom allows a myotomy to be performed in patients with previous surgical myotomy with a modest increase in technical difficulty while preserving efficacy, by easily avoiding the area of previous surgical manipulation.[15–17] Moreover, because the myotomy is performed without disruption of the diaphragmatic hiatus and suspensory ligaments, reflux rates are comparable with that of LHM with partial wrap.[12,18]

ACCESSORIES AND EQUIPMENT FOR PERORAL ENDOSCOPIC MYOTOMY

The endoscopic accessories and electrosurgical unit (ESU) settings used in POEM are variable among centers and are selected from among the armamentarium of standard accessories of endoscopic submucosal dissection (ESD), the parent technique of POEM, shown in **Table 1** and **Fig. 1**. There is little evidence demonstrating superiority of any one particular accessory over another. The two most commonly used knives are the Triangle Tip knife (Olympus Medical Systems, Tokyo, Japan) and the T-Type HybridKnife (ERBE, Tübingen, Germany), with sporadic use of the Hook Knife (Olympus Medical Systems), Insulated tip knife2 (IT-2 knife) (Olympus Medical Systems), and Dual Knife (Olympus Medical Systems) (listed in decreasing frequency) by a small number of centers with low/modest volumes of POEMs. In a randomized trial comparing the two commonly used knives, the Triangle Tip knife and the Hybrid-Knife, in 100 patients receiving POEM, the HybridKnife resulted in a shorter procedure time by 13 minutes (22.9 ±6.7 minutes vs 35.9 ±11.7 minutes; $P<.0001$) and fewer minor intraprocedural bleeding episodes (3.6 ±1.8 vs 6.8 ±5.2; $P<.0001$).[19] An animal study comparing the Short ST hood (Fujifilm, Tokyo, Japan) with a regular cylindrical hood for submucosal tunneling demonstrated that the Short ST hood resulted in decreased procedure time by facilitating quicker entry into the submucosal space.[20]

INDICATIONS
Achalasia

Excellent safety and efficacy data for POEM have accumulated over the past 7 years and continue to mount. In lieu of formal guidelines, based on the current evidence and expert consensus, POEM can be considered as the first-line treatment of all achalasia at expert centers.[21] Contraindications for POEM include severe coagulopathy, submucosal fibrosis preventing tunnel formation, and severe cardiopulmonary disease precluding general anesthetic.[22]

Diffuse Esophageal Spasm and Hypercontractile Esophagus

With its established success with achalasia, POEM indications have expanded to include diffuse esophageal spasm (DES) and hypercontractile esophagus.[23] Because of the lower incidence of these disorders, the data are not as extensive as that for achalasia. In addition, there is debate regarding the inclusion of the LES in the myotomy. Currently, the authors' practice is to include the LES in the myotomy for 3 reasons. The first and most important is that these motility disorders frequently require extended myotomies often of 20 cm or more. With long myotomies, contraction vigor is significantly reduced, typically resulting in iatrogenic ineffective esophageal motility. In some patients, the remaining contraction vigor is inadequate to completely propel the food bolus across the preserved LES, resulting in worsening of symptoms. Second, although contentious, DES and hypercontractile esophagus have been shown to progress to achalasia.[24,25] If this occurs in patients in whom the LES is spared, patients will develop symptoms and require additional treatment. Finally, despite the increased risk of reflux with LES inclusion in the myotomy, the risk of complicated or proton pump inhibitor (PPI)–refractory reflux seems diminutive based on current data.[26] However, because of the low incidence of DES and hypercontractile esophagus, multicenter collaboration is required to develop an evidence-based methodology for POEM application to these motility disorders.

TECHNIQUE

To minimize the risk of aspiration during intubation, endoscopy is first performed under conscious sedation to suction residual debris from the esophagus. After intubation, the esophagus and GEJ are examined to identify the trachea, left main bronchus, aortic arch, spine, GEJ, and abnormal contractions (**Fig. 2**). The entry site

Table 1
Equipment and accessories used in peroral endoscopic myotomy

Insufflation	**CO_2 regulation unit (UCR) with extralow flow tubing MAJ-1816 (Olympus Medical Systems, Tokyo, Japan)**
	CO_2 Efficient Endoscopic Insufflator (ERBE Tubingen, Germany)
ESU	**Vio 300D/200D (ERBE)**
ERBE VIO300D/ VIO200D	**Triangle Tip knife (Olympus Medical Systems)**
	MI: Endocut I effect 1, duration 1, interval 3
	T: Spray Coag effect 2, 50 W
	M: Selective use of MI and T settings
	H: Spray Coag effect 2, 50 W (TT knife-minor bleeding or small vessels)
	Soft Coag effect 5, 80 W (Coagrasper, moderate/severe bleeding or large vessels)
	T-Type Hybrid knife (ERBE Tubingen, Germany)[a]
	MI: Endocut Q Effect 3, duration 1, interval 4
	T: Endocut Q Effect 3, duration 1, interval 4
	M: Endocut Q Effect 3, duration 1, interval 4
	H: Forced Coag Effect 2, 60 W (T-Type HybridKnife, minor bleeding or small vessels)
	Forced Coag Effect 2, 50 W (Coagrasper, moderate/severe bleeding or large vessels)
Distal attachment	**Fujifilm short ST Hood DH-28GR (Fujifilm, Tokyo, Japan)**
	Oblique cap MH-588 (Olympus Medical Systems)
	Tapered Cap D-201–11,802 (Olympus Medical Systems)
Endoscopic knife	**Triangle Tip knife KD 640L (Olympus Medical Systems)**
	T-Type HybridKnife 20, 150–060 (ERBE)
	Hook Knife KD-620LR (Olympus Medical Systems)
	Insulated tip knife2 KD-611L (Olympus Medical Systems)
	Dual Knife KD-650L (Olympus Medical Systems)
Hemostasis	**Coagulation forceps (Olympus Coagrasper FD-411QR)**
Submucosal injectate	**Half normal saline + 5% dextrose in water (0.45NS + D5W)**
	Saline (HybridKnife does not use viscous injectates for injection via the tip of the knife)
	Glycerol mixture (10% glycerol and 5% fructose)
	Saline + alginate mixture
	Hydroxypropyl methylcellulose + mesna
Submucosal injectate adjuncts	**Indigo carmine**
	Methylene blue
	Epinephrine (*adverse events reported*)
Hemostatic clips	**Quick Clip 2 HX201LR-135L (Olympus Medical Systems)**
	EZ-CLIP HX-110Q (Olympus Medical Systems)
	Resolution Clips M00522610 (Boston Scientific, Marlborough, MA)
Endoscopic suturing device	OverStitch Endoscopic Suturing System *ESS-G02–160* (Apollo Endosurgery, Austin, TX)
Injection catheters	**Injection Needle NM 400L-0425 (Olympus Medical Systems)**
	Spray catheter PW-5V-1 (Olympus Medical Systems)
Overtube	**Flexible Overtube MD-48518 (Sumitomo Bakelite, Tokyo, Japan)**
	Guardus Overtube (US Endoscopy, Mentor, OH)
Decompression	**14G IV angiocath catheter**
	Veress needle

Bold text represents the equipment used by the authors.

Abbreviations: CO_2, carbon dioxide; H, hemostasis; IV, intravenous; M, myotomy; MI, mucosal incision; T, tunneling.

[a] Settings used by Zhou et al[17].

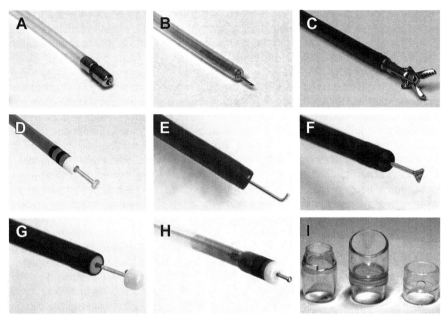

Fig. 1. Accessories used in POEM: (*A*) Spray catheter PW-5V-1 used off label not as injection device for nonpuncture contact submucosal injection once within the tunnel; (*B*) Injection Needle NM 400L-0425; (*C*) Coagrasper Hemostatic Forceps FD-411QR; (*D*) T-Type HybridKnife 20,150 to 060; (*E*) Hook Knife KD-620LR; (*F*) Triangle Tip knife KD 640L; (*G*) Insulated tip knife2 KD-611L; (*H*) Dual Knife KD-650L; (*I*) Hoods from left to right: short ST Hood DH-28GR, Oblique cap MH-588, Tapered Cap D-201 to 11,802. (*Courtesy of* [*A, B, C, E, F, G, H, I* (Oblique cap MH-588; Tapered Cap D-201-11802)] Olympus Medical Systems, Tokyo, Japan, with permission; and [*D*] ERBE, Tübingen, Germany, with permission; and [*I* (short ST Hood DH-28GR)] Fujifilm, Tokyo, Japan.)

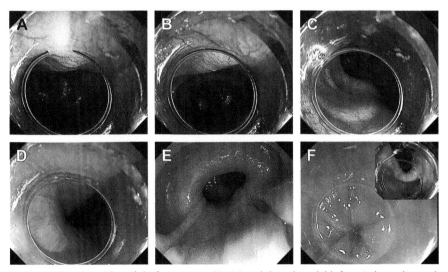

Fig. 2. Landmarks to identify before mucosal incision: (*A*) trachea, (*B*) left main bronchus arch, (*C*) spine, (*D*) aortic arch, (*E*) abnormal contraction, (*F*) GEJ in forward and retroflexed views.

is chosen and submucosal injection, mucosal incision, and submucosal entry are performed (**Fig. 3**, Video 1). After submucosal entry, the tunnel is extended distally via the ESD technique up to 2 to 3 cm into the gastric cardia. In **Table 2**, the various indicators of location within the submucosal tunnel are listed. The most precise and reliable method to confirm the location of the distal extent of the tunnel involves using a second ultraslim gastroscope inserted into the submucosal tunnel (or native lumen) with subsequent transillumination (**Fig. 4**).[27] In performing a selective circular muscle myotomy, the circular muscle bundles are cut gradually until the longitudinal muscle is identified and the intermuscular space can be accessed. Then the endoscopic knife is advanced into the intermuscular space, and the circular bundles are hooked and cut. At the GEJ, the tissue planes become less well delineated and the working space is reduced. Therefore, at the GEJ the myotomy should progress in an extremely controlled meticulous manner to avoid mucosal damage or laceration of perforating gastric arteries. It should be noted that there are alternative myotomy techniques that have been reported. One widely applied technique by the Shanghai group and other centers consists of full-thickness myotomy rather than circular-layer-only myotomy.[28] Recently a group from Harbin, China reported a technique that consists of simultaneous dissection of the submucosa and muscularis rather than first completing the submucosal tunnel and then performing the myotomy.[29] After completion of the myotomy and confirmation of hemostasis, prophylactic antibiotic is instilled into the tunnel and the mucosal entry site is closed with 4 to 6 clips. Alternative closure methods include over-the-scope clips (OTSCs, OVESCO, Tübingen, Germany), fully covered self-expanding metal stents (FCSEMS), endoscopic suturing devices, and a combination of PolyLoops (Olympus Medical Systems, Tokyo, Japan) with clips.[30–36]

ADVERSE EVENTS

POEM has proven to be a very safe procedure despite the working field being adjacent to multiple vital structures. There have been no reported mortalities or emergent

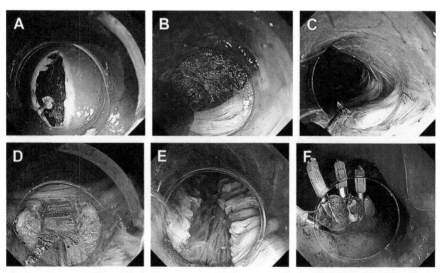

Fig. 3. Steps in POEM: (*A*) mucosal incision after submucosal injection, (*B*) submucosal tunneling, (*C*) completed tunnel, (*D*) circular muscle myotomy, (*E*) completed myotomy, (*F*) closure with clips.

Table 2
Signs indicating location within the submucosal tunnel

Sign (Location)	Usefulness
Insertion depth	Moderate
Palisade vessels (distal esophagus)	Moderate
Narrowing of submucosal tunnel (GEJ)	Moderate
Tight circular muscle bundles (LES)	High[a]
Increased vascularity and capaciousness (gastric cardia)	High[a]
Visibility of contrast during luminal view of cardia (gastric cardia)	High[a]
Transillumination double scope technique (gastric cardia)	High

[a] Most helpful as indicated by the International Per Oral Endoscopic Myotomy survey.[22]

conversions to open surgery despite more than 5000 procedures performed globally. Reported adverse events include bleeding, mucosal injury, mediastinitis (radiologic), peritonitis, pneumonia, tunnel infection, capnoperitoneum, capnomediastinum, capnothorax, capnopericardium, thoracic effusions, and atelectasis. Fortunately, serious adverse events are very rare; most adverse events are mucosal injury or tense pneumoperitoneum, which are generally managed easily without clinical consequence. This review is a detailed review of the most common and relevant adverse events, as more comprehensive reviews of all adverse events are already available.[37]

Insufflation-Related Adverse Events

Insufflation-related adverse events compose a significant proportion of the adverse events.[38] It is obligatory that pure carbon dioxide (CO_2) insufflation is used, as with the use of air insufflation there is an increased incidence and severity of insufflation related complications.[39] The potential insufflation-related adverse events include subcutaneous emphysema, capnoperitoneum, capnomediastinum, capnothorax, and capnopericardium. There is one report of tension capnopericardium occurring during POEM as the result of an unrecognized defect in the pericardium made during the

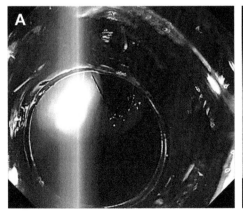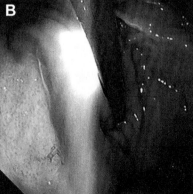

Fig. 4. Transillumination double scope method demonstrating the position of the distal tunnel: (*A*) ultraslim gastroscope in the tunnel and regular gastroscope in the stomach; (*B*) regular gastroscope in tunnel and ultraslim gastroscope in stomach.

myotomy. This resulted in the development of tension capnopericardium causing cardiac arrest. After cardiopulmonary resuscitation, the patient made a full recovery and was discharged 8 days later without sequelae.[40] Tense capnoperitoneum is the most commonly encountered insufflation-related adverse event that requires intervention, with an overall incidence of about 20%.[38] A key factor in insufflation-related adverse events is the volume of gas insufflated, which depends on the flow rate of CO_2 and total insufflation time dictated by operator insufflation. Insufflation-related adverse can be minimized with the use of low-flow or extralow-flow CO_2. This point was demonstrated by Familiari and colleagues[41] in a series of 100 POEMs whereby in the first 79 cases in which medium- or high-flow CO_2 was used the incidence of tense capnoperitoneum was 36.7%, whereas for the remaining 21 cases, low-flow CO_2 tubing was used and no events of tense capnoperitoneum occurred. In a series of 220 POEMs by Ramchandani and colleagues,[42] the first 100 cases used low-flow CO_2 resulting in an incidence of tense pneumoperitoneum of 28%. For the subsequent 120 cases, extralow flow was used and pneumoperitoneum rates decreased to 10%. Thus, using low-flow or extralow-flow CO_2 with judicious insufflation is recommended as it may minimize the incidence of clinically significant insufflation-related adverse events. However, it should be note that the magnitude of the decrease in the incidence of tense pneumoperitoneum in these series is likely amplified by the fact that the higher-flow CO_2 was used early in the operators' learning curve when operative times were likely longer and judicious use of insufflation less skillful.

Mucosal Perforation

The overall incidence of mucosal perforation is less than 10% and generally decreases with increasing operator experience.[11,21,43–45] Techniques used to close the mucosal perforations include hemostatic clips, endoscopic suturing with OverStitch (Apollo Endosurgery, Austin, TX), fibrin sealants, FCSEMS, and a combination of endoloops with clips.[46–48] In case series reporting mucosal perforation, only one patient with perforation had a treatment failure (post-POEM Eckardt >3).[49] In addition, although accidental mucosal perforations have been reported by numerous published POEM series at various relatively low frequencies, there are only 2 reports of patients who required laparoscopic/thoracoscopic intervention in the immediate postoperative period because of leaks.[13,49] Most mucosal perforations are closed endoscopically without alteration to the postprocedure course. Thus, in sum, mucosal perforations are infrequent and are typically endoscopically managed safely and effectively without sequelae.

Bleeding

Major bleeding with POEM has been exceptionally rare. There is one report of severe intraprocedural bleeding.[50] This bleeding occurred at the authors' center during the gastric myotomy phase in which a perforating artery was severed. The severed artery was eventually visualized and coagulated; however, the patient did require transfusion. The procedure was completed successfully without any further adverse events. This case is the only case of severe intraprocedural bleeding encountered in more than 1000 POEMs at the authors' center, yielding a significant intraprocedural bleeding incidence of less than 0.1%. Significant delayed bleeding is also rare, with only 7 cases reported in the literature. In a series of 428 POEMs, Li and colleagues,[51] experienced a delayed bleeding rate of 0.7% (3 cases). All 3 cases required emergent endoscopy; 2 had bleeding sites identified within the tunnel, and hemostasis was achieved with coagulation forceps. In the other case, the bleeding site could not be identified and a Sengstaken-Blakemore tube was placed within the esophageal lumen for 24 hours. In all 3 cases, definitive hemostasis was achieved with no long-term sequelae. Minami and colleagues reported 2 cases of delayed bleeding in a series of 28 patients, and both resolved with conservative management without requiring endoscopy or transfusion.[52] In a series of 100 patients, Sharata and colleagues[35] described one delayed intratunnel hemorrhage that was managed conservatively with readmission and transfusion but without the need for other intervention. Benech and colleagues[53] reported the development of a 34 mm × 110-mm hematoma 24 hours after POEM in a patient on antiplatelet therapy. The patient was managed conservatively and discharged 8 days later without sequelae. Thus, severe intraprocedural and delayed bleeding with POEM are remarkably rare and when encountered have been managed successfully without deleterious consequences.

EFFICACY

Treatment success for achalasia has been defined by an Eckardt score of 3 or less. Objective measures that correlate with clinical success include timed barium esophagram (TBE), integrated relaxation pressure (IRP), distensibility, and LES pressure (LESP). Adequate emptying on TBE after pneumatic dilation and Heller myotomy has been shown to correlate well with clinical treatment success as well as sustained clinical response within 1 year, whereas poor emptying correlates with LES dysfunction and recurrence within 1 year.[54–57] A post-therapy IRP less than 15 mm Hg (for Sierra design transducers) correlates well with clinical response and adequate emptying on TBE.[58,59] Distensibility, a physical measurement of the GEJ, also reliably correlates with esophageal emptying and clinical response.[60–62] Based on all these available parameters (Eckardt score, TBE, IRP, LESP, and distensibility), POEM has demonstrated consistent efficacy clinically, manometrically, and functionally.[35,42,49,63,64] There are now 20 series totaling more than 2000 patients, with follow-up ranging from 6 months to more than 2 years, with most reporting 90% or greater sustained efficacy (**Table 3**). However, exceptions are the 5-center European International Prospective Multicenter Study with 82% clinical efficacy at 1 year[65] and the 3-center study (Hamburg, Rome, Portland) by Werner and colleagues[66] in which there was an initial 96% treatment success and after a 2-year follow-up there was a decrease to 78% sustained success. The exact cause of increased symptom recurrence in these two trials is unclear; however, it is likely due to learning curve issues. In the European MCT, 5 centers contributed their earliest cases totaling only 70 patients; in the Werner study, 50% of patients with symptom recurrence were among the first 10 cases performed at each of the 3 centers (including Hamburg, which also participated in the European Multicenter trial). The technical basis for this result is likely due to inadequate or incomplete myotomy at the GEJ, which is the most common cause of recurrent symptoms after myotomy whether performed laparoscopically or perorally.[67–69] The tunneling and myotomy from the GEJ to the gastric cardia are the most technically demanding and clinically important aspects of the POEM procedure. Hence, formal training/proctoring by an expert during the learning curve (estimated range 20–60 cases)[43,44,70] to prevent a high incidence of inadequate myotomy and subsequent high rate of symptom recurrence is important. In the rare case of persistent or recurrent symptoms after POEM, repeat POEM can be successfully performed with excellent clinical results. Li and colleagues[69] performed repeat POEM in 15 patients with persistent or recurrent symptoms at a mean of 13.5 months (range 4–37 months) after the primary POEM. Clinical success (Eckardt score to ≤3) was achieved in 100% of patients at a mean follow-up of 11.3 months.

Table 3
Outcomes of peroral endoscopic myotomy series with 30 or more patients with 6 or more months of follow-up

Study	Location	N	Age (y) (Range)	Prior Treatment (%)	Sigmoid Achalasia (%)	Operating Time (min) (Range)	Myotomy Length (cm) (Range)	Mean Follow-up (mo)	Efficacy[a] (%)	GERD[b] (%)	Minor/Major Adverse Events[c] n/n (%/%)
Li et al,[28] 2013	Shanghai, China	238	39.8 (NA)	41.6	7.6	45.7 (NA)	10.2 (NA)	8.5	95.0	18.6	63/0 (26/0)[d]
Cai et al,[19] 2014	Shanghai, China	100	40.9 (18–72)	24	8	29.9 (NA)	10.8 (7–13)	11.5	96.5	10	6/0 (6/0)
Ling et al,[87] 2014	Nanjing, China	87	41.6 (18–66)	0	NA	42 (NA)	NA	14.4	97.7	5.7	2/0 (2.3/0)
Sharata et al,[35] 2014	Portland, Oregon, United States	100	58 (18–83)	35	NA	128 (45–215)	8 (4–23)	16	98	38.2	17/1 (17/1)
Teitelbaum et al,[88] 2014	Chicago, IL, United States	41	45 (NA)	10	NA	110 (NA)	9 (NA)	15	92	59	22/1 (53.6/2.4)
Ling et al,[89] 2014	Nanjing, China	51	42.9 (NA)	41.2	NA	38.4 (NA)	9.9 (NA)	13.9	NA	7.8	2/0 (3.9/0)
Stavropoulos et al,[45] 2014	Mineola, United States	100	52 (17–93)	42	20	106 (39–240)	12 (3–26)	13.3	97	24	32/0 (32/0)[f]
Chen et al,[86] 2015	Nanjing, China	45	46.3 (26–72)	22	NA	73.8 (NA)	9.56 (NA)	24	100	6.7	3/0 (6.7/0)
Hu et al,[90] 2015	Shanghai, China	32	43.6 (18–72)	71.9	100	63.7 (22–130)	10.3 (7–14)	30	96.8	18.8	15/0 (46.9/0)[d]
Ju et al,[91] 2015	Qingdao, China	112	48 (18–59)	NA	NA	NA	NA (10–12)	12	100	18.9	8/0 (7.1/0)
Ramchandani et al,[42] 2015	Hyderabad, India	220	39 (9–74)	41.4	20.5	88 (38–180)	12 (6–19)	13.4	92	16	77/0 (35/0)

Lu et al,[92] 2015	Hangzhou, China	50	42.8 (14–70)	16	NA	55.4 (30–120)	10.5 (NA)	7.3	96	0	0/0 (0/0)
Duan et al,[93] 2015	Changsha, China	123	42.1 (NA)	14.6	8.9	59.6 (NA)	10.5 (NA)	21	98.4	1.6	14/0 (11.3/0)
Inoue et al,[50] 2015	Tokyo, Japan	500	43 (32–58)	40.6	15.4	90 (70.8–119)	14 (12–16)	12–24[e]	91	19.4	16/0 (3.2/0)
Hoppo et al,[94] 2015	Pittsburgh, PA, United States	35	56.9 (23–86)	33.3	8.6	185 (107–327)	13 (6–22)	7	87	NA	20/0 (57/0)
Werner et al,[66] 2015	Multicenter	80	44.9 (9–88)	40	NA	103.4 (54–220)	12.7	29	78.5	37.5	16/0 (20/0)
Jones et al,[74] 2015	Ohio, United States	43	53.5 (NA)	NA	NA	103 (NA)	15 (NA)	6	98[g]	58	15/0 (34.9/0)
Tang et al,[95] 2015	Beijing, China	67	38.2 (16–68)	32.8	NA	60.8 (30–180)	9.7 (7–15)	12	93.9	5.97	2/0 (2.9/0)
Familiari et al,[41] 2016	Rome, Italy	100	48.4 (NA)	24	7	83 (49–140)	12 (7–17)	11	94.5	53.4	33/0 (33/0)
Total	—	2124	—	—	—	—	—	16.2	91	20	365/2 (17.2/0.09)

Abbreviations: GERD, gastroesophageal reflux disease; NA, data not available.

a Eckardt 3 or less.

b Evidence of GERD by 24 pH, endoscopy, or GERD questionnaire.

c Minor = Clavien-Dindo grade I to IIIa; Major = Clavien Dindo grade IIIb to V. Asymptomatic radiologic findings NOT included. Subcutaneous emphysema, pneumoperitoneum mucosal injury included ONLY if intervention required.

d Air insufflation used in some cases.

e 1- to 2-year follow-up was available on 74% of patients.

f All mucosal damage included.

g Non-Eckardt score used.

REFLUX

The heightened emphasis and concern regarding reflux after POEM has thus far not been substantiated, with a sparsity of reflux-related adverse events in the literature at now maximum follow-up periods of 5 to 7 years and mean follow-up periods of 2 to 3 years in pioneering centers and no reports so far of PPI-refractory reflux. To date, there has been one reported case of a peptic stricture that was successfully managed with balloon dilation. The patient was lost to follow-up and subsequently presented 22 months after POEM with recurrent dysphagia and was discovered to have a peptic stricture.[66] Posttreatment reflux has been inconsistently reported in the achalasia literature. In a systematic review and meta-analysis of LHM published in 2009, the incidence of reflux was 8.8%.[71] Similar to LHM, the incidence of reflux in POEM was 10.9% in a systematic review and meta-analysis published in 2014.[38] However, the reported incidences of reflux among studies included were based on variable definitions that included mostly subjective data, such as positive scores on self-assessment questionnaires and patient self-reporting of reflux symptoms, and only scant objective data, such as abnormal acid exposure on 24-hour esophageal pH testing and esophagitis on endoscopy. In the 2011 European randomized achalasia trial comparing pneumatic dilation with LHM, which used 24-hour esophageal pH testing, the reflux rates for LHM and pneumatic dilation were 23% and 15% ($P = .28$), respectively.[72] In a comparative study by Bhayani and colleagues[12] of 64 LHM versus 37 POEM reflux was assessed with 24-hour esophageal pH testing in 31 out of 64 of the LHMs and 23 out of 37 of the POEMs, demonstrating no statistically significant difference in reflux incidence (LHM 32% vs POEM 39%; $P = .7$). In a somewhat uneven comparison, Kumagai and colleagues[18] observed gastroesophageal reflux disease (GERD) symptoms in 7 out of 42 POEM patients (16.7%) compared with abnormal acid exposure in 7 of the 24 LHM patients who underwent pH testing (29%). A low correlation has been found between post-POEM reflux symptoms and abnormal acid exposure on 24-hour esophageal pH testing. In 2015, Familiari and colleagues[73] showed that only 42% of post-POEM patients with esophagitis had reflux symptoms. Similarly, Jones and colleagues[74] demonstrated that post-POEM, 50% of asymptomatic patients had abnormal acid exposure. Based on the current evidence on reflux incidence, including 24-h esophageal pH testing, esophagitis on endoscopy, validated GERD questionnaires and patient self-reporting, clinically significant acid reflux after POEM seems comparable with rates in the 20% to 40% range reported in high quality studies assessing GERD after LHM with Dor or Toupet fundoplication. Therefore, there is indeed a moderate risk of reflux after POEM; however, the risk seems to be fairly similar to that of surgical myotomy with an antireflux procedure. In addition, the risk of reflux-associated adverse events or reflux refractory to PPI is minimal so far. However, this important issue is continuing to evolve, as we are now having an exponential growth of the procedure with rapidly expanding data from many centers.

PERORAL ENDOSCOPIC MYOTOMY VERSUS LAPAROSCOPIC HELLER MYOTOMY

There have been no randomized trials comparing POEM versus LHM; however, currently 2 registered randomized trials are due for completion between 2017 and 2019.[75,76] There have been 8 studies comparing POEM with LHM that have demonstrated POEM typically results in shorter procedure time, hospital stay and days to return to regular activities, decreased blood loss, and postprocedure pain, all with at least equivalent clinical efficacy and reflux rates.[12–14,18,49,77–79] In a systematic review and meta-analysis that included 19 studies, POEM was as least as effective as LHM for the treatment of achalasia.[38] A comparative study by Kumbhari and colleagues[14] examined the outcomes for type III achalasia in 49 POEMs and 26 LHMs. POEM had a significantly higher clinical success rate (POEM 98.0% vs LHM 80.8%; $P = .01$), longer myotomy (POEM 16 cm vs LHM 8 cm; $P<.01$), shorter procedure time (POEM 102 minutes vs LHM 264 minutes; $P<.01$), and fewer adverse events (POEM 6% vs LHM 27%; $P<.01$). In cases of previous failed myotomy or recurrence of symptoms after surgical myotomy, POEM has a clinical success rate of more than 90% and the advantage of freedom to select the myotomy position, avoiding areas of known surgical manipulation, scarring, and fibrosis, which is not possible with LHM.[15–17]

RISK OF INFECTION AND IMPLICATIONS FOR OTHER TRANSESOPHAGEAL NATURAL ORIFICE TRANSLUMINAL ENDOSCOPIC SURGERY PROCEDURES

The fear of life-threatening mediastinitis was a major concern at the onset of POEM; as a result, all endoscopic devices were sterilized with ethylene oxide gas. Despite sterilization, the endoscope was introduced through a nonsterile oropharynx. Subsequently, with the observation that no clinically significant infections occurred despite the lack of sterility with entry through the oropharynx, the seemingly futile sterilization practice was discontinued without any adverse events in subsequent cases. However, all patients are given prophylactic antibiotics intravenously and topically through direct instillation into the submucosal tunnel. In addition, good oral hygiene is strongly encouraged before POEM, with some operators advocating the use of an oral chlorhexidine rinse and eradication of esophageal candidiasis if present. The prophylactic antibiotics seem to be effective given the thousands of POEM procedures performed without reports of mediastinal sepsis or major peritonitis.[26] There is one case of localized peritonitis that was managed conservatively with antibiotics and one report of a retroperitoneal abscess that required drainage via interventional radiology.[80,81] There have been 3 reports of esophageal leaks, none of which developed serious infectious adverse events; one was managed conservatively with antibiotics and thoracic drainage, whereas the other two required laparoscopic or thoracoscopic drainage.[13,49] Thus, contrary to surgical dogma, the risk of infection with POEM has been remarkably low. The paucity of mediastinitis or peritonitis associated with POEM despite peritoneal and mediastinal exposure with a nonsterile endoscope should alleviate some angst related to the risk of infection with transesophageal NOTES for applications such as mediastinoscopy. The low risk of infection-related adverse events in transesophageal NOTES has also been supported by minimal infection-related adverse events with live animal models undergoing transesophageal thoracoscopy with lung biopsy and mediastinoscopy with nodal excision.[82–84] In a randomized survival study in a porcine model, Córdova and colleagues[85] compared NOTES mediastinoscopy with conventional video-assisted mediastinoscopy. There was no statistically significant difference between groups in the occurrence of bacteremia, mediastinitis, or abscesses. Based on experience with POEM and multiple animal studies, the risk of severe infection with transesophageal NOTES seems to be modest and should not pose an overwhelming barrier to further development of transesophageal peritoneal/mediastinal NOTES.

SUMMARY

Since it was first introduced in 2008, POEM has been increasingly performed and accepted worldwide for the treatment of achalasia and spastic esophageal motility disorders. POEM has permitted safe and effective esophageal cardiomyotomy for spastic esophageal motility disorders with the capacity to tailor the position and length of the myotomy to the clinical setting, contrary to LHM, which is limited in myotomy position and length. POEM has demonstrated excellent safety and long-term clinical efficacy. For DES and hypercontractile esophagus, the inclusion of the LES in the myotomy is controversial. However, inclusion of the LES in the myotomy may prevent subsequent symptom development due to ineffective esophageal motility or disease progression to achalasia. POEM has demonstrated that with the administration of prophylactic antibiotics, entrance into the sterile mediastinum/peritoneum with a nonsterile endoscope has a negligible risk of causing serious infection. POEM has also demonstrated that procedural innovation without dependence on technological innovation can generate dramatic clinical advancement. Thus, although necessary, device innovation should not overshadow procedural innovation in NOTES development.

SUPPLEMENTARY DATA

Supplementary data related to this article can be found at http://dx.doi.org/10.1016/j.giec.2015.12.002.

REFERENCES

1. Heller E. Extramukose kardioplastik beim chronischen kardiospasmus mit dilatation des oesophagus. Mitt Grenzgeb Med Chir 1914;27:141–9.
2. Zaaijer JH. Cardiospasm in the aged. Ann Surg 1923;77:615–7.
3. Ellis F Jr, Olsen AM, Holman CB, et al. Surgical treatment of cardiospasm (achalasia of the esophagus): considerations of aspects of esophagomyotomy. J Am Med Assoc 1958;166:29–36.
4. Ortega JA, Madureri V, Perez L. Endoscopic myotomy in the treatment of achalasia. Gastrointest Endosc 1980;26:8–10.
5. Shimi S, Nathanson LK, Cuschieri A. Laparoscopic cardiomyotomy for achalasia. J R Coll Surg Edinb 1991;36:152–4.
6. Pellegrini C, Wetter LA, Patti M, et al. Thoracoscopic esophagomyotomy. Initial experience with a new approach for the treatment of achalasia. Ann Surg 1992;216:291–6 [discussion: 296–9].
7. Kalloo AN, Singh VK, Jagannath SB, et al. Flexible transgastric peritoneoscopy: a novel approach to diagnostic and therapeutic interventions in the peritoneal cavity. Gastrointest Endosc 2004;60:114–7.
8. Marescaux J, Dallemagne B, Perretta S, et al. Surgery without scars: report of transluminal cholecystectomy in a human being. Arch Surg 2007;142:823–6 [discussion: 826–7].
9. Zorrón R, Filgueiras M, Maggioni LC, et al. NOTES. Transvaginal cholecystectomy: report of the first case. Surg Innov 2007;14:279–83.
10. Pasricha PJ, Hawari R, Ahmed I, et al. Submucosal endoscopic esophageal myotomy: a novel experimental approach for the treatment of achalasia. Endoscopy 2007;39:761–4.
11. Inoue H, Minami H, Kobayashi Y, et al. Peroral endoscopic myotomy (POEM) for esophageal achalasia. Endoscopy 2010;42:265–71.
12. Bhayani NH, Kurian AA, Dunst CM, et al. A comparative study on comprehensive, objective outcomes of laparoscopic Heller myotomy with per-oral endoscopic myotomy (POEM) for achalasia. Ann Surg 2014;259:1098–103.
13. Ujiki MB, Yetasook AK, Zapf M, et al. Peroral endoscopic myotomy: a short-term comparison with the standard laparoscopic approach. Surgery 2013;154:893–7 [discussion: 897–900].

14. Kumbhari V, Tieu AH, Onimaru M, et al. Peroral endoscopic myotomy (POEM) vs laparoscopic Heller myotomy (LHM) for the treatment of type III achalasia in 75 patients: a multicenter comparative study. Endosc Int Open 2015;3:E195–201.
15. Onimaru M, Inoue H, Ikeda H, et al. Peroral endoscopic myotomy is a viable option for failed surgical esophagocardiomyotomy instead of redo surgical Heller myotomy: a single center prospective study. J Am Coll Surg 2013;217:598–605.
16. Vigneswaran Y, Yetasook AK, Zhao JC, et al. Peroral endoscopic myotomy (POEM): feasible as reoperation following Heller myotomy. J Gastrointest Surg 2014;18:1071–6.
17. Zhou PH, Li QL, Yao LQ, et al. Peroral endoscopic remyotomy for failed Heller myotomy: a prospective single-center study. Endoscopy 2013;45:161–6.
18. Kumagai K, Tsai JA, Thorell A, et al. Per-oral endoscopic myotomy for achalasia. Are results comparable to laparoscopic Heller myotomy? Scand J Gastroenterol 2015;50:505–12.
19. Cai MY, Zhou PH, Yao LQ, et al. Peroral endoscopic myotomy for idiopathic achalasia: randomized comparison of water-jet assisted versus conventional dissection technique. Surg Endosc 2014;28:1158–65.
20. Aihara H, Kumar N, Ryan MB, et al. Mo1538 a novel endoscopic tapered-tip CAP significantly reduces time for endoscopic submucosal tunneling. Gastrointest Endosc 79:AB475–6.
21. Stavropoulos SN, Desilets DJ, Fuchs KH, et al. Per-oral endoscopic myotomy white paper summary. Gastrointest Endosc 2014;80:1–15.
22. Stavropoulos SN, Modayil RJ, Friedel D, et al. The International Per Oral Endoscopic Myotomy Survey (IPOEMS): a snapshot of the global POEM experience. Surg Endosc 2013;27:3322–38.
23. Khashab MA, Messallam AA, Onimaru M, et al. International multicenter experience with peroral endoscopic myotomy for the treatment of spastic esophageal disorders refractory to medical therapy (with video). Gastrointest Endosc 2015; 81(5):1170–7.
24. Paterson WG, Beck IT, Da Costa LR. Transition from nutcracker esophagus to achalasia. A case report. J Clin Gastroenterol 1991;13:554–8.
25. Fontes LH, Herbella FA, Rodriguez TN, et al. Progression of diffuse esophageal spasm to achalasia: incidence and predictive factors. Dis Esophagus 2013;26: 470–4.
26. Bechara R, Ikeda H, Inoue H. Peroral endoscopic myotomy: an evolving treatment for achalasia. Nat Rev Gastroenterol Hepatol 2015;12:410–26.
27. Grimes KL, Inoue H, Onimaru M, et al. Double-scope per oral endoscopic myotomy (POEM): a prospective randomized controlled trial. Surg Endosc 2015. [Epub ahead of print].
28. Li QL, Chen WF, Zhou PH, et al. Peroral endoscopic myotomy for the treatment of achalasia: a clinical comparative study of endoscopic full-thickness and circular muscle myotomy. J Am Coll Surg 2013;217:442–51.
29. Liu B-R, Song J-T, Omar Jan M. Video of the month. Am J Gastroenterol 2015; 110:499.
30. Yang D, Draganov PV. Closing the gap in POEM. Endoscopy 2013;45:677.
31. Stavropoulos SN, Modayil R, Friedel D. Current applications of endoscopic suturing. World J Gastrointest Endosc 2015;7:777–89.
32. Saxena P, Chavez YH, Kord Valeshabad A, et al. An alternative method for mucosal flap closure during peroral endoscopic myotomy using an over-the-scope clipping device. Endoscopy 2013;45:579–81.

33. Yang D, Zhang Q, Draganov PV. Successful placement of a fully covered esophageal stent to bridge a difficult-to-close mucosal incision during peroral endoscopic myotomy. Endoscopy 2014;46(Suppl 1 UCTN):E467–8.
34. Kumta NA, Mehta S, Kedia P, et al. Peroral endoscopic myotomy: establishing a new program. Clin Endosc 2014;47:389–97.
35. Sharata AM, Dunst CM, Pescarus R, et al. Peroral endoscopic myotomy (POEM) for esophageal primary motility disorders: analysis of 100 consecutive patients. J Gastrointest Surg 2015;19(1):161–70.
36. Zhang Y, Wang X, Fan Z. Reclosure of ruptured incision after peroral endoscopic myotomy using endoloops and metallic clips. Dig Endosc 2014;26:295.
37. Chandrasekhara V, Desilets D, Falk GW, et al. The American Society for Gastrointestinal Endoscopy PIVI (Preservation and Incorporation of Valuable Endoscopic Innovations) on peroral endoscopic myotomy. Gastrointest Endosc 2015;81:1087–100.e1.
38. Talukdar R, Inoue H, Reddy DN. Efficacy of peroral endoscopic myotomy (POEM) in the treatment of achalasia: a systematic review and meta-analysis. Surg Endosc 2015;29(11):3030–46.
39. Ren Z, Zhong Y, Zhou P, et al. Perioperative management and treatment for complications during and after peroral endoscopic myotomy (POEM) for esophageal achalasia (EA) (data from 119 cases). Surg Endosc 2012;26:3267–72.
40. Banks-Venegoni AL, Desilets DJ, Romanelli JR, et al. Tension capnopericardium and cardiac arrest as an unexpected adverse event of peroral endoscopic myotomy (with video). Gastrointest Endosc 2015;82(6):1137–9.
41. Familiari P, Gigante G, Marchese M, et al. Peroral endoscopic myotomy for esophageal achalasia: outcomes of the first 100 patients with short-term follow-up. Ann Surg 2016;263(1):82–7.
42. Ramchandani M, Nageshwar Reddy D, Darisetty S, et al. Peroral endoscopic myotomy for achalasia cardia: a single center experience of over 200 consecutive patients: treatment analysis and follow up. Dig Endosc 2016;28(1):19–26.
43. Kurian AA, Dunst CM, Sharata A, et al. Peroral endoscopic esophageal myotomy: defining the learning curve. Gastrointest Endosc 2013;77:719–25.
44. Teitelbaum EN, Soper NJ, Arafat FO, et al. Analysis of a learning curve and predictors of intraoperative difficulty for peroral esophageal myotomy (POEM). J Gastrointest Surg 2014;18:92–8 [discussion: 98–9].
45. Stavropoulos SN, Moyadil RJ, Brathwaite CE, et al. Mo1530 per oral endoscopic myotomy (POEM) for achalasia: large single-center 4-year series by a gastroenterologist with emphasis on objective assessment of emptying, GERD, LES distensibility and post-procedural pain. Gastrointest Endosc 2014;79:AB472–3.
46. Ling T, Pei Q, Pan J, et al. Successful use of a covered, retrievable stent to seal a ruptured mucosal flap safety valve during peroral endoscopic myotomy in a child with achalasia. Endoscopy 2013;45(Suppl 2 UCTN):E63–4.
47. Modayil R, Friedel D, Stavropoulos SN. Endoscopic suture repair of a large mucosal perforation during peroral endoscopic myotomy for treatment of achalasia. Gastrointest Endosc 2014;80:1169–70.
48. Li H, Linghu E, Wang X. Fibrin sealant for closure of mucosal penetration at the cardia during peroral endoscopic myotomy (POEM). Endoscopy 2012;44(Suppl 2 UCTN):E215–6.
49. Hungness ES, Teitelbaum EN, Santos BF, et al. Comparison of perioperative outcomes between peroral esophageal myotomy (POEM) and laparoscopic Heller myotomy. J Gastrointest Surg 2013;17:228–35.

50. Inoue H, Sato H, Ikeda H, et al. Per-oral endoscopic myotomy: a series of 500 patients. J Am Coll Surg 2015;221:256–64.
51. Li Q-L, Zhou PH, Yao LQ, et al. Early diagnosis and management of delayed bleeding in the submucosal tunnel after peroral endoscopic myotomy for achalasia (with video). Gastrointest Endosc 2013;78:370–4.
52. Minami H, Isomoto H, Yamaguchi N, et al. Peroral endoscopic myotomy for esophageal achalasia: clinical impact of 28 cases. Digestive endoscopy: official journal of the Japan Gastroenterological Endoscopy Society 2014;26:43–51.
53. Benech N, Pioche M, O'Brien M, et al. Esophageal hematoma after peroral endoscopic myotomy for achalasia in a patient on antiplatelet therapy. Endoscopy 2015;47(Suppl 1):E363–4.
54. Andersson M, Lundell L, Kostic S, et al. Evaluation of the response to treatment in patients with idiopathic achalasia by the timed barium esophagogram: results from a randomized clinical trial. Dis Esophagus 2009;22:264–73.
55. Torquati A, Richards WO, Holzman MD, et al. Laparoscopic myotomy for achalasia: predictors of successful outcome after 200 cases. Ann Surg 2006;243: 587–91 [discussion: 591–3].
56. Vaezi MF, Baker ME, Achkar E, et al. Timed barium oesophagram: better predictor of long term success after pneumatic dilation in achalasia than symptom assessment. Gut 2002;50:765–70.
57. Ghoshal UC, Kumar S, Saraswat VA, et al. Long-term follow-up after pneumatic dilation for achalasia cardia: factors associated with treatment failure and recurrence. Am J Gastroenterol 2004;99:2304–10.
58. Ghosh SK, Pandolfino JE, Rice J, et al. Impaired deglutitive EGJ relaxation in clinical esophageal manometry: a quantitative analysis of 400 patients and 75 controls. Am J Physiol Gastrointest Liver Physiol 2007;293:G878–85.
59. Nicodeme F, de Ruigh A, Xiao Y, et al. A comparison of symptom severity and bolus retention with Chicago classification esophageal pressure topography metrics in patients with achalasia. Clin Gastroenterol Hepatol 2013;11:131–7 [quiz: e15].
60. Kwiatek MA, Pandolfino JE, Hirano I, et al. Esophagogastric junction distensibility assessed with an endoscopic functional luminal imaging probe (EndoFLIP). Gastrointest Endosc 2010;72:272–8.
61. Pandolfino JE, de Ruigh A, Nicodème F, et al. Distensibility of the esophagogastric junction assessed with the functional lumen imaging probe (FLIP) in achalasia patients. Neurogastroenterol Motil 2013;25:496–501.
62. Rohof WO, Hirsch DP, Kessing BF, et al. Efficacy of treatment for patients with achalasia depends on the distensibility of the esophagogastric junction. Gastroenterology 2012;143:328–35.
63. Chiu PW, Wu JC, Teoh AY, et al. Peroral endoscopic myotomy for treatment of achalasia: from bench to bedside (with video). Gastrointest Endosc 2013;77: 29–38.
64. Verlaan T, Rohof WO, Bredenoord AJ, et al. Effect of peroral endoscopic myotomy on esophagogastric junction physiology in patients with achalasia. Gastrointest Endosc 2013;78:39–44.
65. Von Renteln D, Fuchs KH, Fockens P, et al. Peroral endoscopic myotomy for the treatment of achalasia: an international prospective multicenter study. Gastroenterology 2013;145:309–11.e1–3.
66. Werner YB, Costamagna G, Swanström LL, et al. Clinical response to peroral endoscopic myotomy in patients with idiopathic achalasia at a minimum follow-up of 2 years. Gut 2015. [Epub ahead of print].

67. Zaninotto G, Costantini M, Portale G, et al. Etiology, diagnosis, and treatment of failures after laparoscopic Heller myotomy for achalasia. Ann Surg 2002;235: 186–92.
68. Loviscek MF, Wright AS, Hinojosa MW, et al. Recurrent dysphagia after Heller myotomy: is esophagectomy always the answer? J Am Coll Surg 2013;216:736–43 [discussion: 743–4].
69. Li QL, Yao LQ, Xu XY, et al. Repeat peroral endoscopic myotomy: a salvage option for persistent/recurrent symptoms. Endoscopy 2016;48(2):134–40.
70. Patel KS, Calixte R, Modayil RJ, et al. The light at the end of the tunnel: a single-operator learning curve analysis for per oral endoscopic myotomy. Gastrointest Endosc 2015;81(5):1181–7.
71. Campos GM, Vittinghoff E, Rabl C, et al. Endoscopic and surgical treatments for achalasia: a systematic review and meta-analysis. Ann Surg 2009;249:45–57.
72. Boeckxstaens GE, Annese V, des Varannes SB, et al. Pneumatic dilation versus laparoscopic Heller's myotomy for idiopathic achalasia. N Engl J Med 2011; 364:1807–16.
73. Familiari P, Greco S, Gigante G, et al. Gastro-esophageal reflux disease after peroral endoscopic myotomy (POEM). Analysis of clinical, procedural and functional factors, associated with GERD and esophagitis. Dig Endosc 2016;28(1):33–41.
74. Jones EL, Meara MP, Schwartz JS, et al. Gastroesophageal reflux symptoms do not correlate with objective pH testing after peroral endoscopic myotomy. Surg Endosc 2015. [Epub ahead of print].
75. Hospital U.o.S.P.G. Laparoscopy Heller myotomy with fundoplication associated versus peroral endoscopic myotomy. In: ClinicalTrials.gov [Internet]. Bethesda (MD): National Library of Medicine (US); 2014.
76. Rösch T. Endoscopic versus laparoscopic myotomy for treatment of idiopathic achalasia: a randomized, controlled trial. In: ClinicalTrials.gov [Internet]. Bethesda (MD): National Library of Medicine (US); 2012.
77. Teitelbaum EN, Soper NJ, Pandolfino JE, et al. An extended proximal esophageal myotomy is necessary to normalize EGJ distensibility during Heller myotomy for achalasia, but not POEM. Surg Endosc 2014;28:2840–7.
78. Teitelbaum EN, Boris L, Arafat FO, et al. Comparison of esophagogastric junction distensibility changes during POEM and Heller myotomy using intraoperative FLIP. Surg Endosc 2013;27:4547–55.
79. Chan SM, Wu JC, Teoh AY, et al. Comparison of early outcomes and quality of life after Laparoscopic Heller's cardiomyotomy to per oral endoscopic myotomy for treatment of achalasia. Dig Endosc 2016;28(1):27–32.
80. Inoue H, Ikeda H, Onimaru M, et al. 54 Clinical results in 300 cases of POEM for esophageal achalasia a single institute registered prospective study. Gastrointest Endosc 77:AB121–2.
81. Yang S, Zeng MS, Zhang ZY, et al. Pneumomediastinum and pneumoperitoneum on computed tomography after peroral endoscopic myotomy (POEM): postoperative changes or complications? Acta Radiol 2015;56(10):1216–21.
82. Gee DW, Willingham FF, Lauwers GY, et al. Natural orifice transesophageal mediastinoscopy and thoracoscopy: a survival series in swine. Surg Endosc 2008; 22:2117–22.
83. Turner BG, Gee DW, Cizginer S, et al. Endoscopic transesophageal mediastinal lymph node dissection and en bloc resection by using mediastinal and thoracic approaches (with video). Gastrointest Endosc 2010;72:831–5.
84. Liu YH, Chu Y, Wu YC, et al. Feasibility of endoscopic transoral surgical lung biopsy in a live canine model. Surg Innov 2012;19:162–70.

85. Córdova H, Cubas G, Boada M, et al. Adverse events of NOTES mediastino-scopy compared to conventional video-assisted mediastinoscopy: a randomized survival study in a porcine model. Endosc Int Open 2015;3(6):E571–6.
86. Chen X, Li QP, Ji GZ, et al. Two-year follow-up for 45 patients with achalasia who underwent peroral endoscopic myotomy. Eur J Cardiothorac Surg 2015;47(5): 890–6.
87. Ling TS, Guo HM, Yang T, et al. Effectiveness of peroral endoscopic myotomy in the treatment of achalasia: a pilot trial in Chinese Han population with a minimum of one-year follow-up. J Dig Dis 2014;15:352–8.
88. Teitelbaum EN, Soper NJ, Santos BF, et al. Symptomatic and physiologic out-comes one year after peroral esophageal myotomy (POEM) for treatment of acha-lasia. Surg Endosc 2014;28(12):3359–65.
89. Ling T, Guo H, Zou X. Effect of peroral endoscopic myotomy in achalasia patients with failure of prior pneumatic dilation: a prospective case-control study. J Gastroenterol Hepatol 2014;29:1609–13.
90. Hu JW, Li QL, Zhou PH, et al. Peroral endoscopic myotomy for advanced acha-lasia with sigmoid-shaped esophagus: long-term outcomes from a prospective, single-center study. Surg Endosc 2015;29(9):2841–50.
91. Ju H, Ma Y, Liang K, et al. Function of high-resolution manometry in the analysis of peroral endoscopic myotomy for achalasia. Surg Endosc 2015. [Epub ahead of print].
92. Lu B, Li M, Hu Y, et al. Effect of peroral esophageal myotomy for achalasia treat-ment: a Chinese study. World J Gastroenterol 2015;21:5622–9.
93. Duan T, Zhou J, Tan Y, et al. 180 Peroral endoscopic myotomy for severe acha-lasia: the comparison of full-thickness myotomy and circular myotomy. Gastroint-est Endosc 2015;81:AB118.
94. Hoppo T, Thakkar SJ, Schumacher LY, et al. A utility of peroral endoscopic myot-omy (POEM) across the spectrum of esophageal motility disorders. Surg Endosc 2016;30(1):233–44.
95. Tang X, Gong W, Deng Z, et al. Comparison of conventional versus Hybrid knife peroral endoscopic myotomy methods for esophageal achalasia: a case-control study. Scand J Gastroenterol 2015;51:1–7.

Per-Oral Pyloromyotomy (POP)

An Emerging Application of Submucosal Tunneling for the Treatment of Refractory Gastroparesis

Carter Lebares, MD[a], Lee L. Swanstrom, MD, FACS, FASGE[b],*

KEYWORDS

- Pyloroplasty • Pyloromyotomy • Gastroparesis • POEM • POP
- Endoscopic pylormyotomy

KEY POINTS

- Disruption of the pylorus improves symptoms of gastroparesis.
- Per-oral pyloromyotomy is a minimally invasive approach that shows good efficacy in the treatment of refractory gastroparesis.
- The POEM tunneling technique provides good access to the pylorus.
- Early data shows correction of gastric emptying in a significant percentage of patients.

INTRODUCTION

A growing body of literature supports the use of laparoscopic pyloroplasty as a minimally invasive treatment of refractory gastroparesis that has failed conservative measures and for benign gastric outlet obstruction. Endoscopic pyloric dilation, stent placement, and Botox have been described for similar indications, but often with transient or mixed results. With wider acceptance of endoscopic submucosal dissection and per-oral endoscopic myotomy (POEM) as a viable treatment for achalasia, it is not surprising that a similar tunneling approach would be applied to dysfunctions of the pylorus resulting in poor gastric emptying. Per-oral pyloromyotomy (POP) has recently been proposed as an endoscopic alternative to surgical pyloroplasty or pylormyotomy because it is less invasive by its nature and potentially more durable than current endoscopic treatments. Using technologies common to POEM, POP involves the creation of a submucosal tunnel followed by division of the pyloric sphincter muscles. Here the physiologic basis of pyloric disruption for various gastric disorders as

[a] University of California San Francisco, San Francisco, California; [b] Institute of Image-guided Minimally Invasive Surgery, Institut Hospitalo universitaire, University of Strasbourg, 1, Place de l' Hopital, 67900 Strasbourg, France
* Corresponding author.
E-mail address: lswanstrom@gmail.com

Gastrointest Endoscopy Clin N Am 26 (2016) 257–270
http://dx.doi.org/10.1016/j.giec.2015.12.012
1052-5157/16/$ – see front matter © 2016 Elsevier Inc. All rights reserved.

well as the development of POP, its potential indications, the precise steps in this highly skill-dependent technique, and early data in humans is reviewed.

THE PYLORUS AND PYLORIC DISRUPTION

The pylorus is frequently involved in benign digestive disorders, including gastric outlet obstruction and gastroparesis (delayed gastric emptying in the absence of mechanical obstruction). One of the most common examples of this is congenital hypertrophic pyloric stenosis. This idiopathic condition has a population incidence of 2 to 4 per 1000 live births and presents with gastric obstructive symptoms (vomiting and failure to feed) at a very early age. For more than 100 years, it has been effectively palliated by the division of the abnormally hypertrophic pyloric sphincter. Today, pediatric pyloromyotomy is 99% effective at relieving patient symptoms and is increasingly performed laparoscopically.[1] In the adult population, gastric outlet obstruction is most commonly due to reactive pyloric stenosis—usually secondary to chronic peptic ulcer disease or caustic ingestion. As a purely mechanical problem, this diagnosis and its treatment are fairly straightforward and, if unresponsive to medical therapy including endoscopic dilation, responds well to surgical emptying treatments such as a pyloroplasty or distal gastrectomy. More importantly, pyloric dysfunction is implicated in the rather ill-defined category of gastroparesis. Gastroparesis, defined as a delay in gastric emptying not related to a mechanical outlet obstruction, can be idiopathic, diabetic, or postsurgical. Pyloric disruption has been used for this diagnosis with varying degrees of success.[2]

Surgical pyloroplasty has been successfully used to treat benign gastric outlet obstruction for decades, and it at least theoretically makes sense. Pyloroplasty (per the Heineke-Mikulicz method)[3] involves longitudinal division of the full thickness of the pyloric ring, thereby obliterating the cause of obstruction. This division is followed by transverse closure of the full-thickness defect, thereby assuring a geometrically enlarged lumen. An alternative procedure is a pyloromyotomy, which involves the longitudinal division of the serosa and muscular layers of the distal stomach, pylorus, and proximal duodenal bulb, leaving the mucosa intact. The choice of whether one uses a pyloromyotomy or a pyloroplasty depends somewhat on the procedure; for example, the current standard of care for congenital hypertrophic pyloric stenosis in children is pyloromyotomy, but the usual treatment of gastric outlet related to peptic ulcer disease is a pyloroplasty plus vagotomy (or antrectomy).[4–7] Following esophagectomy with gastric interposition, benign gastric outlet obstruction (which affects approximately 15% of patients) has been described as benefitting from surgical pyloroplasty or pyloromyotomy, although it can also be treated with endoscopic balloon dilation.[8–11] Pyloric disruption by endoscopic balloon dilation can also be used to treat obstruction from chronic ulcers or caustic stricture,[12–14] although in these settings definitive treatment often requires surgery. Endoscopic self-expanding metallic stents are another intriguing possibility for treating both benign pyloric stenosis and gastroparesis. Studies to date are small and uncontrolled, but several have demonstrated symptomatic improvement and/or reduced gastric-emptying times with transpyloric stenting.[15,16] Unfortunately, this technique is plagued by the issue of migration, which currently hinders any long-term use of stents.[17]

Regarding gastroparesis, the role of pyloric disruption has only recently come to the fore with a growing body of literature citing benefit in this context. Gastroparesis is historically an ill-defined and highly complex disease. It is thought to stem from a combination of damage to the vagus nerve or myenteric plexus, reduced hormone secretion (motilin and grehlin), and diminished growth factors required by the Interstitial Cells of Cajal (the gastric pacemakers). Atony of the corpus, continuous spasm of the pyloric ring, and desynchronization between stomach, duodenum, and pylorus are often described. Because of the complex pathophysiology of gastroparesis, it is not surprising that symptoms correlate poorly with gastric emptying, resulting in multiple subtypes of the disease.[18,19] Diagnosis requires the presence of chronic symptoms (either nausea, vomiting, early satiety, postprandial fullness, or upper abdominal pain) typically assessed via the validated Gastroparesis Cardinal Symptom Index, GCSI,[20] delayed gastric emptying, as evidenced by scintigraphy, and a contrast study ruling-out mechanical obstruction. Symptoms, which directly influence the patient's quality of life, are currently used to assess treatment success. Even in this quagmire of a poorly defined, complex disorder with modest overall incidence (1.8%–4% in the general population), treating gastroparesis is still worthwhile. Patients are significantly debilitated; the economic burden is profound, and the incidence of gastroparesis-related hospitalizations has increased 158% between 1995 and 2004.[19,21]

Dietary modification and symptom control with antinausea and antiemetic medications remain first-line therapy. Failing these, prokinetics often are next. Metoclopramide, the only US Food and Drug Administration (FDA)-approved medication for gastroparesis treatment in the United States, currently carries a black-box warning of tardive dyskinesia, and prolonged use is associated with tachyphylaxis.[22] Gastric electrical stimulation is currently FDA-approved on protocol (humanitarian device exemption) for diabetic and idiopathic gastroparesis.[23] Benefits have been found in relieving nausea and vomiting, with conflicting results regarding the effect on gastric emptying.[24] A major issue with this device is its high cost and orphan device status, which makes it difficult to access in North America.

Endoscopic intrapyloric injection of botulinum toxin A, which was promising in initial open-label studies,[25–28] has since demonstrated no difference from placebo in 2 randomized controlled trials.[29,30] As a result, The American Gastroenterological Society no longer recommends intrapyloric botulinum toxin injections in the treatment of gastroparesis.[31]

As stated earlier, both antral and pyloric dysfunctions have been demonstrated in the pathogenesis of gastroparesis. Although improved gastric emptying does not *consistently* correlate with improved symptoms, it is known that improved gastric emptying *frequently* correlates with improved symptoms in children and adults.[32] It is also known that pyloroplasty has a long history as an effective and permanent gastric drainage procedure in the context of mechanical obstruction and elective vagotomy.[2] Moreover, as early as 2007, foregut surgeons began reporting improved gastric emptying and substantially improved nonreflux symptoms in gastrointestinal reflux disease (GERD) patients who had received pyloroplasty in conjunction with fundoplication.[33,34] Currently, several groups perform simultaneous laparoscopic fundoplication and pyloroplasty as routine practice in patients meeting the diagnostic criteria for both GERD and gastroparesis.[35] A similar synergy has been seen with the addition of laparoscopic pyloroplasty to the use of the gastric stimulator.[36]

CURRENT EVIDENCE FOR LAPAROSCOPIC PYLOROPLASTY AND GASTROPARESIS

Evidence-based medicine might dictate that laparoscopic pyloroplasty should be the primary treatment of gastroparesis. Hibbard and colleagues[37] published a retrospective, single-center review of prospectively collected data. Twenty-eight patients with refractory gastroparesis (25% diabetic) underwent laparoscopic Heineke-Mikulicz pyloroplasty or, in 2 patients, a laparoscopic-assisted pyloroplasty using a transoral circular stapler. Patients with prior or concomitant gastric surgery were excluded. Refractory gastroparesis was defined by classic symptoms *and* an abnormal gastric-emptying study in the absence of mechanical obstruction. By 3-month follow-up, 92%

of patients reported improved or resolved symptoms ($P \leq .013$, albeit not assessed by GCSI). Half the patients had a postoperative gastric-emptying study, which was normalized in 71% ($P = .001$). Fourteen percent of patients had early recurrent symptoms, resulting in subsequent interventions (3 gastric stimulation, 1 fundoplication). Nevertheless, these results were striking enough to inspire several similar studies in rapid succession.

In another retrospective review by Toro and colleagues,[34] 50 gastroparetic patients (10% diabetic) also underwent laparoscopic Heineke-Mikulicz pyloroplasty. Major differences in this study were inclusion of patients with prior or concomitant foregut surgery (68% and 64%, respectively) and the use of the GCSI to evaluate symptoms postoperatively. Although long-term follow-up is also unavailable, 2-month follow-up showed similar rates of symptom improvement and improved gastric-emptying times (82% and 96%, respectively, both $P<.001$). More than half of the patients (54%) had normalized gastric-emptying times, and there was no incidence of dumping syndrome after pyloroplasty. Of note, the 5 diabetics included in the study had substantial improvement in gastric-emptying times, suggesting that pyloroplasty is indeed effective even in this patient population.

Mancini and colleagues[35] retrospectively evaluated the effects of laparoscopic and open pyloroplasty in 46 patients with gastroparesis (30% diabetic). Patients with prior gastric surgery, including stimulator placement, were excluded. Preoperative and postoperative evaluations involved the GCSI and gastric-emptying scintigraphy with follow-up of at least 12 months. Improved gastric emptying was found in 90% of patients, with 60% demonstrating normalized emptying values ($P = .001$). Symptoms were assessed preoperatively and postoperatively for 41 patients, all of whom demonstrated statistically significant improvement (mean difference = -2.3, $P<.005$). This study confirmed the efficacy of surgical pyloroplasty for treating gastroparetic symptoms and gut dysfunction, including in diabetics.

Shada and colleagues[38] provided more definitive evidence by examining pyloroplasty as first-line surgical therapy for refractory gastroparesis in a retrospective review of 177 patients, 58% of whom had concurrent fundoplication for presumed overflow reflux. Overall, 90% of gastroparetic patients had concurrent surgery of some kind (Heller myotomy, paraesophageal hernia repair, percutaneous endoscopic gastrostomy [PEG], or J tube). Gastroparesis was defined by scintigraphy, endoscopic visualization of retained food after prolonged NPO (nothing by mouth) status, or clinical symptoms suspicious for vagal nerve injury after complex foregut surgery. In fact, 13 patients had normal gastric-emptying scintigraphy times, but were highly symptomatic with retained solid food found repeatedly on endoscopy. Postoperative scintigraphy was performed in almost half the patients (n = 70), 85% of whom had improved emptying times and 77% of whom had normalized ($P = .001$). In place of the GCSI, a standardized Symptom Severity Scale was used for evaluating symptoms. Of the 9 major symptoms queried, all showed statistically significant improvement at 1 month ($P = .0001$) except early satiety ($P = .14$). Of interest, all symptoms showed small increases between the 3- and 6-month evaluation, underscoring the need for long-term follow-up in this complex patient population. It should be noted that 11% of patients went on to another surgical treatment (gastrectomy or gastric stimulator) due to severe, refractory symptoms.

In summary, for nearly 2 decades pyloroplasty has been shown to improve gastric emptying, yet it has only recently been evaluated as a primary treatment for gastroparesis. To date, findings are promising, suggesting that surgical pyloroplasty is as safe and effective (if not more so) as any other available treatment option for medically refractory gastroparesis. It is now clear that surgical pyloroplasty does not preclude subsequent or concomitant interventions if needed.

THE EVOLUTION OF PER-ORAL PYLOROPLASTY

With the increasing acceptance of POEM for the treatment of achalasia,[39,40] it was hypothesized early on that an analogous procedure could be used to address diseases of the pylorus, perhaps replicating the results of surgical pyloroplasty in the treatment of benign gastric outlet obstruction and gastroparesis. POP was proposed as a less invasive potential alternative. Using different nomenclature and slightly different techniques, this idea has been explored for more than a decade.

In 2001, Hagiwara and colleagues[41] reported results from 5 adults with postoperative pyloric stenosis who had persistent obstruction after treatment with oral prokinetics and repeated endoscopic balloon dilation. Endoscopically, 2 to 3 radial incisions were made through mucosa and muscle using a needle knife. These incisions were extended from antrum to duodenal bulb followed by low-pressure balloon dilation for 15 to 20 minutes. Patients returned for repeat endoscopic balloon dilation after 1 week. No complications were reported, and all patients remained obstruction-free (based on esophagogastroduodenoscopy, symptoms, and barium swallow) at 10- to 26-month follow-up.

In 2005, Ibarguen-Secchia[42] published a single-center pilot study examining outcomes in children with congenital pyloric stenosis.[42] In this population of patients, the practice of pyloromyotomy has a long, well-vetted and successful history. The investigator, an accomplished endoscopist, proposed that an endoscopic approach might allow these patients to avoid general anesthesia and return to oral intake more quickly. Ten infants (7 boys), between 3 and 7 weeks old, underwent endoscopic pylotomyotomy for congenital pyloric stenosis under conscious sedation. Using either a needle knife (7) or standard sphincterotome (3), 2 incisions were made at the pylorus, one anterior and one posterior, first through the mucosa and then through the circular muscle fibers. Muscle division was continued until longitudinal fibers were seen. Mucosotomies were not closed. All patients were taking per os fluids within 2 hours, and 80% were discharged home the same day. The remaining patients were kept overnight because of persistent vomiting, which subsequently resolved. Follow-up occurred between 6 months and 2 years, and all patients continued to do well. Zhang and colleagues[43] reported similar outcomes with the same technique in 8 children. In this study, 1 postoperative patient developed persistent vomiting after 1 month of resolved symptoms. Repeat endoscopic pyloromyotomy was performed, and the patient was symptom free thereafter. Zhang's remaining patients were similarly doing well at follow-up from 2 to 9 months after the operation.

Endoscopic submucosal tunneling and esophageal myotomy were first demonstrated in animals by Pasricha and colleagues[44] 3 years before Inoue reported on his POEM technique in man. The experiment involved 4 pigs and a submucosal tunnel made after incising the mucosa 5-cm lower esophageal sphincter. The submucosal space was developed with electrocautery, and the gastroscope was introduced into this submucosal space. After creating a tunnel, the circular muscle fibers of the distal esophagus were then divided by needle knife and the mucosotomy closed with clips. There were no complications before sacrifice at 5 days. Manometry performed on postprocedural day 5 showed that average LES pressures had fallen from 16.4 mm Hg to 6.7 mm Hg.

The feasibility of applying this tunneling technique to the pylorus was first described in animals by Kawai and colleagues[45] in 2012. Four pigs underwent submucosal tunneling followed by endoscopic pylomyotomy. The median resting pressure of the pyloric sphincter was reduced by 63% immediately following the procedure, and a 50% reduction was maintained at 2-week reassessment (just before sacrifice). Chaves and colleagues,[46] in another animal study, did not measure sphincter resting pressure, but rather evaluated sphincter division post-mortem. They report similar results in their 6 pigs, which underwent a nearly identical procedure.

PER-ORAL PYLOROPLASTY DATA IN HUMANS

The first human case of endoscopic pyloromyotomy via a submucosal tunnel (initially referred to as "G-POEM" but more commonly referred to as "POP") was a case report by Khashab and colleagues.[47] This case report described the feasibility of the technique in a young woman with severe, refractory gastroparesis secondary to type I diabetes. She was not a candidate for gastric stimulation (due to other health issues); she refused all surgery, and transpyloric stents had failed because of repeated migration. The endoscopic pyloromyotomy was performed by Haruhiro Inoue using the principles he established for POEM. There were no complications. Initial postprocedural evaluation showed on-going delay in gastric emptying, but notably improved symptoms, which persisted at 12-week follow-up. One month later, a similar case report was published by Chaves and colleagues[48] involving a patient with postsurgical gastroparesis as defined by symptoms and scintigraphy. There were no immediate complications, but no follow-up information was provided.

The first prospective series of patients to undergo POP with midterm follow-up and statistical analysis of results was reported by Shlomovitz and colleagues[49] in 2015. Seven female patients with refractory gastroparesis (2 postsurgical, 5 idiopathic) underwent POP along with a concomitant foregut procedure under institutional review board (IRB) protocol. Six patients had concomitant laparoscopic fundoplication or cholecystectomy, allowing the POP procedure to be done under laparoscopic observation. The seventh patient had endoluminal fundoplication and POP without laparoscopy. Two patients in this early series had major complications. The first complication was bleeding on postoperative day 14 that required readmission and endoscopic control for bleeding at the site of the mucosotomy. This complication was attributed to noncompliance with the standard postoperative proton pump inhibitor (PPI) regimen and subsequent development of a bleeding gastric ulcer at the mucosal incision site. The second complication was the development of nocosomial pneumonia, which required a 6-day hospital stay. One patient had no improvement in symptoms and later underwent laparoscopic pyloroplasty, also with no improvement of symptoms. The remaining 6 patients reported improved symptoms at 3-month follow-up via the gastroparesis symptom monitor worksheet (Medtronic, Minneapolis, MN, USA). However, only improvements in nausea and epigastric burning were statistically significant. Five patients had repeat gastric-emptying studies at 3-month follow-up, showing improved or normalized values in 4 patients.

PATIENT SELECTION

Any intervention in the case of gastroparesis should occur only after exhaustion of all medical options. **Fig. 1** describes the treatment algorithm the author uses to determine who might be a candidate for POP.

PER-ORAL PYLOROPLASTY TECHNIQUE

The operative technique for POP follows the same basic principles as described by Inoue in the context of POEM for achalasia[38] (**Fig. 2**). There are some important

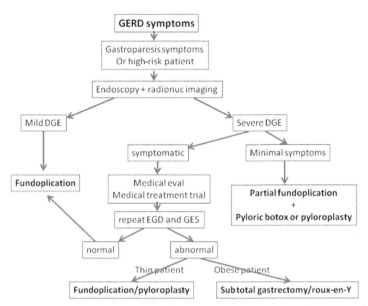

Fig. 1. Treatment algorithm for suspected gastroparesis. EGD, esophagogastroduodenoscopy; GES, gastric emptying study.

differences to consider in the setting of endoscopic pyloromyotomy. Control of the endoscope is difficult in the distal stomach. There are no clear demarcations between the muscle layers of the antrum and pylorus, and the duodenum has thin and fragile mucosal and muscular layers. There are also multiple large blood vessels both intramural and extramural that may be encountered. For these reasons, POP should not be an interventional endoscopist's first foray into submucosal tunneling in the upper gastrointestinal (GI) tract.

However, once ready, the technique is as follows:

Preoperative workup should proceed as described above. Standard antibiotic prophylaxis and a single 8-mg dose of dexamethasone (to limit mucosal swelling) are

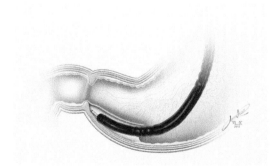

Fig. 2. Operative technique for POP. (*From* Chaves DM, de Moura EG, Mestieri LH, et al. Endoscopic pyloromyotomy via a gastric submucosal tunnel dissection for the treatment of gastroparesis after surgical vagal lesion. Gastrointest Endosc 2014;80(1):164; with permission.)

administered preoperatively. Under general anesthesia, the patient is positioned supine, and upper endoscopy is performed with a high-definition forward-viewing gastroscope (GIF-H180; Olympus, Tokyo, Japan). The stomach is lavaged as needed and carefully surveyed. A 50-cm gastric overtube (Guardus Overtube-Gastric; US Endoscopy, Mentor, OH, USA) is placed to add stability to the endoscope and secured externally with tape. After fitting the gastroscope with an angled, transparent dissection cap, a mucosotomy site is selected 3 to 5 cm from the pylorus on the posterior greater curve side of the stomach (7:00 o'clock position). This position offers a compromise between the natural track of the endoscope along the greater curve, and the large perforating blood vessels from the gastroepiploics that enter the stomach at the 9:00 o'clock position. A mucosal lift is performed with standard lifting solution (500 mL of normal saline mixed with 0.5 mL of 1:1000 epinephrine and 3–4 drops of methylene blue).

A 1.5-cm longitudinal mucosal incision is made in the cushion, using a triangle tip knife (Olympus), using an Endocut Q mode, Effect 2 (ERBE, Tubingen, Germany). To create the tunnel, spray coagulation (60W Effect 2; ERBE) is used. If there is difficulty introducing the scope into the submucosal plane, a 15-mm biliary extraction balloon (Cook Medical, Bloomington, IN, USA) can be inserted into the submucosal plane, inflated, and then pulled halfway into the dissection cap as the scope is advanced into the submucosal plane. There should be frequent and liberal use of lifting solution during tunnel creation, using the distal injection port of the biliary extraction balloon. This maneuver physically and visually enhances the correct dissection plane in the submucosal level 3 (sm3) layer. Keeping the dissection immediately adjacent to the gastric muscle aids in orientation and keeps most of the submucosal layer attached to the otherwise very fragile gastric mucosa. Encountered blood vessels can be coagulated with the triangle tip knife if they are no larger in diameter than the shaft of the knife itself (**Fig. 3**). Larger vessels require use of the coagulation forceps. The tunnel is continued until just past the pyloric ring, into the most proximal duodenal bulb. Because of the thinness of the duodenal wall, no attempt is made to tunnel onto the duodenum itself. To maintain scope orientation and to assess progress, periodically exit the tunnel and observe from the luminal side. Mucosa overlying the tunnel will appear slightly blanched (**Fig. 4**).

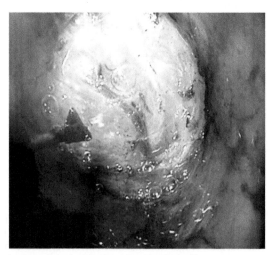

Fig. 3. Blood vessels coagulated with the triangle tip knife.

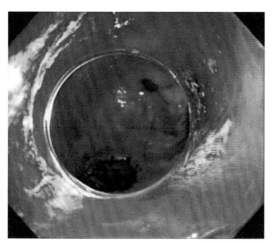

Fig. 4. Mucosa overlying the tunnel will appear slightly blanched. (*From* Shlomovitz E, Pescarus R, Cassera MA, et al. Early human experience with per-oral endoscopic pyloromyotomy (POP). Surg Endosc 2015;29:543–51; with permission.)

Upon completing the tunnel, the myotomy is started 2 cm proximal to the pylorus and proceeds in a proximal-to-distal fashion (**Fig. 5**). The myotomy is also performed with the triangle tip knife, but with settings adjusted to spray coagulation, 40W Effect 2 (ERBE) for hemostasis and Endocut Q for fine dissection. In this step, unlike in POEM, all muscle layers are divided down to the serosa with the division continuing distally

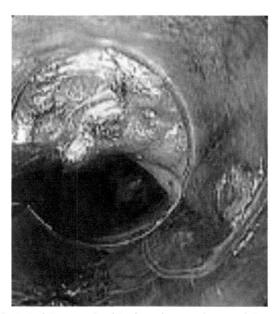

Fig. 5. Myotomy is started 2 cm proximal to the pylorus and proceeds in a proximal-to-distal fashion. (*From* Soares RV, Swanstrom LL. Endoscopic approaches to gastroparesis. Curr Opin Gastroenterol 2015;31(5):368–73; with permission.)

until the musculature visibly thins. This division signals the transition from pyloric bar to duodenal musculature and is another place to proceed with great caution because of the perpendicular position of duodenal mucosa at this level (**Fig. 6**). At completion of the myotomy, it is important to inspect for hemostasis within the tunnel and for mucosal injury within the gastroduodenal lumen. Bleeding should be addressed with coagulation if possible, and any inadvertent mucosal injury should be addressed with inverting endoscopic clips. Finally, the mucosotomy at the tunnel entry site is closed with clips or endoscopic suturing, as preferred.

Following the procedure, the author's standard practice is to admit the patient for overnight observation. Diet is held until an upper GI series is performed the next day confirming adequate drainage and no leak. The patient is then started on a clear liquid diet and transitioned to a puree/soft diet the following day. This diet is continued for 1 week to avoid dislodging the clips. High-dose PPI (40 mg twice a day) is started following the procedure and continued for a period of 6 weeks. It is important to stress to patients the importance of the PPI regimen as the author has had one patient return with an upper GI bleed because of ulceration at the mucosotomy site. Patients are seen at 2 weeks and again at 6 months after the operation when endoscopy and a gastric-emptying study are repeated.

OUTCOMES

Since the original publication with 7 patients,[49] the author has performed an additional 6 cases for a total of 13 POP procedures. Indications included idiopathic gastroparesis in 8, postesophagectomy delayed gastric emptying in 3, and 2 postfundoplication gastroparetics presumably due to vagal nerve damage. Six patients had a concomitant laparoscopic procedure (Nissen or cholecystectomy) as part of the original IRB study protocol. An additional patient had an endoluminal sutured fundoplasty for GERD. Operative data are listed in **Table 1**.

Overall, symptoms were improved or eliminated in 92% of patients at short-term follow-up. One patient had no improvement and went on to have a laparoscopic pyloroplasty with still no improvement. Five patients had marked improvement with nausea/vomiting symptom scores of 0 or 1; 6 had moderate improvement with scores of 2, and 1 had a postoperative score of 3 (4 preoperative) but was able to get off of

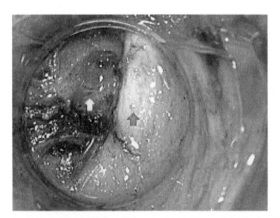

Fig. 6. The perpendicular position of duodenal mucosa. (*From* Khashab MA, Stein E, Clarke JO. Gastric peroral endoscopic myotomy for refractory gastroparesis: first human endoscopic pyloromyotomy (with video). Gastrointest Endosc 2013;78(5):764–8; with permission.)

Table 1
Results from current clinical experience with per-oral pyloroplasty in Portland

Operative time	127 (88–146) min
Operative complications	2 (15%)
Postoperative readmission for nausea/vomiting	3 (23%)
Postoperative complication (GI bleed)	1 (8%)
Length of stay	1.5 (0–6) d
Blood loss	11 (0–120) cc
Symptoms improved or eliminated	12 (92%)

enteral feeds and have a PEG tube removed. Eight patients have had their 6-month endoscopy and gastric emptying study (GES). There was no retained food (0/8), a dilated pylorus (7/8), and 6 patients had a normal 4-hour emptying and 2 had improved but still abnormal emptying (10% at 4 hours, 17% at 4 hours). Twelve of the 13 were moderately or very happy to have had the procedure.[50]

SUMMARY

Despite the newness of the POP technique, and the limited data available for assessing its true impact on gastroparesis or benign gastric outlet obstruction, the early data seem to indicate that this will be a promising addition to the treatment options for this very difficult patient group. Experimental work has already begun to help refine the technique, with hopes of clarifying efficacy and better understanding indications. Considering the heterogeneity of causes and presentations of gastroparetics, it makes sense that subsets of patients are likely to benefit from POP, but dependable methods for determining these groups are required for POP to achieve a prominent role in the care algorithm for gastroparesis.

REFERENCES

1. Acker SN, Garcia AJ, Ross JT, et al. Current trends in the diagnosis and treatment of pyloric stenosis. Pediatr Surg Int 2015;31(4):363–6.

2. Søreide K. Pyloroplasty for benign gastric outlet obstruction–indications and techniques. Scand J Surg 2006;95:11–6.

3. Rachlin L. Vagotomy and Heineke-Mikulicz pyloroplasty in the treatment of pyloric stenosis. Am Surg 1970;36(4):251–3.

4. Wang YR, Richter JE, Dempsey DT. Trends and outcomes of hospitalizations for peptic ulcer disease in the United States, 1993 to 2006. Ann Surg 2010;251:51.

5. Fineberg HV, Pearlman LA. Surgical treatment of peptic ulcer in the United States. Trends before and after the introduction of cimetidine. Lancet 1981;1:1305–7.

6. Schwesinger WH, Page CP, Sirinek KR, et al. Operations for peptic ulcer disease: paradigm lost. J Gastrointest Surg 2001;5:438–43.

7. Smith JW, Mathis T, Benns MV, et al. Socioeconomic disparities in the operative management of peptic ulcer disease. Surgery 2013;154(4):672–8.

8. Antonoff MB, Puri V, Meyers BF, et al. Comparison of pyloric intervention strategies at the time of esophagectomy: is more better? Ann Thorac Surg 2014; 97(6):1950–7.

9. Lanuti M, de Delva PE, Wright CD, et al. Post-esophagectomy gastric outlet obstruction: role of pyloromyotomy and management with endoscopic pyloric dilatation. Eur J Cardiothorac Surg 2007;31(2):149–53.

10. Gaur P, Swanson SJ. Should we continue to drain the pylorus in patients undergoing an esophagectomy? Dis esophagus 2014;27(6):568–73.

11. Urschel JD, Blewett CJ, Young JE, et al. Pyloric drainage (pyloroplasty) or no drainage in gastric reconstruction after esophagectomy: a meta-analysis of randomized controlled trials. Dig Surg 2002;19:160–4.

12. Kochhar R, Sethy PK, Nagi B, et al. Endoscopic balloon dilatation of benign gastric outlet obstruction. J Gastroenterol Hepatol 2004;19:418–22.

13. Kochhar R, Dutta U, Sethy PK, et al. Endoscopic balloon dilation in caustic-induced chronic gastric outlet obstruction. Gastrointest Endosc 2009;69(4):800–5.

14. Kochhar R, Kochhar S. Endoscopic balloon dilation for benign gastric outlet obstruction in adults. World J Gastrointest Endosc 2010;2(1):29–35.

15. Khasab MA, Besharati S, Ngamruengphong S. Refractory gastroparesis can be successfully managed with endoscopic transpyloric stent placement and fixation (with video). Gastrointest Endosc 2015;82(6):1106–9.

16. Choi WJ, Park JJ, Park J, et al. Effects of the temporary placement of a self-expandable metallic stent in benign pyloric stenosis. Gut Liver 2013;7(4):417–22.

17. Clarke JO, Sharaiha RZ, Kord Valeshabad A, et al. Through-the-scope transpyloric stent placement improves symptoms and gastric emptying in patients with gastroparesis. Endoscopy 2013;45(Suppl 2 UCTN):E189–90.

18. Pasricha PJ, Parkman HP. Gastroparesis: definitions and diagnosis. Gastroenterol Clin North Am 2015;44(1):1–7.

19. Wang YR, Fisher RS, Parkman HP. Gastroparesis-related hospitalizations in the United States: trends, characteristics, and outcomes, 1995-2004. Am J Gastroenterol 2008;103:313–22.

20. Revicki DA, Rentz AM, Dubois D, et al. Gastroparesis Cardinal Symptom Index (GCSI): development and validation of a patient reported assessment of severity of gastroparesis symptoms. Qual Life Res 2004;13:833–44.

21. Enweluzo C. Gastroparesis: a review of current and emerging treatment options. Clin Exp Gastroenterol 2013;5(6):161–5.

22. Rao AS, Camilleri M. Review article: metoclopramide and tardive dyskinesia. Aliment Pharmacol Ther 2010;31:11–9.

23. Lal N, Livemore S, Dunne D, et al. Gastric electrical stimulation with the Enterra System: a systematic review. Gastroenterol Res Pract 2015;2015:762972.

24. Heckert J, Sankineni A, Hughes WB, et al. Gastric electric stimulation for refractory gastroparesis: a prospective analysis of 151 patients at a single center. Dig Dis Sci 2015;61(1):168–75.

25. Miller LS, Szych GA, Kantor SB, et al. Treatment of idiopathic gastroparesis with injection of botulinum toxin into the pyloric sphincter muscle. Am J Gastroenterol 2002;97:1653–60.

26. Ezzeddine D, Jit R, Katz N, et al. Pyloric injection of botulinum toxin for treatment of diabetic gastroparesis. Gastrointest Endosc 2002;55:920–3.

27. Woodward MN, Spicer RD. Intrapyloric botulinum toxin injection improves gastric emptying. J Pediatr Gastroenterol Nutr 2003;37:201–2.

28. Bromer MQ, Friedenberg F, Miller LS, et al. Endoscopic pyloric injection of botulinum toxin A for the treatment of refractory gastroparesis. Gastrointest Endosc 2005;61:833–9.

29. Arts J, Holvoet L, Caenepeel P, et al. Clinical trial: a randomized-controlled cross-over study of intrapyloric injection of botulinum toxin in gastroparesis. Aliment Pharmacol Ther 2007;26:1251–8.
30. Friedenberg FK, Palit A, Parkman HP, et al. Botulinum toxin A for the treatment of delayed gastric emptying. Am J Gastroenterol 2008;103:416–23.
31. Camilleri M, Parkman HP, Shafi MA, et al, American College of Gastroenterology. Clinical guideline: management of gastroparesis. Am J Gastroenterol 2013;108: 18–37.
32. Hasler WL. Gastroparesis: pathogenesis, diagnosis and management. Nat Rev Gastroenterol Hepatol 2011;8(8):438–53.
33. Van Sickle KR, McClusky DA, Swafford VA, et al. Delayed gastric emptying in patients undergoing antireflux surgery: analysis of a treatment algorithm. J Laparoendosc Adv Surg Tech A 2007;17:7–11.
34. Toro JP, Lytle NW, Patel AD, et al. Efficacy of laparoscopic pyloroplasty for the treatment of gastroparesis. J Am Coll Surg 2014;218(4):652–6.
35. Mancini SA, Angelo JL, Peckler Z, et al. Pyloroplasty for refractory gastroparesis. Am Surg 2015;81(7):738–46.
36. Sarosiek I, Forster J, Lin Z, et al. The addition of pyloroplasty as a new surgical approach to enhance effectiveness of gastric electrical stimulation therapy in patients with gastroparesis. Neurogastroenterol Motil 2013;25:134–80.
37. Hibbard ML, Dunst CM, Swanström LL. Laparoscopic and endoscopic pyloro-plasty for gastroparesis results in sustained symptom improvement. J Gastrointest Surg 2011;15(9):1513–9.
38. Shada AL, Dunst CM, Pescarus R, et al. Laparoscopic pyloroplasty is a safe and effective first-line surgical therapy for refractory gastroparesis. Surg Endosc 2015. [Epub ahead of print].
39. Inoue H, Minami H, Kobayashi Y, et al. Peroral endoscopic myotomy (POEM) for esophageal achalasia. Endoscopy 2010;42(4):265–71.
40. NOSCAR POEM White Paper Committee, Stavropoulos SN, Desilets DJ, et al. Per-oral endoscopic myotomy white paper summary. Gastrointest Endosc 2014;80(1):1–15.
41. Hagiwara A, Sonoyama Y, Togawa T, et al. Electrosurgical incisions plus balloon dilatation for postoperative pyloric stenosis. Gastrointest Endosc 2001;53(4): 504–8.
42. Ibarguen-Secchia E. Endoscopic pyloromyotomy for congential pyloric stenosis. Gastrointest Endosc 2005;61(4):598–600.
43. Zhang YX, Nie YQ, Xiao X, et al. Treatment of congenital hypertrophic pyloric stenosis with endoscopic pyloromyotomy. Zhonghua Er Ke Za Zhi 2008;46:247–51.
44. Pasricha PJ, Hawari R, Ahmed I, et al. Submucosal endoscopic esophageal myotomy: a novel experimental approach for the treatment of achalasia. Endoscopy 2007;39(9):761–4.
45. Kawai M, Peretta S, Burckhardt O, et al. Endoscopic pyloromyotomy: a new concept of minimally invasive surgery for pyloric stenosis. Endoscopy 2012; 44(2):169–73.
46. Chaves DM, Gusmon CC, Mestieri LH, et al. A new technique for performing endoscopic pyloromyotomy by gastric submucosal tunnel dissection. Surg Laparosc Endosc Percutan Tech 2014;24(3):e92–4.
47. Khashab MA, Stein E, Clarke JO. Gastric peroral endoscopic myotomy for refractory gastroparesis: first human endoscopic pyloromyotomy (with video). Gastrointest Endosc 2013;78(5):764–8.

48. Chaves DM, de Moura EG, Mestieri LH, et al. Endoscopic pyloromyotomy via a gastric submucosal tunnel dissection for the treatment of gastroparesis after surgical vagal lesion. Gastrointest Endosc 2014;80(1):164.
49. Shlomovitz E, Pescarus R, Cassera MA, et al. Early human experience with peroral endoscopic pyloromyotomy (POP). Surg Endosc 2015;29:543–51.
50. Soares RV, Swanstrom LL. Endoscopic approaches to gastroparesis. Curr Opin Gastroenterol 2015;31(5):368–73.

Submucosal Tunneling Endoscopic Resection (STER) and Other Novel Applications of Submucosal Tunneling in Humans

Bing-Rong Liu, MD, PhD*, Ji-Tao Song, MD

KEYWORDS

- Endoscopic resection • Subepithelial tumors • Submucosal endoscopy
- Natural orifice transluminal endoscopic surgery

KEY POINTS

- STER seems to be an effective therapy for treatment of small and medium size gastrointestinal tumors originating from the muscularis propria.
- Common complications of STER are gas-related, most of which resolve with conservative treatment without surgical intervention.
- New applications of submucosal tunneling technique continue to be developed and further clinical applications in the future are anticipated.

INTRODUCTION

The submucosal tunneling technique, originally developed at the Mayo Clinic, was described as submucosal endoscopy with a mucosal flap safety valve.[1] It has been shown to be a technically feasible access method for natural orifice transluminal endoscopic surgery (NOTES).[2–4] The submucosal tunneling technique was subsequently adapted for endoscopic esophageal myotomy for the treatment of achalasia in humans, known as per oral endoscopic myotomy (POEM).[5–8] During the POEM procedure, the submucosal tunnel becomes the working space for partial esophageal

The authors contributed equally to this work.

Competing Interests: The authors have no financial relationships relevant to this publication to disclose.

Department of Gastroenterology and Hepatology, The Second Affiliated Hospital of Harbin Medical University, No. 246 Xuefu Road, Nangang District, Harbin 150086, People's Republic of China

* Corresponding author.

E-mail address: liubingrong@medmail.com.cn

myotomy. Inspired by this technique, Xu and workers[9] used a submucosal tunnel as the working space for endoscopic resections and called the technique submucosal tunneling endoscopic resection (STER). We refer to this as tunneling endoscopic muscularis dissection because it allows precise dissection and resection of tumors as deep as the muscularis propria.[10] This article summarizes the current applications of STER for subepithelial tumors and describes other related uses of submucosal tunneling.

SUBMUCOSAL TUNNELING ENDOSCOPIC RESECTION
Indications

STER for subepithelial tumors is generally limited to tumors less than 3.5 cm in diameter because subepithelial tumors greater than 3.5 cm are technically difficult to retrieve from the submucosal tunnel and mouth because of the limited size of the esophageal submucosal tunnel. Large tumors may also result in poor endoscopic visualization because of the mass effect. A few cases of resection of subepithelial tumor greater than 3.5 cm have been reported, although some were removed by piecemeal resection[11] and some had a minimum diameter less than 3.5 cm.[12,13] Tumor size is an important indicator of gastrointestinal stromal tumor (GIST) risk of malignancy,[14] and en bloc resection is preferred because piecemeal resection results in tumor capsule rupture and thus violates an important principle of cancer surgery.[15] Piecemeal resection of benign lesions, such as leiomyomas, is considered acceptable but because the histology of a subepithelial tumor often cannot be accurately diagnosed by endoscopic ultrasound (EUS)-guided aspiration or other endoscopic biopsy techniques before operation and considering the technical difficulties mentioned previously, we recommend the 3.5-cm limit rule be followed.

In terms of location, STER is suitable for tumors originating from the muscularis propria layer of the esophagus or cardia and for many tumors located in the greater curvature of the distal gastric body. However, because it is difficult to create a gastric submucosal tunnel for tumors in the deep fundus or lesser curvature of the gastric body and antrum often the only choice is endoscopic direct full-thickness resection in a retroflexed fashion.[16] For subepithelial tumors arising from muscularis propria in the circular funnel-like cardia area within 8 cm of the gastroesophageal junction, a transcardiac endoscopic tunneling technique is generally a feasible, safe, and easy therapeutic approach from below the cardia.[17] Hu and colleagues[18] also reported that STER was a feasible, safe, and effective method for treating rectal subepithelial tumor originating from the muscularis propria layer.

Preparation and Equipment

Before the procedure, routine EUS and esophageal computed tomography (CT) are performed to determine the size, possible layer of origin, margin, and growth pattern of the subepithelial tumors and to provide information regarding anatomic features of the adjacent structures. In our center, we perform a special esophageal inflatable CT scan in which air is infused into the esophageal lumen through a previously inserted nasoesophageal tube during chest CT scan.[19] Esophageal inflatable CT scan provides superior visualization of the relationship between the subepithelial tumor and the esophageal wall and offers the advantage of a multiazimuthal observation in one plane. Other investigators have also confirmed that CT is especially useful to complement and validate the EUS findings and provides comprehensive and accurate information for confirmation of the use of an endoscopic therapeutic approach.[20] STER procedures are performed under general anesthesia with tracheal intubation. In most cases, a carbon dioxide insufflator is used for carbon dioxide (CO_2) gas insufflation during the procedure. CO_2 has advantages compared with room air including fast diffusion and rapid absorption reducing the incidence of clinically important cutaneous emphysema, mediastinal emphysema, and pneumothorax.[21]

Technique/Procedures

The first step is creation of a submucosal tunnel to expose the tumor. After submucosal injection of a solution of epinephrine in saline (1:100,000) and/or indigo carmine, a 2-cm longitudinal mucosal incision is made with a Hook knife, which is our preference, or other similar knife without insulated tip approximately 5 cm proximal to the lesion. For gastric lesions 3 cm is sufficient because of elasticity of gastric wall. A submucosal tunnel is then created between mucosal and muscular layers using endoscopic submucosal dissection technique while advancing toward the tumor. Submucosal tunneling is extended beyond the tumor to secure sufficient working space for tumor resection at the most difficult distal side of the tumor. It is important not to perforate the mucosa during submucosal tunneling because preserving the integrity of the digestive tract mucosa prevents leakage of the gastrointestinal (GI) contents into the body cavity and promotes early wound healing.[22] Repeated injections of saline solution are especially helpful to differentiate the mucosal layer from the tumor mass and to avoid unexpected mucosal injury.

The second step is tunneling endoscopic enucleation of the subepithelial tumor from the muscularis propria. Endoscopic enucleation is performed within the submucosal tunnel by dissecting the tumor away from any connecting muscle fibers. For tumors involving the deep layers of the muscularis propria, circumferential full-thickness muscularis propria resection is performed using the endoscopic knife and even snare resection if necessary. The highest priority during the procedure is safe and complete resection of the tumor, without disruption of the tumor capsule. The tumor is finally removed via the submucosal tunnel. The resection site and tunnel is examined for remnant tumor and bleeding. En bloc resection is defined as the presence of an intact fibrous capsule of resected tumor and the absence of any remnant of tumor observed at endoscopy. Recently, we had success by using a single tunnel to resect multiple esophageal subepithelial tumors originating from the muscularis propria layer (**Fig. 1**).

Finally, closure of mucosal incision at the tunnel entry site is accomplished with endoclips or other endoscopic closure devices. At the end of the procedure, before withdrawal of the endoscope, careful endoscopic inspection is performed to confirm the integrity of mucosal overlying the tunnel.

Postoperative Care and Follow-Up

All patients are admitted for inpatient hospital observation. Proton pump inhibitors and broad-spectrum antibiotics are prescribed for 3 days. The patients are monitored for chest distress, dyspnea, and blood oxygen saturation. If necessary, temporary chest tube drainage is performed. Commonly, patients are given nothing by mouth on postoperative Day 1. Liquid diet is started on Day 2. An endoscopic examination is done 3 days after the initial procedure to evaluate the condition of the mucosa followed by barium swallow radiography to check for leakage. If both tests are normal, a regular soft diet is initiated. Postoperative pathologic examination includes examination of the lesion margins, cell type, and mitotic count per 50 high-power fields and immunohistochemical staining for CD117, CD34, smooth muscle actin, desmin, and S-100 markers. For incompletely resected GISTs with medium or high risk of malignancy, secondary surgery or imatinib treatment is recommended. Follow-up includes clinic visits to assess for delayed complications, repeat standard

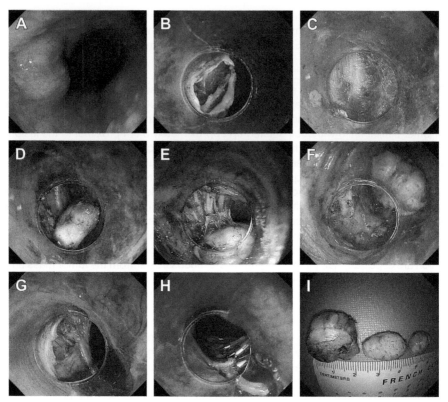

Fig. 1. Submucosal tunneling endoscopic resection for multiple esophageal subepithelial tumors originating from the muscularis propria. (*A*) Endoscopic view of the esophageal subepithelial tumors. (*B*) The mucosal incision at the tunnel entry site. (*C*) Submucosal tunneling. (*D*) Dissection of the first tumor from surrounding tissue within the submucosal space. (*E*) Dissection of the second tumor from surrounding tissue within the same submucosal tunnel. (*F*) Endoscopic dissection of the third tumor. (*G*) Deep muscular layer defect after tumor resection. (*H*) Closure of the mucosal incision at the tunnel entry site. (*I*) The three resected subepithelial tumors.

endoscopy, and EUS 2 months after procedures and then annually. For moderate- and high-risk GISTs, cross-sectional imaging is also performed at 6- to 12-month intervals for 3 to 5 years and then annually as is recommended after surgical resection of such tumors.[23]

Outcomes

Although most subepithelial tumors are benign, some have malignant potential, especially GISTs originating from the muscularis propria.[24] Resection of these tumors provides a definitive diagnosis and may be curative. Several studies have evaluated the use of the submucosal tunneling technique to resect subepithelial tumors (**Table 1**).[9,10,17,25–31] The en bloc resection rate was 83.3% to 100%. In the initial case series, two of nine (22%) patients required conversion to open surgery. Both of these patients had tumors that were too large (60 mm and 75 mm, respectively) for safe endoscopic removal because of a loss of endoscopic overview.[25] All subepithelial tumors had detailed histopathologic diagnosis including those with piecemeal resection. To date, no postresection recurrences have been reported. However,

Table 1
Recent publications of submucosal tunneling endoscopic resection for gastrointestinal subepithelial tumors originating from the muscularis propria layer

Ref	No. Cases (Tumors)	Location	Mean Tumor Size (mm)	Pathology	Mean Operating Time (min)	En Bloc Resection Rate, n (%)	Complications	Follow-Up Time (mo) and Recurrence
Xu et al[9]	15 (15)	9 esophagus, 3 cardia, 2 body, 1 autrum	19	5 GISTs, 9 leiomyomas, 1 glomus tumor	78.7	15 (100)	1 Pp, 1 Pt, 1 SE	3.9 None
Inoue et al[25]	7 (7)	3 esophagus, 4 cardia	18.6	1 GIST, 5 leiomyomas, 1 aberrant pancreas	152.4	7 (100)	None	5.5 None
Gong et al,[26] 2012	12 (12)	8 esophagus, 4 cardia	19.5	7 GISTs, 5 leiomyomas	48.3	10 (83.3)	2 Pt and SE	—
Liu et al[10]	12 (12)	7 esophagus, 5 cardia	18.5	2 GISTs, 9 leiomyomas, 1 schwannoma	78.3	12 (100)	8 ME and SE, 4 Pt, 3 Pp, 2 PE	7.1 None
Wang et al[27]	80 (83)	67 esophagus, 16 cardia	23.2	15 GISTs, 68 leiomyomas	61.2	81 (97.6)	2 SE, 1 Pt, 1 MP, 3 chest pain	10.2 None
Ye et al,[28] 2014	85 (85)	60 esophagus, 16 cardia, 9 stomach	19.2	19 GISTs, 65 leiomyomas, 1 calcifying fibrous tumor	57.2	85 (100)	6 Pt, 8 SE, 4 Pp	8 None
Lu et al[17]	18 (19)	19 fundus	20.1	13 GISTs, 6 leiomyomas	75.1	19 (100)	2 Pp	5 None
Li et al,[29] 2015	32 (32)	3 fundus close to cardia, 12 corpus close to cardia, 6 lesser curvature of corpus, 11 greater curvature of antrum	23	11 GISTs, 18 leiomyomas, 1 calcifying fibrous tumor, 1 glomus tumor, 1 schwannoma	51.8	32 (100)	1 bleeding, 6 Pp, 3 Pt and SE	28 None
Wang et al[30]	57 (57)	57 esophagogastric junction	21.5	7 GISTs, 46 leiomyomas, 2 schwannoma, 1 lipoma, 1 granular cell tumor	47	57 (100)	12 ME and SE, 5 Pt, 3 Pp, 2 PE	12 None
Zhou et al,[31] 2015	21 (21)	21 esophagogastric junction	23	6 GISTs, 15 leiomyomas	62.9	21 (100)	9 ME and SE	12 None

Abbreviations: GIST, gastrointestinal stromal tumor; ME, mediastinal emphysema; MP, mucosal perforation; PE, pleural effusion; Pp, pneumoperitoneum; Pt, pneumothorax; SE, subcutaneous emphysema.

long-term follow-up studies regarding outcome are needed to better evaluate the long-term success of the procedure. The largest retrospective study enrolled 290 patients with subepithelial tumors originating from the muscularis propria of the upper GI tract and was reported at the US Digestive Disease Week in 2014.[32] The available data are consistent with the notion that STER is an effective and a safe method for upper-GI submucosal tumors with diameter size less than 35 mm. The overall rates of en bloc resection and piecemeal resection were 95.4% and 4.6%, respectively, and local recurrences and distant metastasis have not been reported in follow-up. Tumor size and shape significantly affect the en bloc rate with large size and irregular shape being associated with more difficult procedures, an increased risk of requiring piecemeal resection, and were significant contributors to STER-related complications.

Adverse Events and Their Management

During STER, air frequently leaks from the GI lumen, especially in patients who have a full-thickness muscularis propria defect after tumor removal. The most common adverse events in published series[9,10,17,25–31] were gas-related and were more common with tumors originating from the deep muscularis propria layer; most resolved with conservative treatment without secondary infection or long-term consequences. Temporary thoracic drainage was rarely required. Because carbon dioxide is rapidly absorbed and exhaled through the lungs, its use is essential to reduce gas-related complications. In our study of 12 patients, subcutaneous and mediastinal emphysema occurred in eight (66.7%), pneumothorax in four (33.3%), and pneumoperitoneum in three (25%). All seven cases where the tumor involved the deep layers of the muscularis propria were associated with mediastinal and subcutaneous emphysema, pneumothorax, and/or pneumoperitoneum. In contrast, only one out of the five cases where the tumor involved only the superficial muscularis propria experienced a small amount of mediastinal and subcutaneous emphysema.[10] Only one case of postprocedural emphysema (12.5%) required subcutaneous puncture; all others resolved spontaneously. Among the four cases of pneumothorax (three unilateral, one bilateral), only one case (25.0%) required placement of a chest tube; the other three cases (75.0%) had a self-limiting course. All cases of pneumoperitoneum and pleural effusion resolved after conservative management without any secondary infections. No patient developed delayed hemorrhage or chronic fistula. Mucosal scars at the esophageal incision site were observed in all patients by follow-up endoscopy 2 months after the procedures. The mean follow-up time was 7.1 ± 4.3 (range, 2–15) months. Xu and colleagues[33] reviewed adverse events in 290 patients with subepithelial tumors originating from the muscularis propria of the upper GI tract who underwent STER and reported mucosal tears in three cases (1.0%), large hemorrhage (blood loss more than 200 mL) in five (1.7%), subcutaneous emphysema in 61 (21.0%), pneumothorax in 22 (7.5%), pneumoperitoneum in 15 (5.2%), minimal pleural effusion accompanied with minimal bilateral lung inflammation in 49 (16.9%), esophageal-pleural fistula in one (0.3%), and secondary esophageal diverticulum in two (0.6%). Most complications after STER resolved with conservative management without surgical intervention or long-term consequences. Only 11 (3.8%) required transient thoracic drainage.

Current Controversies/Future Considerations

Although STER is a promising approach for endoscopic diagnosis and therapy for subepithelial tumors, it is time-consuming. Most procedure time is consumed creating the submucosal tunnel and dissecting the tumor from the attached submucosal and muscular fibers. A novel dissecting gel has recently been described and may provide a new platform for submucosal tunneling.[34] The gel resulted in pure submucosal dissection. Dissection of muscular fibers was still required to remove subepithelial tumors originating from the muscularis propria. Leiomyomas, schwannoma, and lipoma are benign without recurrence potential. However, low-risk GISTs have been known to recur 10 years after resection suggesting that long-term follow-up may be required.[35] The ideal follow-up strategies after tunneling endoscopic resection are still unknown.[36] Follow-up of intermediate- to high-risk patients with GISTs should be at shorter intervals than for low-risk patients. In general, we consider that follow-up strategies after tunneling endoscopic resection should be based on the accurate histopathologic diagnosis of the subepithelial tumor.

OTHER NEW APPLICATIONS OF THE SUBMUCOSAL TUNNELING TECHNIQUE
Esophago-Cardial-Gastric Tunneling Peritoneoscopy

NOTES peritoneoscopy can potentially replace laparoscopic peritoneoscopy for diagnosis of intra-abdominal diseases, such as unexplained ascites and for staging of malignancies,[37,38] because it offers potential benefits of minimal pain, shorter hospital stays, and optimal cosmesis compared with conventional open or laparoscopic surgery.[39,40] Inspired by the clinical practice of transcardiac endoscopic tunneling resection technique, our team developed the esophago-cardial-gastric tunneling (ECGT) access to enter the peritoneal cavity for peritoneoscopy using an in vivo dog model to evaluate its feasibility and safety.[41] The potential advantages of ECGT access include straight insertion without mechanical limitations, reliable healing, and easy closure (**Fig. 2**). After the experimental study, one patient with unexplained ascites underwent ECGT peritoneoscopy without incident. Accurate histopathologic information was obtained with the final diagnosis of peritoneal tuberculosis. ECGT peritoneal access may be a promising technique for diagnostic peritoneoscopy.

Endoscopic Esophageal Epiphrenic Diverticulum Inversion

Esophageal epiphrenic diverticula are uncommon and currently surgical therapy is technically challenging such that it is currently used only when symptoms are incapacitating or if life-threatening respiratory complications occur.[42] A review of 25 published series reported a postoperative morbidity of 21%. The most severe complication was suture leakage, which occurred in 15%.[43] We reported a case of an epiphrenic diverticulum being successfully managed by endoscopic diverticulum inversion using the submucosal tunneling technique (**Fig. 3**).[44] First, a submucosal tunnel was created approximately 5 cm proximal to the epiphrenic diverticulum. When the endoscope reached the diverticulum, the muscular layer defect was observed in the submucosal space and the endoscope could be advanced into the mediastinal cavity through the defect. The mucosa of the epiphrenic diverticulum was separated completely from surrounding tissue at the level of the submucosa using a combination of blunt and electrocautery dissection. After complete dissection of the mucosa, the endoscope was retracted into the esophageal lumen and the epiphrenic diverticulum inversion was performed using suction. The inversed diverticular mucosa was then ligated using a nylon loop. Finally, the mucosal entry incision was closed with endoclips as is done with the POEM procedure. The patient developed fever after the procedure, but the body temperature returned to normal the next day. The white blood cell was mildly elevated (12.8 × 10^9/L). Liquid diet was resumed after 1 week. Follow-up endoscopy after 10 months showed the obvious reduction of the epiphrenic diverticulum and mucosal healing. The patient's preoperative symptoms were relieved completely at follow-up

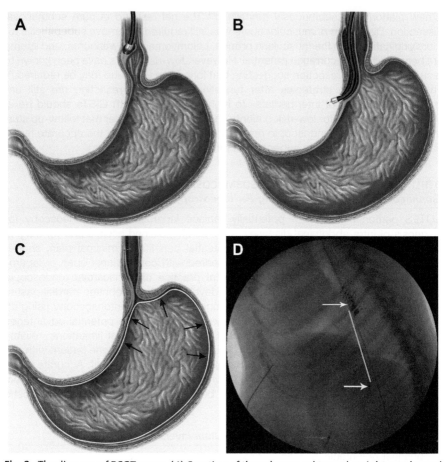

Fig. 2. The diagram of ECGT access. (*A*) Creation of the submucosal tunnel at right esophageal wall approximately 5 cm proximal to the esophagogastric junction. (*B*) Submucosal tunneling 3 to 5 cm distal to the esophagogastric junction and seromuscular incision at the end of the tunnel for advancing the scope to peritoneal cavity. (*C*) Gastric mucosal integrity was maintained after the procedure (*black arrow*) and the esophageal mucosal incision was closed by clips; the gastric seromuscular exit site was separated from esophageal mucosal entry by lower esophageal sphincter contractions. (*D*) Radiographic view of the ECGT access trace: endoscopic clips mark the esophageal mucosal entry site (*white arrow*), the gastric exit (*yellow arrow*), the greater curvature (*red arrow*), and ECGT peritoneal access direction (*green line*).

suggesting that symptomatic epiphrenic diverticulum can be successfully managed with endoscopic diverticulum inversion using the submucosal tunneling technique. Another group has reported a somewhat different tunnel-based technique in two patients with esophageal diverticular. Giant mid-esophageal diverticula were successfully treated by POEM.[45] Additional studies are needed.

SUMMARY

The submucosal tunneling technique was originally developed to provide safe access to the peritoneal cavity for NOTES procedures. With this technique, the submucosal tunnel becomes the working space for partial myotomy and tumor

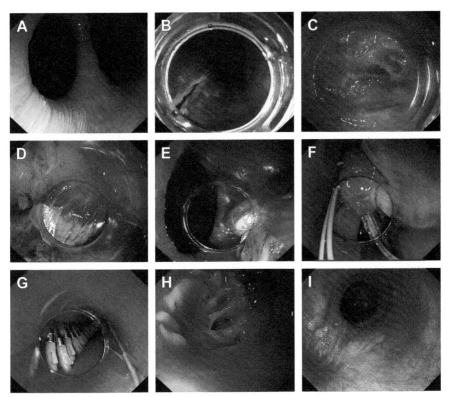

Fig. 3. Endoscopic esophageal epiphrenic diverticular inversion and reduction by using the submucosal tunneling technique. (*A*) Endoscopic view of the 5-cm epiphrenic diverticulum. (*B*) Endoscopy showing the mucosal incision 5 cm proximal to the diverticulum. (*C*) Submucosal tunnel advance toward the diverticulum. (*D*) Submucosal dissection within the diverticulum lumen. (*E*) Intratunnel views of the muscular defect underlying the diverticulum. (*F*) Luminal view of the inversion of the diverticular mucosa and ligation by using a nylon loop. (*G*) Closure of the mucosal tunnel entry site. (*H*) Follow-up endoscopy after 1 month showed the regenerating healing mucosa and the reduced diverticulum lumen. (*I*) Follow-up endoscopy after 10 months showed the obvious reduction of the diverticulum lumen and complete mucosal healing.

resection. The submucosal space has come to represent the "third space" distinguished from GI lumen (first space) and peritoneal cavity (second space). New applications continue to be developed and further clinical applications in the future are anticipated.

ACKNOWLEDGMENTS

The authors thank all those who helped them during this work. A special acknowledgment is shown to David Y. Graham, who gave help and assisted in correcting for language, grammar, and syntax.

REFERENCES

1. Sumiyama K, Gostout CJ, Rajan E, et al. Submucosal endoscopy with mucosal flap safety valve. Gastrointest Endosc 2007;65:688–94.

2. Sumiyama K, Tajiri H, Gostout CJ. Submucosal endoscopy with mucosal flap safety valve (SEMF) technique: a safe access method into the peritoneal cavity and mediastinum. Minim Invasive Ther Allied Technol 2008;17:365–9.

3. Pauli EM, Moyer MT, Haluck RS, et al. Self-approximating transluminal access technique for natural orifice transluminal endoscopic surgery: a porcine survival study (with video). Gastrointest Endosc 2008;67:690–7.

4. Yoshizumi F, Yasuda K, Kawaguchi K, et al. Submucosal tunneling using endoscopic submucosal dissection for peritoneal access and closure in natural orifice translumi-nal endoscopic surgery: a porcine survival study. Endoscopy 2009;41:707–11.

5. Inoue H, Minami H, Kobayashi Y, et al. Peroral endoscopic myotomy (POEM) for esophageal achalasia. Endoscopy 2010;42:265–71.

6. von Renteln D, Inoue H, Minami H, et al. Peroral endoscopic myotomy for the treatment of achalasia: a prospective single center study. Am J Gastroenterol 2012;107:411–7.

7. Talukdar R, Inoue H, Reddy DN. Efficacy of peroral endoscopic myotomy (POEM) in the treatment of achalasia: a systematic review and meta-analysis. Surg Endosc 2015;29(11):3030–46.

8. Wei M, Yang T, Yang X, et al. Peroral esophageal myotomy versus laparoscopic Heller's myotomy for achalasia: a meta-analysis. J Laparoendosc Adv Surg Tech A 2015;25:123–9.

9. Xu MD, Cai MY, Zhou PH, et al. Submucosal tunneling endoscopic resection: a new technique for treating upper GI submucosal tumors originating from the muscularis propria layer (with videos). Gastrointest Endosc 2012;75:195–9.

10. Liu BR, Song JT, Kong LJ, et al. Tunneling endoscopic muscularis dissection for subepithelial tumors originating from the muscularis propria of the esophagus and gastric cardia. Surg Endosc 2013;27:4354–9.

11. Tan YY, Zhou YQ, Zhang J, et al. Submucosal tunnel endoscopic resection for upper gastrointestinal submucosal tumors originating from muscularis propria layer measuring ≥35 mm. Gastrointest Endosc 2015;81:AB393.

12. Maydeo A, Sharma A, Bhandari S, et al. Submucosal tunneling and endoscopic resection of a large, esophageal leiomyoma. Gastrointest Endosc 2015;82(5):954.

13. Kumbhari V, Saxena P, Azola A, et al. Submucosal tunneling endoscopic resec-tion of a giant esophageal leiomyoma. Gastrointest Endosc 2015;81:219–20.

14. Joensuu H. Risk stratification of patients diagnosed with gastrointestinal stromal tumor. Hum Pathol 2008;39:1411–9.

15. Joensuu H, Hohenberger P, Corless CL. Gastrointestinal stromal tumour. Lancet 2013;382:973–83.

16. Lu J, Jiao T, Li Y, et al. Heading toward the right direction–solution package for endoscopic submucosal tunneling resection in the stomach. PLoS One 2015; 10:e0119870.

17. Lu J, Zheng M, Jiao T, et al. Transcardiac tunneling technique for endoscopic submucosal dissection of gastric fundus tumors arising from the muscularis propria. Endoscopy 2014;46:888–92.

18. Hu JW, Zhang C, Chen T, et al. Submucosal tunneling endoscopic resection for the treatment of rectal submucosal tumors originating from the muscular propria layer. J Cancer Res Ther 2014;(10 Suppl):281–6.

19. Liu BR, Liu BL, Zhan L, et al. The value of air insufflation CT on diagnosis of esophageal submucosal tumors. Gastroenterology 2013;144:S-612.

20. Chu Y, Qiao X, Gao X, et al. Combined EUS and CT for evaluating gastrointestinal submucosal tumors before endoscopic resection. Eur J Gastroenterol Hepatol 2014;26:933–6.

21. Ren Z, Zhong Y, Zhou P, et al. Perioperative management and treatment for complications during and after peroral endoscopic myotomy (POEM) for esophageal achalasia (EA) (data from 119 cases). Surg Endosc 2012;26:3267–72.

22. Zhang Y, Ye LP, Mao XL. Endoscopic treatments for small gastric subepithelial tumors originating from muscularis propria layer. World J Gastroenterol 2015; 21:9503–11.

23. Demetri GD, von Mehren M, Antonescu CR, et al. NCCN Task Force report: update on the management of patients with gastrointestinal stromal tumors. J Natl Compr Canc Netw 2010;8:S1–41.

24. Sepe PS, Brugge WR. A guide for the diagnosis and management of gastrointestinal stromal cell tumors. Nat Rev Gastroenterol Hepatol 2009;6:363–71.

25. Inoue H, Ikeda H, Hosoya T, et al. Submucosal endoscopic tumor resection for subepithelial tumors in the esophagus and cardia. Endoscopy 2012;44:225–30.

26. Gong W, Xiong Y, Zhi F, et al. Preliminary experience of endoscopic submucosal tunnel dissection for upper gastrointestinal submucosal tumors. Endoscopy 2012;44:231–5.

27. Wang H, Tan Y, Zhou Y, et al. Submucosal tunneling endoscopic resection for upper gastrointestinal submucosal tumors originating from the muscularis propria layer. Eur J Gastroenterol Hepatol 2015;27:776–80.

28. Ye LP, Zhang Y, Mao XL, et al. Submucosal tunneling endoscopic resection for small upper gastrointestinal subepithelial tumors originating from the muscularis propria layer. Surg Endosc 2014;28:524–30.

29. Li QL, Chen WF, Zhang C, et al. Clinical impact of submucosal tunneling endoscopic resection for the treatment of gastric submucosal tumors originating from the muscularis propria layer (with video). Surg Endosc 2015; 29(12):3640–6.

30. Wang XY, Xu MD, Yao LQ, et al. Submucosal tunneling endoscopic resection for submucosal tumors of the esophagogastric junction originating from the muscularis propria layer: a feasibility study (with videos). Surg Endosc 2014;28:1971–7.

31. Zhou DJ, Dai ZB, Wells MM, et al. Submucosal tunneling and endoscopic resection of submucosal tumors at the esophagogastric junction. World J Gastroenterol 2015;21:578–83.

32. Zhang C, Xu MD, Zhou PH, et al. Submucosal tunneling endoscopic resection for submucosal tumors in upper gastrointestinal tract: a feasibility study of 290 consecutive cases. Gastrointest Endosc 2014;79:AB145.

33. Xu MD, Zhou PH, Yao LQ. Peri-operative managements of complications of submucosal tunneling endoscopic resection (STER) for the treatment of upper gastrointestinal submucosal tumors originating from the muscularis propria layer. Gastrointest Endosc 2014;79:AB154.

34. Khashab MA, Saxena P, Valeshabad AK, et al. Novel technique for submucosal tunneling and endoscopic resection of submucosal tumors (with video). Gastrointest Endosc 2013;77:646–8.

35. Kingham TP, DeMatteo RP. Multidisciplinary treatment of gastrointestinal stromal tumors. Surg Clin North Am 2009;89:217–33.

36. Grotz TE, Donohue JH. Surveillance strategies for gastrointestinal stromal tumors. J Surg Oncol 2011;104:921–7.

37. Arun JS, Bingener J. Diagnostic transgastric endoscopic peritoneoscopy for staging of pancreatic and esophageal cancer. Minerva Chir 2012;67:127–40.

38. Bai Y, Qiao WG, Zhu HM, et al. Role of transgastric natural orifice transluminal endoscopic surgery in the diagnosis of ascites of unknown origin (with videos). Gastrointest Endosc 2014;80:807–16.

39. Moris DN, Bramis KJ, Mantonakis EI, et al. Surgery via natural orifices in human beings: yesterday, today, tomorrow. Am J Surg 2012;204:93–102.

40. Fuchs KH, Meining A, von Renteln D, et al. Euro-NOTES status paper: from the concept to clinical practice. Surg Endosc 2013;27:1456–67.

41. Liu BR, Song JT, Kong LJ, et al. Esophago-cardial-gastric tunneling peritoneo-scopy: in vivo dog survival study. J Laparoendosc Adv Surg Tech A 2015; 25(11):920–5.

42. Tedesco P, Fisichella PM, Way LW, et al. Cause and treatment of epiphrenic diverticula. Am J Surg 2005;190:891–4.

43. Hirano Y, Takeuchi H, Oyama T, et al. Minimally invasive surgery for esophageal epiphrenic diverticulum: the results of 133 patients in 25 published series and our experience. Surg Today 2013;43:1–7.

44. Liu BR, Song JT, Fan QW. Endoscopic esophageal epiphrenic diverticulum inversion by using the submucosal tunneling technique. Gastrointest Endosc 2015;81: AB180.

45. Mou Y, Zeng H, Wang Q, et al. Giant mid-esophageal diverticula successfully treated by per-oral endoscopic myotomy. Surg Endosc 2016;30(1):335–8.

Endoscopic Full-thickness Resection (EFTR) for Gastrointestinal Subepithelial Tumors

Mingyan Cai, MD[a], Pinghong Zhou, MD, PhD[a],*,
Luís Carvalho Lourenço, MD[b], Danfeng Zhang, MD[a]

KEYWORDS

- Endoscopic full-thickness resection (EFTR) • Subepithelial tumor (SET)
- Operational approach • Outcomes • Indications and contraindications

KEY POINTS

- Endoscopic full-thickness resection (EFTR) is a minimally invasive technique that has produced promising clinical outcomes as a minimally invasive natural orifice transluminal endoscopic surgery approach to the resection of gastrointestinal subepithelial tumors.
- Emerging suturing devices simplify closure of the full-thickness defect produced by EFTR. However, the mainstay closure technique in Asia, where EFTR is mostly performed, is still metallic endoscopic clips.
- Challenges still exist in professional training, device promotion, and development.

 Video content accompanies this article at www.giendo.theclinics.com

INTRODUCTION

Endoscopists have become more and more aggressive in regard to endoscopic resection as they progress from established expertise in endoscopic mucosal resection (EMR)[1–5] to an ever-expanding experience in endoscopic submucosal dissection (ESD)[6–11] techniques for the en bloc resection of superficial gastrointestinal (GI) lesions arising from the mucosal and submucosal layers. New techniques were developed to excavate muscularis propria (MP)-originating subepithelial tumors (SETs).[12–29] These techniques, often referred to as endoscopic submucosal excavation (ESE) or endoscopic muscularis dissection (EMD), are best suited for SETs without any extraluminal growth component. Furthermore, from an oncologic standpoint, these techniques

All authors declare no conflict of interest.
[a] Endoscopy Center and Endoscopy Research Institute, Zhongshan Hospital, Fudan University, 180 Fenglin Road, Shanghai 20032, China; [b] Gastroenterology Department, Hospital Professor Doutor Fernando Fonseca, IC-19, Venteira, Amadora 2720276, Portugal
* Corresponding author. 180 Fenglin Road, Shanghai 200032, China.
E-mail address: ph.zhou@yahoo.com

cannot guarantee a negative resection margin of muscularis-based tumors such as GI stromal tumors (GISTs) because the muscularis is not removed in toto but, instead, subjected to partial excavation. Both of these issues with ESE or EMD can be addressed by endoscopic full-thickness resection (EFTR). EFTR was first described in 1998 by Suzuki and colleagues.[30] Based on experience with EMR using a ligation device, they reported a new technique for the treatment of early GI tumors, namely EFTR with the use of a ligation device (EFTR-L), followed by endoscopic complete defect closure. Later, in 2001, the same group reported the usefulness of this technique for SETs (2 rectal and 1 duodenal neuroendocrine tumors). EFTR-L was used to perform en bloc resection of these lesions that appeared to have been small (size is not provided), potentially 10 mm or less because the lesions were small enough to be suctioned and ligated within the cap of the ligation device. They report using a proprietary device for tissue apposition and closure before resecting the ligated lesions consisting of a detachable metallic snare with an anchoring needle at its tip. In the case of the duodenal lesion, laparoscopic intervention was needed to suture a microperforation.[31] EFTR can be performed with or without laparoscopic assistance. This article focuses on the techniques and outcomes of pure EFTR without laparoscopic assistance. For an overview of device-assisted EFTR with specialized devices, refer to recent reviews.[32,33] (See Kim HH, Uedo N: Hybrid NOTES: Combined Laparo-Endoscopic Full-Thickness Resection Techniques, in this issue.) Furthermore, the focus is on free-hand EFTR, which uses the same implements as ESD but in a way to effect deeper dissection through the muscularis and/or serosa (see later discussion).

INDICATIONS AND CONTRAINDICATIONS FOR ENDOSCOPIC FULL-THICKNESS RESECTION

Over the past 4 to 5 years, EFTR has been in clinical use in a few elite centers with advanced expertise in endoscopic resection but there is still no consensus about indications or suitability of EFTR. EFTR allows complete resection of tumors, hence reduces the risk of residual tumor, and improves accuracy of pathologic diagnosis and staging. Sumiyama and Gostout[34] proposed that the EFTR technique can be used to resect large laterally spreading tumors and submucosal tumors arising from the submucosa or MP. The group at Endoscopy Center of Zhongshan Hospital proposed indications and contraindications of EFTR (**Box 1**).[33]

Though there is no firm consensus on the exact indications, it is universally agreed that the EFTR procedure should only be carried out by very skilled endoscopists who have mastered ESD, the parent technique for all new natural orifice transluminal endoscopic surgery (NOTES) procedures, including EFTR. EFTR is most frequently used in SETs originating from the MP in the upper GI tract. However, recent publications have also demonstrated the feasibility of EFTR for SETs in the lower GI tract.[35–37]

PREOPERATIVE PREPARATIONS

Before the procedure, the patient should have a preparation similar to that required before general GI surgery. The following should be emphasized:

1. Medical staff and endoscopic accessories
   ○ EFTR is a complex procedure and requires at least 2 trained nurses or technicians and an experienced endoscopist. The success of EFTR depends on the operator's technical skill. The EFTR operator must have mastered electrosurgical, hemostatic and closure techniques, and devices to achieve efficient and complete resection while minimizing and appropriately managing adverse events. The

> **Box 1**
> **Indications and contraindications for endoscopic full-thickness resection**
>
> Indications
> 1. Subepithelial GI tumors arising from the MP based on EUS and CT imaging with diameter ≤5 cm; particularly SETs at locations that are difficult to approach with laparoscopic techniques such as the gastroesophageal junction
>
> 2. Recurrence of epithelial neoplasms in a post-EMR or ESD scar or at a surgical resection site
>
> Contraindications
> 1. High surgical risk due to severe comorbid disease, including severe cardiopulmonary disease, blood disorders, coagulation disorders, and anticoagulant or antiplatelet treatment that cannot be interrupted or discontinued
>
> 2. Anesthesia-related contraindications, such as anesthetic drug allergies or pregnancy
>
> 3. Epithelial neoplasms associated with high risk of lymph node metastasis or periprocedural intraperitoneal dissemination of carcinoma cells
>
> 4. SETs with features on preoperative imaging or histology predicting high risk for aggressive behavior

instruments for EFTR are essentially the same as those used for ESD. Occasionally, in EFTR procedures, a dual-channel endoscope (GIF-2T240, Olympus Corporation, Tokyo, Japan) and grasping forceps (FG-8U-1, Olympus Corporation, Tokyo, Japan) can be used to prevent the tumor from falling into the abdominal cavity. For closure of the GI wall defect, in most clinical settings in which advanced suturing devices are not commercially available (as is the case in Asia currently), purse-string closure via metallic clips and Endoloops (MAJ-254 or MAJ-340, Olympus Corporation, Tokyo, Japan) is the most commonly used technique.[38]

2. Multidisciplinary collaboration
   - Complex procedures such as EFTR require multidisciplinary support from various departments including anesthesia, surgery, gastroenterology, pathology, and intensive care.
3. Bowel preparation
   - Good bowel preparation is necessary for EFTR. Dietary modification and oral laxatives (polyethylene glycol) are used to prepare the colon for colonic lesions. Milk and high-sugar foods are not recommended to prevent flatulence. Patients fast for 8 hours before the procedure.
4. Prophylactic antibiotics
   - Half an hour before EFTR, all patients receive intravenous infusion of a third-generation cephalosporin.[39]

OPERATIONAL APPROACH

A transparent cap is usually attached to the tip of scope (D-201–10,704, Olympus Corporation, Tokyo, Japan) to ensure better view, tissue traction, and positioning; and to facilitate hemostasis in case of bleeding.

Herein, only the technique of pure or free-hand EFTR is discussed. The operational approach can be described as follows[40]: (**Fig. 1**, Video 1)

1. After making several marking dots with an electrosurgical knife around the lesion, a mixture solution (100 mL of normal saline, 1 mL of indigo carmine, and 1 mL of

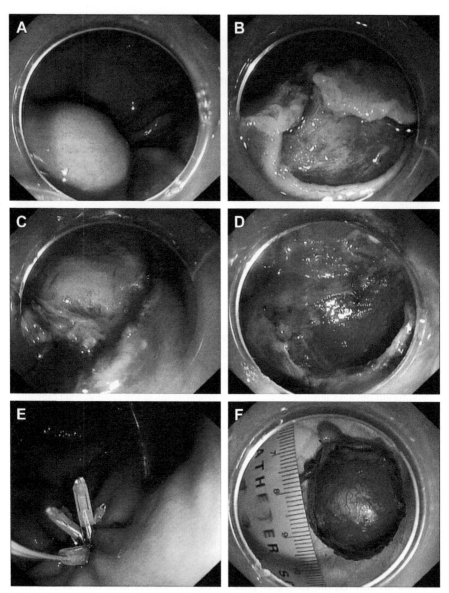

Fig. 1. Endoscopic full-thickness resection for a SET in gastric fundus. (*A*) A SET was located in the gastric fundus. (*B*) The tumor was revealed after mucosal incision. (*C*) Full-thickness resection was performed with an insulated-tip knife. (*D*) The full-thickness wall defect after tumor removal. (*E*) The gastric wall defect was managed by purse-string suture with the combined application of clip and Endoloop. (*F*) The resected specimen was about 3 cm (serosa showing upside).

1:1000 epinephrine solution) is injected into the submucosa. Precutting of the mucosal and submucosal layer around the lesion is performed per typical ESD technique with the usual ESD accessories. To ensure a better view for the ensuing resection of the deeper layers, the mucosa and submucosa covering the luminal aspect of the lesion are sometimes resected with a snare to expose the lesion itself and facilitate margin assessment during the remainder of the resection.

2. A circumferential incision is made through the MP layer around the lesion, again using ESD technique and a Hook knife (KD-620LR, Olympus Corporation, Tokyo, Japan) or other similar ESD knife, depending on operator experience and preference.

3. Due to the close relation between subepithelial GI tumors and the serosal layer that is frequently present, complete resection of the lesion and associated MP while preserving an intact serosal layer is often not possible. Hence, resection of the serosa around the lesion is often inevitable because the MP is being excised by use of the Hook knife or other suitable needle knife (KD-10Q-1, Olympus Corporation, Tokyo, Japan), thus creating an active perforation of the GI wall.

4. Completion of the full-thickness resection of the tumor may require switching from the Hook knife to an insulated-tip knife (KD-610 L, KD-611 L, Olympus Corporation, Tokyo, Japan) to avoid injury of adjacent organs or structures in the peritoneal or chest cavities in the absence of laparoscopic overview or assistance. A dual-channel endoscope is sometimes used with a forceps grasping the tumor before the final cut freeing the tumor from the GI wall to avoid having the tumor fall into the peritoneal cavity, which could complicate retrieval. Finally, the tumor, including its surrounding MP and serosa, is removed via the mouth (or anus for lower tract EFTR). During resection, the highest priority is the safe and complete removal of the tumor without interruption of the tumor capsule.

5. Closure of the gastric wall defect in a periphery-to-center manner can be performed simply with standard endoscopic clips when the size of the full-thickness defect is smaller than the width of the open clip. When the diameter of the defect is slightly larger than the width of the open clip, it can be reduced by air suction and then still be managed by standard clips. However, when the defect is larger than 15 to 20 mm, it may be difficult to approximate and close securely with standard through-the-scope clips. Such larger defects can be managed by clips combined with Endoloops (**Fig. 2**) or by the omental-patch method.[41] By this method, the greater omentum is sucked into the gastric cavity and the defect is closed by affixing the omentum to the edges of the defect with standard endoscopic clips.

6. A 20-gauge needle is inserted in right upper quadrant to relieve the pneumoperitoneum during the procedure (**Fig. 3**). Patients are kept nil by mouth after surgery and nursed in semi-Fowlers position. A nasogastric tube is routinely placed to deflate the stomach; in addition, it helps to detect early postprocedural bleeding.

CLINICAL OUTCOMES OF ENDOSCOPIC FULL-THICKNESS RESECTION

Refinements of a relatively new procedure such as EFTR are necessary to provide reliable and safe results. Safety and efficacy for routine application in human beings will require further validation in randomized trials and should be undertaken by a multidisciplinary team of surgeons and endoscopists.

Esophageal Subepithelial Tumors

Submucosal tunneling endoscopic resection (STER) is used to resect esophageal SETs arising from the MP layer,[42–44] yielding good clinical results and deemed preferable to EFTR for lesions located in areas of the GI tract where tunneling is feasible. Thus the data of pure EFTR on esophageal SETs is limited. However, for large esophageal lesions (greater than one-third of the circumference) an STER approach may be difficult or impossible to manage because it is difficult to extract the tumor from the

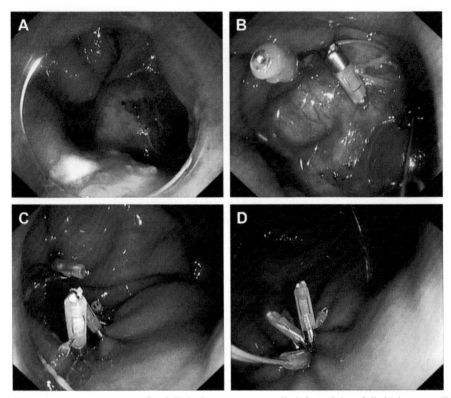

Fig. 2. Purse-string suture of a full-thickness gastric wall defect. (*A*) A full-thickness wall defect after tumor removal. (*B, C*) The purse-string suture was performed by the combined application of clip and Endoloop. The Endoloop was placed above the defect, then the loop clipped with the edge of wall defect, nicely and evenly. (*D*) The defect was tucked underneath the string and the Endoloop tightened to achieve full-thickness closure of the defect.

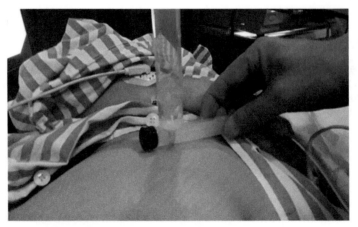

Fig. 3. Air venting by needle puncture during EFTR.

tunnel and the overall dissection is too extensive to allow secure closure via the tunnel approach. At the Endoscopy Center of Zhongshan Hospital, a fully covered retrievable esophageal stent (JSMA, Changzhou, China) is applied, lengths ranging from 60 to 100 mm, to manage the wall defect after EFTR of large SETs with good initial results (data in submission) (**Fig. 4**). The stent has a long string that can be affixed to prevent stent migration and to facilitate endoscopic removal of the stent at 1 to 2 weeks postresection.

Gastric Subepithelial Tumors

Most upper GI SETs are GISTs, which are potentially malignant tumors. National Comprehensive Cancer Network guidelines recommend surgery for suspected GISTs 2 cm or larger and endoscopic surveillance of those smaller than 2 cm. This approach creates a large burden of surgery and endoscopy for small SETs, most of which are low risk.[45] Most of the EFTR reports about clinical outcomes of gastric SETs come from Asian centers, mostly from China. **Table 1** summarizes the clinical outcomes of EFTR for upper GI SETs. The Zhongshan Hospital group reported the first series of EFTR for gastric SETs with a mean tumor sizes of 2.8 cm (1.2–4.5 cm) arising from the MP. The tumors were resected using EFTR technique as previously described and the gastric wall defect was closed with standard through-the-scope

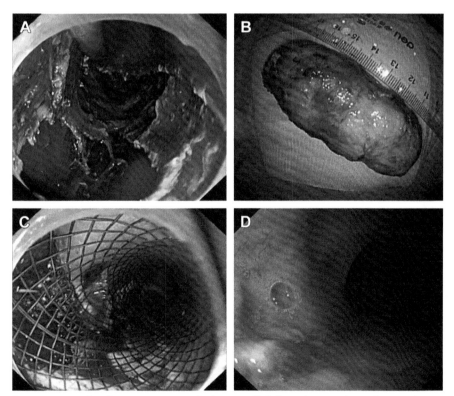

Fig. 4. Stenting for the management of a large wall defect after esophageal EFTR of a SET. (*A, B*) EFTR was performed to dissect an 8 cm leiomyoma. (*C*) A fully covered retrievable esophageal stent was deployed to manage the large wall defect. (*D*) The stent was removed 1 week later and 1 month follow-up gastroscopy showed a well-healed scar.

Table 1
Clinical outcomes of endoscopic full-thickness resection for upper gastrointestinal subepithelial tumors

Authors (Year)	Number of Subjects	Location	Mean Tumor Size (millimeters)	Procedure Time (min)	Suture Technique	En Bloc Resection Rate	Adverse Events	Mean Length of Hospital Stay, Days (Range)	Pathologic Condition	Mean Follow-up Time (mo) and Recurrence (%)
Zhou et al,[40] 2011	26	Stomach	28	105	Clips	100%	0	5.5 (3–8)	16 GIST, 6 leiomyomas, 3 glomus tumors, 1 schwannoma	8, 0
Ye et al,[48] 2014	51	Stomach	24	52	Clips plus Endoloops	98% (50/51)	0	5.9 (3–9)	21 Leiomyomas, 30 GIST	22.4, 0
Huang et al,[47] 2014	35	Stomach	28	90	Clips	100%	5 pneumoperitoneum	6.0 (4–10)	25 GIST, 7 leiomyoma, 2 autonomic nerve tumors	6, 0
Feng et al,[46] 2014	48	Stomach	15.9	59.7	Clips	100%	5 abdominal distention	(4–7) Days not mentioned	43 GIST, 4 leiomyoma, 1 schwannoma	Not mentioned, 0
Yang, et al,[50] 2015	41	Stomach	16.3	78.8	OTSC or clips	100%	1 abdominal pain, 1 dysuria, 1 abdominal pain and fever, 1 nausea and vomiting, 1 pharyngalgia, 1 tenderness of upper abdomen	5.4 Range not mentioned	33 GIST, 4 leiomyomas, 1 NET, 1 ectopic pancreas, 1 schwannoma, 1 hyaline degeneration	—
Guo et al,[49] 2015	23	Stomach	12.1	40.5	OTSC	100%	2 localized peritonitis	3 (2–5)	19 GIST, 4 leiomyoma	3, 0

Abbreviations: NET, neuroendocrine tumor; OTSC, over-the-scope clip.

clips. Complete resection rate was 100% with a mean procedure time of 105 minutes; no major complications were reported.[40]

Three other groups recently confirmed these results in similar studies.[46–48] Another, more recent, retrospective study reported on a similar resection technique in 20 subjects with gastric SETs. In this study, however, the wall defects were closed with clips and Endoloops without severe complications and an en bloc resection rate of 100%.[38] Guo and colleagues[49] used an over-the-scope clip to close the wall defect of EFTR and achieved good results; however, this device is only applicable to lesions less than or equal to 2 cm. Wang and colleagues[51] retrospectively compared the endoscopic resection and laparoscopic resection of nonintracavitary gastric stromal tumors; 31 out of 66 subjects in endoscopic resection group received EFTR. Although EFTR group was embedded in a larger group with ESD and did not have the direct comparison with laparoscopic surgery, the endoscopy group did show superiority in turns of shorter hospital stay, less cost, and reduced postoperative complications.

Duodenal Subepithelial Tumors

There are no series of free-hand EFTR of duodenal lesions due to the difficulty in closing large defects in the duodenum and the high incidence of leaks and severe associated morbidity from duodenal perforations. Likely due to these concerns, only laparoscopy-assisted EFTR has been reported for duodenal carcinoids[52] and device-assisted EFTR with preclosure before resection as, for example, in the recent study by Schmidt and colleagues[53] reviewed in detail in the dedicated article (see Bauder M, Schmidt A, Caca K: Non-exposure, Device-Assisted Endoscopic Full-Thickness Resection, in this issue.) Recently, the corresponding author's group retrospectively studied 374 subjects who underwent endoscopic treatment of duodenal lesions from January 2008 to February 2015. There were 15 pure duodenal EFTRs with fairly good outcomes (data in submission).

Colorectal Subepithelial Tumors

Xu and colleagues[35] reported that EFTR using an ESD-like technique with subsequent metal clip closures is feasible for resection of colonic SETs. No deaths occurred within 30 days, and no recurrence was detected after a median of 18 months follow-up. However, 2 of 16 subjects required laparoscopic closure of the colonic wall defect and 2 subjects developed signs of peritonitis. More data are awaited regarding EFTR of colonic lesions. However, due to the high risk for aggressive behavior in colonic GISTs and carcinoids, EFTR may need to be restricted to smaller lesions. Furthermore, due to the more dire consequences of inadequate closure in the colon relative to the upper GI tract, more secure closure techniques and devices are needed, such as the Ovesco FTR device (GmbH, Tübingen, Germany)[37,54] or endoscopic suturing.[55,56]

SUMMARY AND FUTURE PERSPECTIVES

SETs can be approached easily and without incisions from the mouth or anus using a flexible endoscope, making EFTR the surgical procedure with the lowest degree of invasiveness. Recent developments have brought EFTR into clinical use for selected indications. These developments have again pushed the frontiers of endoluminal resections toward NOTES interventions. There are many merits in extremely minimally invasive surgery, such as reducing the burden (financial, physical, and mental) on patients as well as medical costs.

There are several challenges that need to be addressed before EFTR can enter the mainstream and become widely adopted: (1) the promotion of the emerging suturing and EFTR devices into daily endoscopic practice, (2) the multidisciplinary training of endoscopists to gain both knowledge of gastroenterology and general surgery, and (3) the development of new devices that improve aspects of EFTR that remain inferior to surgical technologies such as novel robust hemostatic devices and staplers.

SUPPLEMENTARY DATA

Supplementary data related to this article can be found online at http://dx.doi.org/10.1016/j.giec.2015.12.013.

REFERENCES

1. Inoue H, Endo M. Endoscopic esophageal mucosal resection using a transparent tube. Surg Endosc 1990;4:198–201.
2. Inoue H, Endo M, Takeshita K, et al. A new simplified technique of endoscopic esophageal mucosal resection using a cap-fitted panendoscope (EMRC). Surg Endosc 1992;6:264–5.
3. Endo M. Endoscopic resection as local treatment of mucosal cancer of the esophagus. Endoscopy 1993;25:672–4.
4. Inoue H, Takeshita K, Hori H, et al. Endoscopic mucosal resection with a cap-fitted panendoscope for esophagus, stomach, and colon mucosal lesions. Gastrointest Endosc 1993;39:58–62.
5. Kudo S. Endoscopic mucosal resection of flat and depressed types of early colorectal cancer. Endoscopy 1993;25:455–61.
6. Oyama T, Tomori A, Hotta K, et al. Endoscopic submucosal dissection of early esophageal cancer. Clin Gastroenterol Hepatol 2005;3:S67–70.
7. Ono H. Endoscopic submucosal dissection for early gastric cancer. Chin J Dig Dis 2005;6:119–21.
8. Kato M. Endoscopic submucosal dissection (ESD) is being accepted as a new procedure of endoscopic treatment of early gastric cancer. Intern Med 2005;44:85–6.
9. Hirasaki S, Tanimizu M, Nasu J, et al. Treatment of elderly patients with early gastric cancer by endoscopic submucosal dissection using an insulated-tip diathermic knife. Intern Med 2005;44:1033–8.
10. Gotoda T. A large endoscopic resection by endoscopic submucosal dissection procedure for early gastric cancer. Clin Gastroenterol Hepatol 2005;3:S71–3.
11. Hirasaki S, Tanimizu M, Moriwaki T, et al. Efficacy of clinical pathway for the management of mucosal gastric carcinoma treated with endoscopic submucosal dissection using an insulated-tip diathermic knife. Intern Med 2004;43:1120–5.
12. Bialek A, Wiechowska-Kozlowska A, Huk J. Endoscopic submucosal dissection of large gastric stromal tumor arising from muscularis propria. Clin Gastroenterol Hepatol 2010;8:e119–20.
13. Chu YY, Lien JM, Tsai MH, et al. Modified endoscopic submucosal dissection with enucleation for treatment of gastric subepithelial tumors originating from the muscularis propria layer. BMC Gastroenterol 2012;12:124.
14. Chun SY, Kim KO, Park DS, et al. Endoscopic submucosal dissection as a treatment for gastric subepithelial tumors that originate from the muscularis propria layer: a preliminary analysis of appropriate indications. Surg Endosc 2013;27:3271–9.
15. He Z, Sun C, Wang J, et al. Efficacy and safety of endoscopic submucosal dissection in treating gastric subepithelial tumors originating in the muscularis

propria layer: a single-center study of 144 cases. Scand J Gastroenterol 2013;48: 1466–73.

16. Lee IL, Lin PY, Tung SY, et al. Endoscopic submucosal dissection for the treatment of intraluminal gastric subepithelial tumors originating from the muscularis propria layer. Endoscopy 2006;38:1024–8.

17. Li L, Wang F, Wu B, et al. Endoscopic submucosal dissection of gastric fundus subepithelial tumors originating from the muscularis propria. Exp Ther Med 2013;6:391–5.

18. Li QL, Yao LQ, Zhou PH, et al. Submucosal tumors of the esophagogastric junction originating from the muscularis propria layer: a large study of endoscopic submucosal dissection (with video). Gastrointest Endosc 2012;75:1153–8.

19. Liu BR, Song JT, Kong LJ, et al. Tunneling endoscopic muscularis dissection for subepithelial tumors originating from the muscularis propria of the esophagus and gastric cardia. Surg Endosc 2013;27:4354–9.

20. Liu BR, Song JT, Qu B, et al. Endoscopic muscularis dissection for upper gastrointestinal subepithelial tumors originating from the muscularis propria. Surg Endosc 2012;26:3141–8.

21. Lu J, Jiao T, Zheng M, et al. Endoscopic resection of submucosal tumors in muscularis propria: the choice between direct excavation and tunneling resection. Surg Endosc 2014;28:3401–7.

22. Meng FS, Zhang ZH, Shan GD, et al. Endoscopic submucosal dissection for the treatment of large gastric submucosal tumors originating from the muscularis propria layer: a single center study. Z Gastroenterol 2015;53:655–9.

23. Reinehr R. Endoscopic submucosal excavation (ESE) is a safe and useful technique for endoscopic removal of submucosal tumors of the stomach and the esophagus in selected cases. Z Gastroenterol 2015;53:573–8 [in German].

24. Shi Q, Zhong YS, Yao LQ, et al. Endoscopic submucosal dissection for treatment of esophageal submucosal tumors originating from the muscularis propria layer. Gastrointest Endosc 2011;74:1194–200.

25. Ye LP, Zhu LH, Zhou XB, et al. Endoscopic excavation for the treatment of small esophageal subepithelial tumors originating from the muscularis propria. Hepatogastroenterology 2015;62:65–8.

26. Zhang S, Chao GQ, Li M, et al. Endoscopic submucosal dissection for treatment of gastric submucosal tumors originating from the muscularis propria layer. Dig Dis Sci 2013;58:1710–6.

27. Zhang Y, Huang Q, Zhu LH, et al. Endoscopic excavation for gastric heterotopic pancreas: an analysis of 42 cases from a tertiary center. Wien Klin Wochenschr 2014;126:509–14.

28. Zhang Y, Ye LP, Zhou XB, et al. Safety and efficacy of endoscopic excavation for gastric subepithelial tumors originating from the muscularis propria layer: results from a large study in China. J Clin Gastroenterol 2013;47:689–94.

29. Zhang Y, Ye LP, Zhu LH, et al. Endoscopic muscularis excavation for subepithelial tumors of the esophagogastric junction originating from the muscularis propria layer. Dig Dis Sci 2013;58:1335–40.

30. Suzuki H, Okuwaki S, Ikeda K, et al. Endoscopic full-thickness resection (EFTR) and waterproof defect closure (ENDC) for improvement of curability and safety in endoscopic treatment of early gastrointestinal malignancies (in Japanese, English abstract). Prog Dig Endosc 1998;52:49–53.

31. Suzuki H, Ikeda K. Endoscopic mucosal resection and full thickness resection with complete defect closure for early gastrointestinal malignancies. Endoscopy 2001;33:437–9.

32. Schmidt A, Meier B, Caca K. Endoscopic full-thickness resection: Current status. World J Gastroenterol 2015;21:9273–85.

33. Zhou PH, Yao LQ, Qin XYE. Endoscopic full-thickness resection (EFTR). In: Atlas of digestive endoscopic resection. Netherlands: Springer; 2014. p. 218–39.

34. Sumiyama K, Gostout CJ. Novel techniques and instrumentation for EMR, ESD, and full-thickness endoscopic luminal resection. Gastrointest Endosc Clin N Am 2007;17:471–85, v–vi.

35. Xu M, Wang XY, Zhou PH, et al. Endoscopic full-thickness resection of colonic submucosal tumors originating from the muscularis propria: an evolving therapeutic strategy. Endoscopy 2013;45:770–3.

36. von Renteln D, Schmidt A, Vassiliou MC, et al. Endoscopic full-thickness resection and defect closure in the colon. Gastrointest Endosc 2010;71:1267–73.

37. Schmidt A, Bauerfeind P, Gubler C, et al. Endoscopic full-thickness resection in the colorectum with a novel over-the-scope device: first experience. Endoscopy 2015;47:719–25.

38. Mitsui T, Goto O, Shimizu N, et al. Novel technique for full-thickness resection of gastric malignancy: feasibility of nonexposed endoscopic wall-inversion surgery (news) in porcine models. Surg Laparosc Endosc Percutan Tech 2013;23: e217–21.

39. Kalloo AN, Singh VK, Jagannath SB, et al. Flexible transgastric peritoneoscopy: a novel approach to diagnostic and therapeutic interventions in the peritoneal cavity. Gastrointest Endosc 2004;60:114–7.

40. Zhou PH, Yao LQ, Qin XY, et al. Endoscopic full-thickness resection without laparoscopic assistance for gastric submucosal tumors originated from the muscularis propria. Surg Endosc 2011;25:2926–31.

41. Hashiba K, Carvalho AM, Diniz G Jr, et al. Experimental endoscopic repair of gastric perforations with an omental patch and clips. Gastrointest Endosc 2001;54:500–4.

42. Xu MD, Cai MY, Zhou PH, et al. Submucosal tunneling endoscopic resection: a new technique for treating upper GI submucosal tumors originating from the muscularis propria layer (with videos). Gastrointest Endosc 2012;75:195–9.

43. Lee CK, Lee SH, Chung IK, et al. Endoscopic full-thickness resection of a gastric subepithelial tumor by using the submucosal tunnel technique with the patient under conscious sedation (with video). Gastrointest Endosc 2012;75:457–9.

44. Ye LP, Zhang Y, Mao XL, et al. Submucosal tunneling endoscopic resection for small upper gastrointestinal subepithelial tumors originating from the muscularis propria layer. Surg Endosc 2014;28:524–30.

45. Stavropoulos SN, Modayil R, Friedel D, et al. Endoscopic full-thickness resection for GI stromal tumors. Gastrointest Endosc 2014;80:334–5.

46. Feng Y, Yu L, Yang S, et al. Endolumenal endoscopic full-thickness resection of muscularis propria-originating gastric submucosal tumors. J Laparoendosc Adv Surg Tech A 2014;24:171–6.

47. Huang LY, Cui J, Lin SJ, et al. Endoscopic full-thickness resection for gastric submucosal tumors arising from the muscularis propria layer. World J Gastroenterol 2014;20:13981–6.

48. Ye LP, Yu Z, Mao XL, et al. Endoscopic full-thickness resection with defect closure using clips and an endoloop for gastric subepithelial tumors arising from the muscularis propria. Surg Endosc 2014;28:1978–83.

49. Guo J, Liu Z, Sun S, et al. Endoscopic full-thickness resection with defect closure using an over-the-scope clip for gastric subepithelial tumors originating from the muscularis propria. Surg Endosc 2015;29(11):3356–62.

50. Yang F, Wang S, Sun S, et al. Factors associated with endoscopic full-thickness resection of gastric submucosal tumors. Surg Endosc 2015;29:3588–93.
51. Wang L, Ren W, Fan CQ, et al. Full-thickness endoscopic resection of nonintracavitary gastric stromal tumors: a novel approach. Surg Endosc 2011;25:641–7.
52. Abe N, Takeuchi H, Shibuya M, et al. Successful treatment of duodenal carcinoid tumor by laparoscopy-assisted endoscopic full-thickness resection with lymphadenectomy. Asian J Endosc Surg 2012;5:81–5.
53. Schmidt A, Meier B, Cahyadi O, et al. Duodenal endoscopic full-thickness resection (with video). Gastrointest Endosc 2015;82:728–33.
54. Schmidt A, Damm M, Caca K. Endoscopic full-thickness resection using a novel over-the-scope device. Gastroenterology 2014;147:740–2.e2.
55. Kantsevoy SV, Bitner M, Hajiyeva G, et al. Endoscopic management of colonic perforations: clips versus suturing closure (with videos). Gastrointest Endosc 2015. [Epub ahead of print].
56. Stavropoulos SN, Modayil R, Friedel D. Current applications of endoscopic suturing. World J Gastrointest Endosc 2015;7:777–89.

Non-Exposure, Device-Assisted Endoscopic Full-thickness Resection

Markus Bauder, MD, Arthur Schmidt, MD, Karel Caca, MD,*

KEYWORDS

- Subepithelial tumors • Endoscopic full-thickness resection • EFTR • GIST
- Over-the-scope • Endoscopic suturing

KEY POINTS

- EFTR after deployment of full-thickness sutures offers a new and effective nonexposure approach for endoscopic resection of subepithelial gastric tumors.
- The novel over-the-scope FTR device is a powerful tool for EFTR of colorectal lesions. The indications for this device may be expanded to include duodenal resections in the future.
- Both techniques may reduce the risk of perforation and subsequent infection or exposure of the peritoneal cavity to luminal contents including neoplastic cells by a "close first – cut later" approach. Further data are needed to confirm this hypothesis.

 Video content accompanies this article at www.giendo.theclinics.com

INTRODUCTION

In most cases subepithelial tumors (SETs) of the gastrointestinal (GI) tract are coincidental findings in routine endoscopy. Although endoscopic ultrasound (EUS) with or without fine-needle aspiration provides essential hints on the nature of such tumors, a definitive diagnosis often cannot be obtained.[1] Particularly if the lesion is suspicious for a gastrointestinal stromal tumor (GIST), endoscopic resection is helpful for the acquisition of a definitive histologic diagnosis and risk

Disclosure: The Department of Gastroenterology and Oncology has received financial support from Ovesco Endoscopy for the coordination and performance of a multicenter trial investigating treatment of recurrent peptic ulcer bleeding using over-the-scope clips. K. Caca and A. Schmidt have received lecture fees from Ovesco Endoscopy for full-thickness resection device training courses.
Department of Gastroenterology and Oncology, Klinikum Ludwigsburg, Medizinische Klinik I, Posilipo-Strasse 1-4, Ludwigsburg 71640, Germany
* Corresponding author.
E-mail address: karel.caca@kliniken-lb.de

stratification. Moreover a histologically confirmed complete resection may spare the necessity of further interventions. Because GISTs often arise from or infiltrate deep into the muscularis propria, endoscopic resection of such tumors with conventional techniques naturally results in or at least harbors a significant risk of GI wall perforation. Therefore secure endoscopic closure techniques are mandatory. There are two possible strategies: the tumor is resected first and defect closure is performed in a second step; or a perforation is prevented by creating serosa-to-serosa apposition underneath the tumor before resection. This article presents two techniques using this "close first–cut later" principle, using a suturing device and a novel over-the-scope device.

ENDOSCOPIC FULL-THICKNESS RESECTION OF GASTRIC SUBEPITHELIAL TUMORS USING THE GERDX SUTURING DEVICE
Indications/Contraindications

For SETs larger than 2 cm that are known GISTs or have EUS morphology suspicious for a GIST resection is recommended by international guidelines.[2–4] Whether SETs smaller than 2 cm that are suspected of being GISTs should be resected or periodically observed remains controversial. Current National Comprehensive Cancer Network guidelines allow periodic follow-up if no high-risk morphology is detected on EUS.[3] Molecular and pathologic analysis of GISTs less than 2 cm showed characteristics of benign behavior. However, there was a dramatic increase in mitotic activity for GISTs greater than 1 cm compared with smaller tumors.[5] Therefore, resection of GISTs greater than 1 cm could be reasonable. Additionally there may be many patients preferring resection to life-long periodic endoscopic follow-up. Therefore a case-by-case decision is needed in cases with GISTs less than 2 cm. Possible indications and contraindications for endoscopic full-thickness resection (EFTR) after transmural suturing are listed in **Table 1**. Performing EUS before EFTR is essential to determine exact tumor size, extramural growth, and regional lymph node status. Furthermore EUS can reliably distinguish lipomas (hyperechoic homogeneous lesions) from potentially malignant lesions. Because of the dimensions of the suturing device its use is limited to gastric lesions.

Recently our group published a retrospective case series of 31 patients who underwent EFTR of gastric SETs. Within this trial tumor sizes up to 40 mm could be resected successfully.[6] Because difficulty to place full-thickness sutures underneath SETs increases with tumor size and thus leads to increased perforation risk we do not recommend resection of tumors larger than 35 mm in diameter with this method.

Table 1	
Indications and contraindications	
Indications	**Contraindications**
Gastric SET with EUS morphology as follows a. Suspected GIST >2 cm b. Suspected GIST <2 cm + high-risk features	Tumor size >35 mm
Symptomatic SET	Large extramural tumor component Signs of systemic spread (eg, suspect locoregional lymphatic nodes, ascites) History of gastric and/or esophageal surgery or stenosis, that impedes the insertion of the EFTR device

Device, Preprocedure Preparation

All patients receive a single-shot antibiotic therapy with intravenous ceftriaxone or ciprofloxacine during the procedure or within 4 hours after the procedure. The following devices have to be prepared:

- The GERDX device (G-Surg, Seeon, Germany), loaded with resorbable, pretied 4-mm sutures and modified expanded polytetrafluoroethylene pledgets (delivered by G-Surg with the device) (**Figs. 1–3**). Loading of the pledgets and sutures in the arms of the device is shown in **Fig. 4**.
- One or two additional pledgets with sutures should be prepared
- 5.8-mm videogastroscope
- Guidewire
- Electrocautery polypectomy snare

Patient positioning

The patient is positioned in left lateral position. Interventions are generally done under deep sedation with propofol and/or midazolam. General anesthesia with endotracheal intubation usually is not necessary. Monitoring of blood pressure, heart rate, and oxygen saturation is mandatory.

Approach

This technique aims at the resection of lesions after application of transmural sutures to secure wall patency and avoiding exposure of the peritoneal cavity to luminal contents. The sutures used for this indication are resorbable (in contrast to the nonresorbable sutures used in the endoscopic antireflux procedure for which this device was originally conceived).

Procedure

1. A guidewire is placed in the gastric antrum. The GERDX device is advanced into the gastric corpus over the wire. To visualize the suturing procedure a 5.8-mm videogastroscope is advanced through the accessory channel of the device by a second endoscopist and the device is advanced to the lesion in either retroflex or straight position depending on tumor localization (**Fig. 6**A).

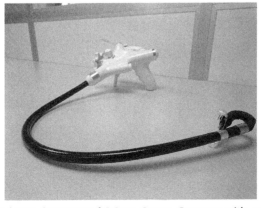

Fig. 1. The GERDX device. (*Courtesy of* G-Surg, Seeon, Germany, with permission.)

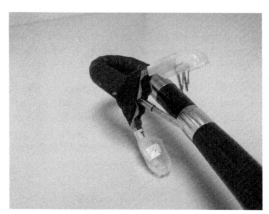

Fig. 2. Tip of the GERDX device with tissue retractor between the arms. (*Courtesy of* G-Surg, Seeon, Germany, with permission.)

2. After opening of the arms of the suturing device (hydraulic mechanism), the tissue retractor is advanced and screwed into the gastric wall at the margin of the tumor. The gastric wall is then retracted into the arms of the suturing device.
3. The arms of the device (preloaded with the previously mentioned pledgets and resorbable sutures) are closed and a full-thickness polytetrafluoroethylene pledgeted suture is placed underneath the tumor to create a serosa-to-serosa apposition (**Fig. 6**C).
4. Steps 1 to 3 are repeated to create an additional suture at the opposing side of the first suture until an intraluminal pseudopolyp has been created (**Figs. 5**A and **6**C). For each suturing process the GERDX device has to be loaded with new pledgets and sutures and inserted again. Usually two full-thickness sutures are sufficient for a tightly apposed gastric wall plication. If necessary, additional sutures may be deployed. In case of uncertainty, EUS may be performed before resection to confirm inclusion of the entire tumor within the inverted plication of the gastric wall (**Fig. 6**D).
5. The pseudopolyp is resected using a monofilament snare above the full-thickness sutures and below the SET (**Fig. 5**B).
6. Afterward inspection of the resection site is mandatory. If necessary, clips are added to close small dehiscences (**Fig. 6**E). Endoscopic hemostasis may be needed in case of bleeding.

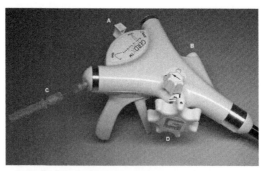

Fig. 3. The handle of the GERDX device. (A) Slide control to open and close arms of the device. (B) Channel for 5.8-mm videogastroscope. (C) Wire of the tissue retractor. (D) Handwheel for tip angulation. (*Courtesy of* G-Surg, Seeon, Germany, with permission.)

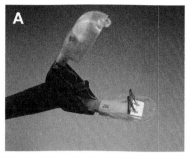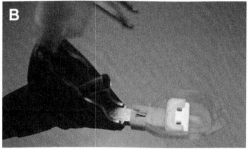

Fig. 4. (*A*) Arm loaded with expanded polytetrafluoroethylene pledget, needle, and pretied suture. (*B*) Opposing arm loaded with expanded polytetrafluoroethylene pledget. (*Courtesy of* G-Surg, Seeon, Germany, with permission.)

7. Subsequently the tumor is retrieved from the stomach for histologic analysis. EUS is performed immediately postresection to confirm complete tumor resection (**Fig. 6**F).

Adverse Events and Management

The most common adverse event is bleeding at the resection site. Furthermore, perforations of the gastric wall can occur if suture position was not correct or if resection was performed underneath the sutures. **Table 2** provides an overview of all adverse events having occurred in our experience.[6] All adverse events could be successfully managed endoscopically. Notably all perforations (N = 3) were detected immediately and closed by deploying another transmural suture with the suturing device, thus qualifying the suturing device for complication management. Bleeding is handled with standard endoscopic strategies, such as the application of clips and/or injection of diluted epinephrine.

Postprocedure Care

Monitoring is continued in a recovery room until the patient is awake and protective reflexes are intact. Standard-dose proton pump inhibitors should be administered

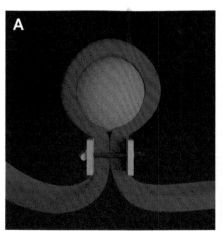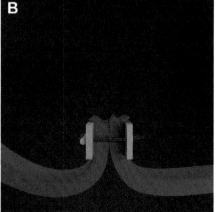

Fig. 5. Schematic illustration of transmural suturing. (*A*) Full-thickness suture with serosa-to-serosa apposition underneath SET. (*B*) After resection GI wall patency is secured by the suture.

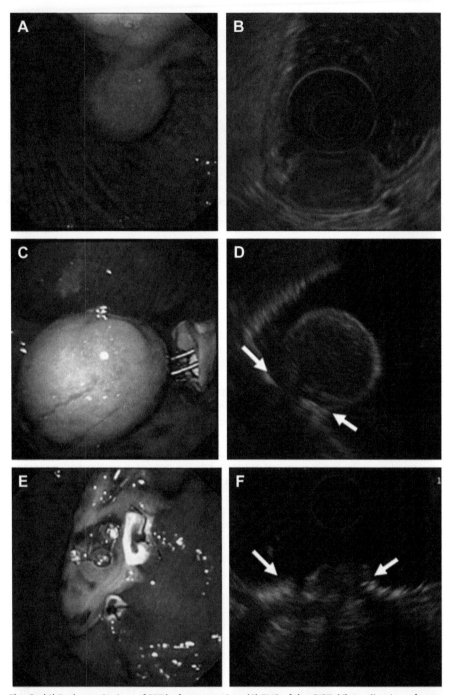

Fig. 6. (A) Endoscopic view of SET before resection. (B) EUS of the GIST. (C) Application of transmural sutures underneath the tumor. (D) EUS showing correctly placed sutures. (E) Inspection of resection site (two transmural sutures, three clips). (F) EUS of resection site to confirm lack of residual tumor. *Arrows*, place of sutures. (*Adapted from* von Renteln D, Schmidt A, Riecken B, et al. Gastric full-thickness suturing during EMR and for treatment of gastric-wall defects(with video). Gastrointest Endosc 2008;67:738–44; with permission.)

Table 2	
List of adverse events in our published experience (N = 31)	
Adverse Events	**Rate of Adverse Event**
Bleeding	12/31 (38.7%)
Perforation	3/31 (9.6%)
Need for surgery	0/31 (0%)

Data from Schmidt A, Bauder M, Riecken B, et al. Endoscopic full-thickness resection of gastric sub-epithelial tumors: a single-center series. Endoscopy 2015;47:156.

for a week. Monitoring red blood count is reasonable. After a fasting period of 24 hours return to normal diet is adapted to patient's symptoms.

Follow-up and Clinical Implications

Because the procedure is not yet widely used, currently there are no international standards for follow-up. Follow-up after histologically confirmed complete tumor resection depends on the histologic diagnosis of the resected specimen and may be done according to the flow chart in **Fig. 7**. Incomplete resection of a GIST should be followed by endoscopic or surgical reresection. Incompletely resected benign SETs may be monitored endoscopically every 1 to 2 years. If no progression or macroscopic recurrence is detected follow-up can be stopped. A histologic diagnosis of GIST requires a subsequent analysis of the mitotic rate and classification according to the Miettinen risk score. Imatinib (Gleevec; Novartis, Basel, Switzerland) therapy should be started for intermediate- or high-risk scores.[7]

Outcomes

The first experiences with this concept were published as small case series by our group in 2008 (N = 1) and 2011 (N = 3).[8,9] In a recent retrospective study of 31 patients undergoing full-thickness resection of gastric SETs by this technique, a complete macroscopic resection and a definite histologic diagnosis could be obtained in all

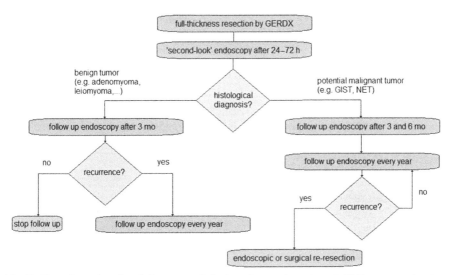

Fig. 7. Flow chart showing follow-up as it is done in our department. NET, neuroendocrine tumor.

cases.[6] Further outcome data are shown in **Table 3**. For most of these patients the Plicator device (NDO Surgical Inc, Mansfield, MA) was used. Because the Plicator device is no longer commercially available, our group has started to use the GERDX suturing device working with the same suturing mechanism.

Current Controversies/Future Considerations

Preliminary data indicate that EFTR of gastric SETs after gastric wall plication via endoluminal application of transmural sutures is feasible, effective, and safe. However, larger prospective studies are needed to confirm these findings. Currently a prospective observational study to gather further data on safety and efficacy of this resection technique is recruiting (FROST [Endoscopic Full Thickness Resection of Gastric Subepithelial Tumors], NCT02488746). Given the lack of larger studies, the surgical approach (eg, laparoscopic wedge resection) is still standard of care. EFTR of GISTs greater than 2 cm can be offered to patients as an individual decision or to patients either unfit or refusing surgery. In 2006, a different technique for EFTR of gastric SETs was presented as an experimental approach: a plication of the gastric wall was created by a stapler device with a flexible shaft before resection.[10] In two patients EFTR of early gastric adenocarcinoma was achieved.[11] However, the stapler technique has not been integrated further into clinical practice because the long (55 mm) and rigid stapler tip was limited in its intraluminal mobility and precision. For instance, the proximal corpus and cardia could not be reached. Designing a more flexible miniaturized version of the stapler device with an integrated countertraction tool could be a solution to this limitation in the future. EFTR may be the next step toward more extended endoscopic oncologic resections; however, EFTR does not allow lymph node resection, therefore raising the question whether tumor resection by this technique involves the risk of subsequent metastatic spread.[12] However, most SETs show benign behavior. Studies comparing laparoscopic wedge resection of GISTs without lymph node dissection with expanded open surgical resection showed no differences in overall survival. In one prospective case series laparoscopic wedge resection even showed a lower recurrence rate.[13,14] These data suggest that lymph node resection is not necessary in GISTs (especially in GISTs <35 mm), thus justifying the use of EFTR in this indication. EUS (including lymph node status assessment) before EFTR is mandatory.

ENDOSCOPIC FULL-THICKNESS RESECTION OF SUBEPITHELIAL TUMORS USING AN OVER-THE-SCOPE DEVICE
Indications/Contraindications

The full-thickness resection device (FTRD; Ovesco, Tuebingen, Germany) has been developed for resection of colorectal lesions, including adenomas and SETs.[15]

Table 3 Outcome data of the case series (N = 31)	
Macroscopically complete resection	31 (100%)
Histologically complete resection	28 (90.3%)
Mean tumor size	20.5 mm (range, 8–48 mm)
Mean follow-up	213 d (range, 1–1737 d)
Local or systemic recurrence	0 (0%)

Data from Schmidt A, Bauder M, Riecken B, et al. Endoscopic full-thickness resection of gastric subepithelial tumors: a single-center series. Endoscopy 2015;47:156.

Recently, resection of duodenal lesions was managed in a small case series as off-label use.[16] The inner diameter of the cap of the device limits the maximum size of the lesion to resect. An exact tumor size limit cannot be stated because resectability depends on the wall thickness, tissue rigidity, and tissue mobility at the resection site. In porcine experiments the maximum size of resected specimen was 40 × 42 mm in the colon.[15] In the largest clinical case series, the maximum size of resected specimen was 40 mm in the colorectum[17] and in a small case series up to the same size in the duodenum.[16] Maximum size of resected SETs was 22 mm. Nevertheless we do not recommend resecting adenomas larger than 30 mm and SETs larger than 20 mm because the resectability cannot be predicted accurately before the procedure. The usually rigid consistency of SETs makes their incorporation into the cap more difficult compared with adenomas. It must be stressed that full-thickness resection in the stomach usually is not possible because of the thickness of the gastric wall. However, superficial resection of small submucosal lesions is possible. In a live porcine model resection of 8-mm strict submucosal lesions was feasible.[18] Because the FTRD system has an outer diameter of 21 mm it is important to stress that peroral insertion of the device and passage through the esophagus is significantly more difficult than in the colorectum. The indications and contraindications are listed in **Table 4**.

Procedure

Device

In comparison with the conventional over-the-scope-clip (OTSC) system, the novel FTRD (**Fig. 8**) is additionally preloaded with a snare that enables resection of the targeted lesion immediately after application of the OTSC. Moreover its cap is longer (23 mm) and larger in inner diameter (13 mm). The preloaded 14-mm OTSC is modified with additional teeth. Subsequently we describe the technique of full-thickness resection of SETs using this novel device.

Preparation

- All patients receive a single-shot antibiotic therapy with intravenous ceftriaxone or ciprofloxacine during the procedure or within 4 hours after the procedure.
- The FTRD system is delivered as a complete set including the device, a cap preloaded with the OTSC and a monofilament snare, a marking probe, and a grasper (see **Fig. 8**A).

Table 4 Indications and contraindications (FTRD)	
Indications	**Contraindications**
Colorectal or duodenal subepithelial tumors	Lesion size >30 mm for adenomas and >20 mm for SETs depending on conditions at resection site
Colorectal or duodenal adenomas • With nonlifting sign • Involving the appendix • Involving a diverticulum	History of surgery/intervention/disease that impedes the insertion of the FTRD (eg, stenosis, adhesions)
Diagnostic full-thickness resections (eg, after incomplete resection of T1 carcinoma, for diagnosis of suspected Hirschsprung disease)	—

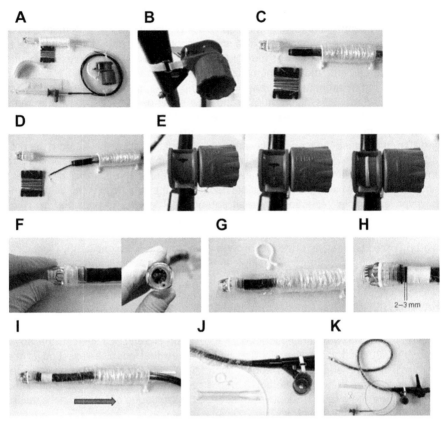

Fig. 8. Assembly of the FTRD system. (*A*) Take parts out of blister. (*B*) Mount handwheel on working channel of endoscope. (*C*) Place endoscope sleeve tube on the endoscope. (*D*) Insert thread retriever, grasp end of thread, and pull thread through the channel. (*E*) Fix the thread at the handwheel and wind it up. (*F*) Place cap onto the endoscope until it reaches stopper. (*G*) Place endoscope sleeve near the cap and remove first plastic clamp. (*H*) Tape end of the sleeve onto the cap with the included tape. Make sure the tape does not touch the white ring. (*I*) Pull sleeve by holding the tube until the end of the scope. (*J, K*) Remove second plastic clamp. Pull out plastic tube and flap it open to remove it from the endoscope. (*Courtesy of* Ovesco Endoscopy, Tuebingen, Germany, with permission.)

- The thread used to trigger the clip release has to be pulled through the working channel of the endoscope with the help of a thread retriever and has to be fixed at the handwheel before mounting the cap on the endoscope (see **Fig. 8**B–E).
- Because the preloaded snare and its release mechanism are located on the outer surface of the endoscope a transparent sheath is needed to cover the whole length of the endoscope (see **Fig. 8**G–J).

Patient positioning At the beginning of the procedure the patient is positioned in left lateral position. After passing the sigmoid colon, the patient can be moved to supine position if necessary. If the FTRD is used for resection in the upper GI tract the patient usually remains in left lateral position. Interventions are generally done under deep sedation with propofol. General anesthesia with endotracheal intubation is usually not necessary. Monitoring of blood pressure, heart rate, and oxygen saturation is mandatory.

Approach This technique aims at the resection of lesions after application of an OTSC to secure wall apposition avoiding exposure of the peritoneal cavity to luminal contents.

Technique/procedure

1. The field of view is limited in comparison with that of a standard colonoscope because of the mounted cap on the FTRD; thus, we recommend marking the target lesion with the high frequency-probe included in the set to facilitate rediscovery of the lesion (Video 1).
2. Having reached the target lesion with the FTRD the lesion is pulled into the cap with the grasper or by using a tissue anchor (Ovesco Endoscopy) (**Figs. 9**B, C and **10**B). It is essential to grasp the lesion at its very center to ensure complete resection. Note that suction should only be used very gently if at all in this step because of the higher risk of pulling extracolonic structures into the cap.
3. The OTSC is deployed underneath the tumor to secure wall apposition before resection (**Fig. 9**D).
4. Subsequently the pseudopolyp that has been created containing the adenoma or SET and surrounding tissue is immediately resected with the preloaded snare above the OTSC. The resected specimen is retrieved in the cap and removed by withdrawing the colonoscope (**Figs. 9**E and **10**D).
5. Inspection of the resection site is mandatory (**Fig. 10**C).

Mean procedure time for steps 1 to 5 was 50 minutes in a case series with 24 patients.[17] If FTRD is used for resection of duodenal lesions steps 1 to 5 remain the same, but it is important to emphasize that insertion of the FTRD through the esophagus has to be performed carefully because of the large outer diameter of the FTRD (21 mm). Balloon dilation or bougienage of the upper esophageal sphincter may be necessary in some cases.

Adverse Events and Management

Potential adverse events are bleeding, perforation, or infection. Both bleeding and perforation can occur at the resection site (immediate or delayed bleeding/perforation) or during advancement of the endoscope with the mounted FTRD. Postpolypectomy syndrome may occur after resection of colorectal lesions. Fixation of extracolonic

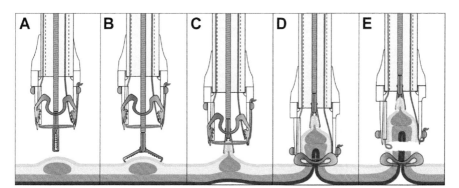

Fig. 9. Schematic illustration of FTRD procedure. (*A, B*) A grasping forceps is advanced through the working channel of the endoscope. (*C*) The target lesion is grasped and pulled into the cap. (*D*) The OTSC is deployed and creates a full-thickness plication of the GI wall. (*E*) The pseudopolyp is resected above the OTSC with the preloaded snare. (*Courtesy of Ovesco Endoscopy, Tuebingen, Germany, with permission.*)

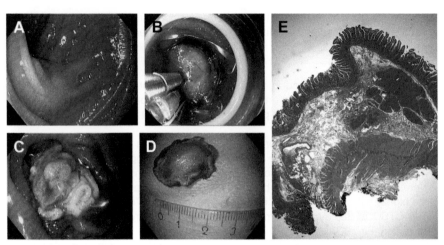

Fig. 10. EFTR of a duodenal SET. (*A*) Duodenal SET before resection. (*B*) The tumor is pulled into the cap by use of a tissue anchor (Ovesco Endoscopy, Tuebingen, Germany). (*C*) Resection site. The OTSC secures wall patency. (*D*) Resected specimen. (*E*) Histology confirming full-thickness resection of duodenal wall including the SET (hematoxylin-eosin, original magnification ×40). Image from Schmidt, et al.[16] (*From* Schmidt A, Meier B, Cahyadi O, et al. Duodenal endoscopic full-thickness resection (with video). Gastrointest Endosc 2015;82:728–33; with permission.)

structures or organs to the colon by the OTSC is a specific complication of the FTRD system. Even if the OTSC is properly closed this can result in delayed perforation. Application of the OTSC at the wrong location (failing to encompass the tumor) and irritation/inflammation of the adjacent healthy tissue by the OTSC are further specific complications. In those cases removal of the OTSC facilitates further endoscopic or surgical intervention. A novel bipolar grasper device (DC Clip Cutter, Ovesco) for removal of OTSC by direct current impulses showed feasibility and efficacy in a recent case series.[19] This device may also facilitate removal of the OTSC if it is still in place on the first follow-up endoscopy to permit uncomplicated site inspection and biopsies if necessary on further follow-up surveillance endoscopies. A list of complications, their frequency in a case series,[17] and their management is provided in **Table 5**. Note that OTSC systems also qualify for complication management, such as hemostasis and defect closure.[20]

Postprocedure Care

Monitoring is to be continued in a recovery room until the patient is awake and protective reflexes are intact. Monitoring of the red blood count and daily abdominal examinations for at least 2 days is reasonable. After 3 to 6 hours, clear liquids are started. The next day return to normal diet is possible in the absence of adverse events. After resection of lesions involving the appendix antibiotic therapy should be extended to a minimum of 4 days to lower the incidence of appendicitis.

Follow-up

Because the procedure is not yet widely used, currently there are no international standards for follow-up. We recommend scheduling patients for the first endoscopic follow-up within 3 to 6 months after resection. Further follow-up should be scheduled individually depending on histology and inspection of the resection site at initial follow-up.

Table 5 Adverse events and their management (FTRD)		
Adverse Event	**Frequency**	**Recommended Management**
Bleeding	1/25 (4%)	• Endoscopic standard hemostasis (eg, injection of epinephrine solution, clip application) • Application of another OTSC • Angiographic or surgical intervention in uncontrollable cases
Perforation (immediate or delayed)	0/25 (0%)	• Application of standard clips or another OTSC • Surgery if endoscopic therapy is not possible • Antibiotics
Postpolypectomy syndrome/infection	2/25 (8%)	• Exclusion of perforation by radiography • Antibiotics
Wrong placement of OTSC/fixation of adjacent tissue by OTSC	0/25 (0%)	• OTSC removal (DC Clip Cutter, Ovesco) • Endoscopic or surgical reintervention

From Schmidt A, Bauerfeind P, Gubler C, et al. Endoscopic full-thickness resection in the colorectum with a novel over-the-scope device: first experience. Endoscopy 2015;47:723; with permission.

Outcomes

Endoscopic resection of GI lesions (including submucosal lesions) by application of an OTSC and subsequent snare resection recently has been described as an effective and safe technique.[20–22] **Table 6** gives an overview of available data. In comparison with endoscopic submucosal dissection, OTSC techniques are less time-consuming, are considered as less technically demanding, and may prevent perforation and exposure of the peritoneal cavity to intraluminal contents. Compared with conventional OTSC systems the new FTRD system provides a technique with time-saving potential because the preloaded OTSC and snare allow clipping and immediate resection without repeated insertion of devices. Moreover, the larger cap size facilitates resection of larger tumors or may increase en bloc resection rate for smaller tumor sizes. In the largest case series available with the novel FTRD a full-thickness resection could be achieved in 87.5% and complete resection was histologically confirmed in 75%.[17] There was no perforation and no major bleeding. The lesions resected in this case series were mainly adenomas. As regards the two submucosal tumors (one leiomyoma and one hamartoma), R0 resection was achieved in both cases without complications.[17] At present there is only one case series reporting on the use of the new device for duodenal lesions. In two nonlifting adenomas and two submucosal tumors (mean tumor size, 28 mm; range, 22–40 mm) macroscopic complete resection was performed. R0 resection was confirmed in three of four cases. Two cases of minor bleeding were controlled endoscopically.[16]

Current Controversies/Future Considerations

Recent data on full-thickness resection of colorectal and duodenal lesions using the novel FTRD device are promising, but further studies are needed and higher case numbers to confirm efficacy and safety. Currently a multicenter prospective study is recruiting to investigate efficacy and safety of EFTR in the colorectum using the FTRD system (ClinicalTrials.gov Identifier: NCT02362126). Concerning EFTR of duodenal lesions a multicenter study is planned. Limitations of the FTRD are the limited field of view through the mounted cap and the limited resection size. Advancing the FTRD through the GI tract is more difficult compared with a standard colonoscope

Table 6
Outcome data (conventional OTSC and FTRD)

Study	Outcome
Mönkemüller et al,[20] 2014 Conventional OTSC system • EFTR of SETs (N = 2)	Overall success rate • EFTR of SETs: 100% Adverse events: 0/16 (0%)
Sarker et al,[21] 2014 (N = 8) Conventional OTSC system in following indication: • EFTR of SET (N = 8) with a mean tumor size of 13.4 mm (range, 9–20 mm)	Macroscopically complete resection: 8/8 (100%) R0 resections: 7/8 (87.5%) Confirmed full-thickness resection: 2/8 (25%) Adverse events: 0/8 (0%)

Fähndrich and Sandmann,[22] 2015 (N = 17)
Conventional OTSC system in following
indications:
• EFTR of SETs (N = 7) with a mean tumor size
of 20.7 mm (range, 10–25 mm)
• EFTR after R1 resection polypectomy (N = 6)
• EFTR of adenoma relapse (N = 3)
Novel FTRD system in following indication:
• EFTR after R1 resection polypectomy (N = 1)
	a. Conventional OTSC
	  Technical success: 15/16 (93.8%)
	  Macroscopically complete resection:
	  15/15 (100%)
	  R0 resection: 15/15 (100%)
	  Confirmed full-thickness resection: 10/15
	  (66.7%)
	  Adverse events: 0/15 (0%)
	b. Novel FTRD system
	  Technical success: 1/1 (100%)
	  Macroscopically complete resection: 1/1
	  (100%)
	  R0 resection: 1/1 (100%)
	  Confirmed full-thickness resection: 1/1
	  (100%)
	  Adverse events: 0/1 (0%)

Valli et al,[23] 2014 (N = 1) Novel FTRD system in following indication: • Adenoma involving diverticulum in the colon	Technical success: 1/1 (100%) Macroscopically complete resection: 1/1 (100%) R0 resection: 1/1 (100%) Confirmed full-thickness resection: 1/1 (100%) Adverse events: 0/1 (0%)
Klare et al,[24] 2015 (N = 1) Novel FTRD system in following indication: • Reresection after R1 resection of a neuro- endocrine tumor in the rectum	Technical success: 1/1 (100%) Macroscopically complete resection: 1/1 (100%) R0 resection: 1/1 (100%) Confirmed full-thickness resection: 1/1 (100%) Adverse events: 0/1 (0%)
Schmidt et al,[16] 2015 (N = 4) Novel FTRD system in following indication: • EFTR of duodenal SETs (N = 2) • EFTR of duodenal nonlifting adenomas (N = 2)	Technical success: 4/4 (100%) Macroscopically complete resection: 4/4 (100%) R0 resection: 3/4 (75%) Confirmed full-thickness resection: 4/4 (100%) Adverse events: 2/4 (50%), minor bleedings in both cases
Schmidt et al,[25] 2014 (N = 3) Novel FTRD system in following indication: • EFTR of recurrent adenomas with nonlifting sign in the colon	Technical success: 3/3 (100%) Macroscopically complete resection: 3/3 (100%) R0 resection: 3/3 (100%) Confirmed full-thickness resection: 3/3 (100%) Adverse events: 0/3 (0%)

(continued on next page)

Table 6 (continued)	
Study	Outcome
Schmidt et al,[17] 2015 (N = 25) Novel FTRD system in following indications: • EFTR of colorectal SETs (N = 2) • EFTR of colorectal adenomas (N = 21) • Diagnostic EFTR after incomplete resection of T1 carcinoma and for Hirschsprung disease (N = 2)	Target lesion reached: 24/25 (96%) Technical success: 20/24 (83.3%) Macroscopically complete resection: 20/24 (83.3%) R0 resection: 18/24 (75%) Confirmed full-thickness resection: 21/24 (87.5%) Adverse events: 3/25 (12%) (for more details see **Table 5**)

Data from Refs.[16,17,20–24]

because of the rigid cap (outer diameter 21 mm) and the transparent sheath covering the whole length of the colonoscope. Further technical modifications (eg, smaller cap size, more flexibility) could facilitate usage of the FTRD use in the upper GI tract.

SUPPLEMENTARY DATA

Supplementary data related to this article can be found at http://dx.doi.org/10.1016/j. giec.2015.12.008.

REFERENCES

1. Eckardt AJ, Adler A, Gomes EM, et al. Endosonographic large-bore biopsy of gastric subepithelial tumors: a prospective multicenter study. Eur J Gastroenterol Hepatol 2012;24:1135–44.
2. ESMO/European Sarcoma Network Working Group. Gastrointestinal stromal tumours: ESMO Clinical Practice Guidelines for diagnosis, treatment and follow-up. Ann Oncol 2014;25(Suppl 3):iii21–6.
3. Von Mehren M, Randall RL, Benjamin RS, et al. Gastrointestinal stromal tumors, version 2.2014. J Natl Compr Canc Netw 2014;12:853–62.
4. Nishida T, Hirota S, Yanagisawa A, et al. Clinical practice guidelines for gastrointestinal stromal tumor (GIST) in Japan: English version. Int J Clin Oncol 2008;13: 416–30.
5. Rossi S, Gasparotto D, Toffolatti L, et al. Molecular and clinicopathologic characterization of gastrointestinal stromal tumors (GISTs) of small size. Am J Surg Pathol 2010;34:1480–91.
6. Schmidt A, Bauder M, Riecken B, et al. Endoscopic full-thickness resection of gastric subepithelial tumors: a single-center series. Endoscopy 2015;47:154–8.
7. Miettinen M, Lasota J. Gastrointestinal stromal tumors: pathology and prognosis at different sites. Semin Diagn Pathol 2006;23:70–83.
8. von Renteln D, Schmidt A, Riecken B, et al. Gastric full-thickness suturing during EMR and for treatment of gastric-wall defects (with video). Gastrointest Endosc 2008;67:738–44.
9. Walz B, von Renteln D, Schmidt A, et al. Endoscopic full-thickness resection of subepithelial tumors with the use of resorbable sutures (with video). Gastrointest Endosc 2011;73:1288–91.
10. Kaehler GF, Langner C, Suchan KL, et al. Endoscopic full-thickness resection of the stomach: an experimental approach. Surg Endosc 2006;20:519–21.

11. Kaehler GF, Collet PH, Grobholz R, et al. Endoscopic full-thickness gastric resection using a flexible stapler device. Surg Technol Int 2007;16:61–5.
12. Meining A. Endoscopic full-thickness resection: the logical step toward more extended endoscopic oncologic resections? Endoscopy 2015;47:101–2.
13. De Vogelaere K, Hoorens A, Haentjens P, et al. Laparoscopic versus open resection of gastrointestinal stromal tumors of the stomach. Surg Endosc 2013;27: 1546–54.
14. Kim KH, Kim MC, Jung GJ, et al. Long term survival results for gastric GIST: is laparoscopic surgery for large gastric GIST feasible? World J Surg Oncol 2012;10:230.
15. Von Renteln D, Kratt T, Rösch T, et al. Endoscopic full-thickness resection in the colon by using a clip-and-cut technique: an animal study. Gastrointest Endosc 2011;74:1108–14.
16. Schmidt A, Meier B, Cahyadi O, et al. Duodenal endoscopic full-thickness resection (with video). Gastrointest Endosc 2015;82:728–33.
17. Schmidt A, Bauerfeind P, Gubler C, et al. Endoscopic full-thickness resection in the colorectum with a novel over-the-scope device: first experience. Endoscopy 2015;47:719–25.
18. Von Renteln D, Rösch T, Kratt T, et al. Endoscopic full-thickness resection of submucosal gastric tumors. Dig Dis Sci 2012;57:1298–303.
19. Schmidt A, Riecken B, Damm M, et al. Endoscopic removal of over-the-scope clips using a novel cutting device: a retrospective case series. Endoscopy 2014;46:762–6.
20. Mönkemüller K, Peter S, Toshniwal J, et al. Multipurpose use of the "bear claw" (over-the-scope-clip system) to treat endoluminal gastrointestinal disorders. Dig Endosc 2014;26:350–7.
21. Sarker S, Gutierrez JP, Council L, et al. Over-the-scope clip-assisted method for resection of full-thickness submucosal lesions of the gastrointestinal tract. Endoscopy 2014;46:758–61.
22. Fähndrich M, Sandmann M. Endoscopic full-thickness resection for gastrointestinal lesions using the over-the-scope clip system: a case series. Endoscopy 2015;47:76–9.
23. Valli PV, Kaufmann M, Vrugt B, et al. Endoscopic resection of a diverticulum-arisen colonic adenoma using a full-thickness resection device. Gastroenterology 2014;147:969–71.
24. Klare P, Burlefinger R, Neu B, et al. Over-the-scope clip-assisted endoscopic full-thickness resection after incomplete resection of a rectal neuroendocrine tumor. Endoscopy 2015;47(Suppl 1):E47–8.
25. Schmidt A, Damm M, Caca K. Endoscopic full-thickness resection using a novel over-the-scope device. Gastroenterology 2014;147:740–2.

Endoscopic Submucosal Dissection (ESD) and Related Techniques as Precursors of "New Notes" Resection Methods for Gastric Neoplasms

CrossMark

Osamu Goto, MD, PhD[a], Hiroya Takeuchi, MD, PhD[b],
Yuko Kitagawa, MD, PhD[b], Naohisa Yahagi, MD, PhD[a],*

KEYWORDS

- Endoscopic submucosal dissection • Laparoscopic endoscopic cooperative surgery
- Nonexposed endoscopic wall-inversion surgery • Sentinel node navigation surgery

KEY POINTS

- Endoscopic submucosal dissection has been established as a curative method of early stage gastrointestinal cancers without lymph node metastasis.
- Endoscopic full-thickness resection would be more feasible with laparoscopic assistance than via a purely endoluminal approach.
- Nonexposed endoscopic and laparoscopic full-thickness resection with possible regional lymphadenectomy can be an ideal approach to the establishment of minimally invasive gastric resection with maximum preservation of the organ.

INTRODUCTION

Gastroscopes first appeared in clinical use in the mid 1950s. Since polypectomy of gastric polyps with an electrocautery snare was performed in the 1960s, a flexible endoscope has been used not only as a diagnostic tool but also for therapeutic purposes. After the development and establishment of endoscopic mucosal resection (EMR) in the 1980s, endoscopic submucosal dissection (ESD) was introduced around

Conflict of Interest: No conflict of interest exists.
[a] Division of Research and Development for Minimally Invasive Treatment, Cancer Center, Keio University School of Medicine, 35 Shinanomachi, Shinjuku-ku, Tokyo 160-8582, Japan;
[b] Department of Surgery, Keio University School of Medicine, Tokyo 160-8582, Japan
* Corresponding author.
E-mail address: yahagi.keio@gmail.com

2000. With the advent of ESD, possible node-negative gastrointestinal cancers can be cured simply via a peroral approach with the flexible endoscope, irrespective of tumor size or submucosal scarring formation under the lesion.

Less-invasive surgical approaches with the flexible endoscope have been continuously explored by enthusiastic endoscopists who are now increasingly interested in moving beyond the submucosal layer. In this article, the current situation of advanced endoscopic techniques beyond ESD is explained after a brief history of ESD, followed by future perspectives.

ENDOSCOPIC SUBMUCOSAL DISSECTION: DAWN OF RADICAL INTRALUMINAL ENDOSCOPIC RESECTION

The previously developed EMR technique had limitations in terms of tumor size and the existence of ulcerative change. Because a snare is used for the resection, the tumor size should always be smaller than that of the snare for en bloc resection.[1–3] Furthermore, when the lesion is accompanied by ulcer formation, the submucosal fibrosis sometimes disturbs en bloc resection because of slipping of the snare. In order to overcome these disadvantages, ESD was developed, whereby a lesion is resected by circumferential mucosal incision and subsequent submucosal dissection under direct visualization.[4–7] By this technique, endoscopists have become capable to cure early cancers very reliably without the help of surgeons if the lesion has an extremely low possibility of lymph node metastasis.[8,9] Several endoscopic devices specifically designed for ESD (eg, IT-Knife [Olympus, Co., Ltd., Tokyo, Japan], Hook Knife [Olympus], Dual knife [Olympus] and so forth) have been invented, and these devices have made this technique more feasible. Although technical difficulty is one of the disadvantages of ESD, this fascinating technique always attracts many therapeutic endoscopists. Therefore, live demonstrations by invited ESD experts or hands-on training in ex vivo/in vivo animal models[10–14] are frequently held in selected institutions around the world. Nowadays, establishment of systematic training methods using isolated animal organs or other modalities are expected to obtain a safe and reliable ESD technique.

ENDOSCOPIC MUSCULAR/FULL-THICKNESS RESECTION: OVER THE SUBMUCOSAL LAYER

Since endoscopists realized that the entire gastrointestinal wall could be cut freely with ESD knives from the inside, they started to explore how far endoscopic resection can be taken. To begin with a challenge to the deeper layers, subepithelial tumors (SETs) became a target. Lee and colleagues[15] tried to resect SETs arising from the muscular layer by dissecting the muscular layer just beneath the tumor, resulting in 75% of complete resection rate without perforation. Hoteya and colleagues[16] selected only SETs arising from the muscularis mucosae and demonstrated favorable outcomes in terms of both complete resection rates and complication rates. Going further, endoscopic full-thickness resection (EFTR), local transmural resection only with a flexible endoscope, was proposed (recognized as one of the natural orifice transluminal endoscopic surgery [NOTES]–related techniques, also known as pure EFTR). After submucosal injection and circumferential mucosal incision around the lesion, seromuscular incision is performed with intentional perforation on the exposed muscular layer. A lesion resected in a full-thickness fashion is retrieved transorally, followed by endoscopic defect closure with hemoclips or other devices. Zhou and colleagues[17] demonstrated the feasibility of this challenging technique; other brave endoscopists, mainly in China, reported acceptable outcomes.[18–21]

However, this technique is associated with several serious problems. First, a secure closure method only by endoluminal endoscopy has not been established so far. The grasping force of commercially available endoclips is too weak to reliably maintain secure closure of the full-thickness wall defect. Over-the-scope clips[22–24] or endoscopic suturing systems[25–27] may solve the problem, but their clinical utility in EFTR is not satisfactorily demonstrated yet. Second, endoscopic manipulation becomes more difficult after the intentional perforation because of the loss of insufflation and partial collapse of the stomach. Third, a blind approach in the phase of intentional perforation and successive seromuscular incision is more difficult and dangerous. For example, in case of bleeding from the abdominal cavity, endoscopic hemostasis from inside the lumen might be impossible. This method is, therefore, questionable in terms of both the feasibility and the safety; it does not seem to have gained widespread acceptance yet. However, some aggressive endoscopists are still trying to overcome these shortcomings and establishing safe and secure EFTR as a pure NOTES technique. For example, Mori and colleagues[28] invented a novel endoscopic device sustaining the collapsing stomach after intentional perforation from the inside as well as a new endoscopic suturing instrument attached to the tip of endoscope for secure closure of the full-thickness defect.[29] Further developments and wider application to humans are expected.

LAPAROSCOPIC ENDOSCOPIC COOPERATIVE SURGERY: A SAFE APPROACH FOR LOCAL RESECTION

To overcome the drawbacks in EFTR, laparoscopic endoscopic cooperative surgery (LECS) or laparoscopy-assisted EFTR (hybrid NOTES) was developed.[30,31] In this procedure, EFTR is performed under laparoscopic assistance and finally the wall defect is closed laparoscopically using linear staplers or a hand-suturing technique. This technique can address all the potential disadvantages previously described for pure EFTR. Using laparoscopic closure, the wall defect can be tightly and securely fastened. Even after intentional perforation of the seromuscular layer, laparoscopic assistance can help to maintain the endoscopic view by exerting traction and suspending the organ from the outside. Surrounding organs or vessels can also be monitored by laparoscopy during EFTR in order not to damage them. Moreover, laparoscopic seromuscular incision using an electrocautery knife or ultrasonically activated coagulating shears after endoscopic seromuscular perforation may save operation time. Hiki and colleagues[30] promoted LECS starting in 2008, and it became accepted as one of the surgical methods covered by the health insurance system in Japan.

However, this promising technique also has an inevitable disadvantage. During the procedure, intentional perforation is required, which may lead to bacterial contamination into the peritoneal cavity and iatrogenic tumor dissemination in case of cancer or an ulcerated SET (eg, ulcerated gastrointestinal stromal tumor). Indeed, free cancer cells are detected in gastric lavage fluid from patients with gastric cancer even at an early stage,[32] although there is room for discussion about the ability of these floating cancer cells to form dissemination foci on the peritoneum. To avoid this theoretic risk, Nunobe and colleagues[33] developed an improved technique of LECS, called inverted LECS. In this technique, the gastric hole is hung up with several strings at the phase of intentional perforation in order not to spill the contents of the stomach. Inverted LECS is, however, still insufficient to avoid iatrogenic tumor seeding or possible port site metastasis because the surface of the neoplasm exposed toward the abdominal cavity might touch the laparoscopic instruments, which could implant tumor cells to other abdominal organs or the abdominal wall during the manipulation.

Therefore, local resection in which transluminal communication is unavoidable should be refrained from, especially for cancers or SETs with ulcer formation. Thus, LECS should be limited only to SETs without ulcer findings.

NONEXPOSED FULL-THICKNESS RESECTION: CHALLENGE TO MINIMALLY INVASIVE PARTIAL GASTRECTOMY FOR CANCERS

How can we do minimally sized local resection without transluminal access? Inoue and colleagues[34] invented a technique of laparoscopic local gastrectomy by pulling a full uninjured mucosal layer including the target lesion toward the outside of the stomach after laparoscopic circumferential seromuscular incision, followed by resection at the bottom of the pulled area with linear staplers, and named this technique the combination of laparoscopic and endoscopic approaches to neoplasia with a nonexposure technique (CLEAN-NET). Using the intact mucosal layer as a safe and clean net to avoid spillage of the gastric contents and contact of laparoscopic instruments with the cancer surface, this method can be applied to SETs regardless of ulcer formation and even cancerous lesions. CLEAN-NET is a relatively simple and time-saving technique. For successful resection in this technique, a critical phase would be setting the resection area by placing markings on the serosal side because the operator cannot resect the lesion under the direct visualization of the target lesion from the inside of the stomach. Especially in cancers, serosal markings must be precisely placed just on the opposite side of the mucosal markings, which are precisely placed endoscopically by close observation of the demarcation line of the tumor.

To resect a target lesion accurately and completely while preserving as much normal tissue as possible, an intraluminal approach would be desirable at the final step of resection because the operator can confirm the demarcation line of the target lesion. Goto and colleagues[35] invented a laparoscopy-assisted, nonexposure technique of EFTR in order to overcome all of these drawbacks mentioned earlier and named it nonexposed endoscopic wall-inversion surgery (NEWS)[36,37] (**Fig. 1**). Under general anesthesia in a spine position, a flexible endoscope is inserted perorally and a laparoscopy port is placed as well as some trocars for laparoscopic devices. Mucosal markings are accurately made endoscopically by close endoscopic observation, followed by laparoscopic serosal markings just on the opposite side of mucosal markings. After circumferential submucosal injection of a hyaluronic acid solution with a small amount of indigo carmine endoscopically, circumferential seromuscular incision is performed laparoscopically until the colored submucosal layer is well exposed. After creating sufficient width of a groove around the lesion, seromuscular hand suturing is performed on the peritoneal side isolating the tumorous area, which is inverted toward the inside of the stomach. Finally, endoscopic circumferential mucosal and submucosal incision is performed with the ESD technique around the inverted lesion. A distinctive feature of this technique is inverting the lesion toward the inside of the stomach by means of laparoscopic seromuscular suturing. In this step, it would be better to insert a spacer (eg, a surgical sponge) between the serosal side of the inverted lesion and the suturing plane to facilitate the subsequent endoscopic mucosal incision. In the endoscopic resection, the inserted spacer works as a vertical end point at the phase of the submucosal incision, a counter-tractor by lifting the lesion, and a protector of the suture line. After introducing this spacer technique to NEWS, we achieved more successful results compared with previous procedures without spacer.

The indication of NEWS is SETs regardless of ulceration and possible node-negative early gastric cancers (EGCs), which would be difficult to resect by ESD. Because a resected lesion must be retrieved transorally, a size limitation exists in

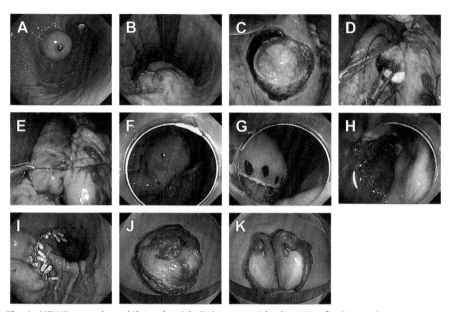

Fig. 1. NEWS procedure. (*A*) A subepithelial tumor with ulcerative findings is located on the anterior wall of middle third of the gastric body. Mucosal markings are placed. (*B*) A hyaluronic acid solution is injected circumferentially into the submucosal layer. (*C*) Using a laparoscopic electrocautery knife, circumferential seromuscular incision and subsequent deeper cut are performed. (*D*) Seromuscular layers are linearly sutured by a laparoscopic hand-suturing technique with the lesion inverted toward the inside of the stomach. Halfway through suturing, a surgical sponge as a spacer is inserted between the suturing plane and the serosal surface of the inverted lesion. (*E*) Seromuscular suturing is finished. (*F*) The lesion is inverted with a spacer. (*G*) Circumferential mucosal incision is started with an endoscopic electrocautery knife along the mucosal markings. (*H*) By subsequent submucosal incision, the stuffed spacer is exposed. (*I*) After the resection, the mucosal edges of the sutured wall defect are closed with endoclips. (*J*) A serosal plane of the resected lesion in a full-thickness fashion. (*K*) The inside of the lesion.

SETs. Practically, the authors apply NEWS to SETs 3 cm or less in size on preoperative diagnosis. However, there is no limitation of size in EGCs because they are not solid. Furthermore, the indication of NEWS can be expanded to possible node-positive EGCs by combining NEWS with sentinel node navigation surgery (SNNS) as described later.

Development of nonexposure techniques aimed at minimally invasive surgery for cancers is still ongoing. Kim and colleagues[38] suggest the efficacy of the full-thickness inversion resection without laparoscopic seromuscular incision in terms of timesaving and avoidance of the risk of perforation from the laparoscopic side. Takizawa and colleagues[39] executed an in vivo animal study and demonstrated feasibility of a wall-inversion method without laparoscopic assistance by creating 2 submucosal tunnels outside the circumferential mucosal incision and getting both together with a large detachable snare. Furthermore, Schmidt and colleagues[40] produced a peroral flexible suturing device and attempted nonexposed EFTR for SETs by suturing the wall at the bottom of the lesion with this novel device creating a pseudopolyp containing the lesion and then cutting the lesion with an endoscopic snare. Even though these techniques are in the initial stages of development, they may prove promising in the future.

LOCAL LYMPHADENECTOMY: EXPANDED INDICATION OF LOCAL ENDOSCOPIC RESECTION FOR POSSIBLE NODE-POSITIVE CANCERS

In applying any minimally invasive partial gastric resection to possible node-positive EGCs, an optimal lymphadenectomy should always be taken into consideration. If EFTR was combined with systematic lymphadenectomy as used in standard gastrectomy (distal gastrectomy or total gastrectomy), postoperative necrosis of the remnant stomach might occur because of excessive resection of feeding arteries, which are removed with surrounding lymph nodes. Accordingly, a few arteries should be preserved for successful EFTR. Several reports describing local resection for a primary lesion combined with local lymphadenectomy have been published so far. Seto and colleagues[41] already demonstrated the feasibility and efficacy of local gastric resection with local lymphadenectomy in 1999. After establishment of ESD, a case of laparoscopy-assisted EFTR with regional lymph node dissection was reported by Abe and colleagues,[42] followed by a Korean study group.[43] In these trials, however, evidence-based lymphadenectomy was not performed. If there is a systematic strategy on the selection of dissected lymph node areas, more secure minimally invasive surgery will be realized without concern about postoperative necrosis or recurrence of cancer in the remaining lymph nodes. In this regard, SNNS may offer an ideal solution.[44] Sentinel node theory, which is already clinically introduced in skin cancers and breast cancers, is a concept that postulates that if no metastasis exists in sentinel nodes, the first-order lymph nodes draining the area of a primary lesion, no further metastasis is expected in other lymph nodes. Kitagawa and colleagues[45] suggested the possible utility of SNNS in EGC with an extremely favorable accuracy of 99% in the prediction of lymph node metastasis using sentinel node biopsy. By combining this concept with nonexposure EFTR techniques, an ideal minimally invasive, function-preserving partial gastric resection with evidence-based minimal lymphadenectomy would be achievable.[46] Therefore, the authors started a clinical trial regarding feasibility and efficacy of NEWS combined with SNNS for EGCs in 2014.[47] Currently, the indication of NEWS plus sentinel node basin dissection is determined as cases satisfied with all of the following conditions[45]: cT1N0M0 EGC 4 cm in size, no prior treatment, single lesion; the number of sentinel node basins (lymphatic areas including sentinel nodes separated by the distribution of 5 feeding arteries) is one or 2 contiguous ones; intraoperative pathologic diagnosis reveals that sentinel nodes have no metastasis. Accumulation of cases and analysis of long-term outcomes are expected in the near future.

FUTURE PERSPECTIVES

Establishment of the ESD technique has had a great influence on therapeutic endoscopists including stimulating interest toward the development of EFTR. Currently, cooperation between flexible endoscopy and rigid laparoscopy may be the optimal option to guarantee safe and secure EFTR. When the indication of EFTR is expanded to epithelial cancers, a nonexposed EFTR technique and minimal lymphadenectomy may be the optimal approach (**Fig. 2**). However, many issues await definitive resolution, for example, how the resection area should be determined for R0 resection in possible node-positive cancers,[48] whether minimally sized partial gastric resection can maintain patients' quality of life, whether minimal lymphadenectomy such as SNNS can achieve radical cure in the long-term, and so forth.

The most important consideration is that the benefit always be for patients. The authors hope that therapeutic endoscopists become aggressive not only in advancing endoluminal surgery but also in investigating the clinical efficacy and patients' benefit.

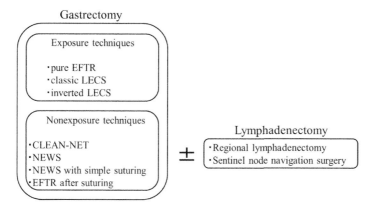

Fig. 2. Current status of full-thickness resection using flexible endoscopy for gastric neoplasms. Exposure techniques can be applied mainly to SETs without ulceration. For SETs with ulceration and cancers, nonexposure techniques are recommended. Especially for cancer with possible lymph node metastasis, nonexposure techniques should be accompanied with localized lymphadenectomy.

REFERENCES

1. Cao Y, Liao C, Tan A, et al. Meta-analysis of endoscopic submucosal dissection versus endoscopic mucosal resection for tumors of the gastrointestinal tract. Endoscopy 2009;41:751–7.
2. Park YM, Cho E, Kang HY, et al. The effectiveness and safety of endoscopic submucosal dissection compared with endoscopic mucosal resection for early gastric cancer: a systematic review and meta-analysis. Surg Endosc 2011;25: 2666–77.
3. Lian J, Chen S, Zhang Y, et al. A meta-analysis of endoscopic submucosal dissection and EMR for early gastric cancer. Gastrointest Endosc 2012;76: 763–70.
4. Ono H, Kondo H, Gotoda T, et al. Endoscopic mucosal resection for treatment of early gastric cancer. Gut 2001;48:225–9.
5. Yamamoto H, Kawata H, Sunada K, et al. Successful en-bloc resection of large superficial tumors in the stomach and colon using sodium hyaluronate and small-caliber-tip transparent hood. Endoscopy 2003;35:690–4.
6. Oyama T, Tomori A, Hotta K, et al. Endoscopic submucosal dissection of early esophageal cancer. Clin Gastroenterol Hepatol 2005;3:S67–70.
7. Yahagi N, Uraoka T, Ida Y, et al. Endoscopic submucosal dissection using the Flex and the Dual knives. Tech Gastrointest Endosc 2011;13:74–8.
8. Gotoda T, Yanagisawa A, Sasako M, et al. Incidence of lymph node metastasis from early gastric cancer: estimation with a large number of cases at two large centers. Gastric Cancer 2000;3:219–25.
9. Hirasawa T, Gotoda T, Miyata S, et al. Incidence of lymph node metastasis and the feasibility of endoscopic resection for undifferentiated-type early gastric cancer. Gastric Cancer 2010;13:267–70.
10. Gotoda T, Ho KY, Soetikno R, et al. Gastric ESD: current status and future directions of devices and training. Gastrointest Endosc Clin N Am 2014;24:213–33.
11. González N, Parra-Blanco A, Villa-Gómez M, et al. Gastric endoscopic submucosal dissection: from animal model to patient. World J Gastroenterol 2013;19:8326–34.

12. Parra-Blanco A, González N, González R, et al. Animal models for endoscopic training: do we really need them? Endoscopy 2013;45:478–84.
13. Bok GH, Cho JY. ESD hands-on course using ex vivo and in vivo models in South Korea. Clin Endosc 2012;45:358–61.
14. Tanaka S, Morita Y, Fujita T, et al. Ex vivo pig training model for esophageal endoscopic submucosal dissection (ESD) for endoscopists with experience in gastric ESD. Surg Endosc 2012;26:1579–86.
15. Lee IL, Lin PY, Tung SY, et al. Endoscopic submucosal dissection for the treatment of intraluminal gastric subepithelial tumors originating from the muscularis propria layer. Endoscopy 2006;38:1024–8.
16. Hoteya S, Iizuka T, Kikuchi D, et al. Endoscopic submucosal dissection for gastric submucosal tumor, endoscopic sub-tumoral dissection. Dig Endosc 2009;21: 266–9.
17. Zhou PH, Yao LQ, Qin XY, et al. Endoscopic full-thickness resection without laparoscopic assistance for gastric submucosal tumors originated from the muscularis propria. Surg Endosc 2011;25:2926–31.
18. Feng Y, Yu L, Yang S, et al. Endolumenal endoscopic full-thickness resection of muscularis propria-originating gastric submucosal tumors. J Laparoendosc Adv Surg Tech A 2014;24:171–6.
19. Huang LY, Cui J, Lin SJ, et al. Endoscopic full-thickness resection for gastric submucosal tumors arising from the muscularis propria layer. World J Gastroenterol 2014;20:13981–6.
20. Shi Q, Chen T, Zhong YS, et al. Complete closure of large gastric defects after endoscopic full-thickness resection, using endoloop and metallic clip interrupted suture. Endoscopy 2013;45:329–34.
21. Ye LP, Yu Z, Mao XL, et al. Endoscopic full-thickness resection with defect closure using clips and an endoloop for gastric subepithelial tumors arising from the muscularis propria. Surg Endosc 2014;28:1978–83.
22. von Renteln D, Vassiliou MC, Rothstein RI. Randomized controlled trial comparing endoscopic clips and over-the-scope clips for closure of natural orifice transluminal endoscopic surgery gastrotomies. Endoscopy 2009;41: 1056–61.
23. Schlag C, Wilhelm D, von Delius S, et al. EndoResect study: endoscopic full-thickness resection of gastric subepithelial tumors. Endoscopy 2013;45: 4–11.
24. Guo J, Liu Z, Sun S, et al. Endoscopic full-thickness resection with defect closure using an over-the-scope clip for gastric subepithelial tumors originating from the muscularis propria. Surg Endosc 2015;29(11):3356–62.
25. Ikeda K, Fritscher-Ravens A, Mosse CA, et al. Endoscopic full-thickness resection with sutured closure in a porcine model. Gastrointest Endosc 2005;62: 122–9.
26. von Renteln D, Schmidt A, Riecken B, et al. Gastric full-thickness suturing during EMR and for treatment of gastric-wall defects (with video). Gastrointest Endosc 2008;67:738–44.
27. Chiu PW, Phee SJ, Wang Z, et al. Feasibility of full-thickness gastric resection using master and slave transluminal endoscopic robot and closure by Overstitch: a preclinical study. Surg Endosc 2014;28:319–24.
28. Mori H, Rafiq K, Kobara H, et al. Innovative noninsufflation EFTR: sufficient endoscopic operative field by mechanical counter traction device. Surg Endosc 2013; 27:3028–34.

29. Mori H, Kobara H, Fujihara S, et al. Feasibility of pure EFTR using an innovative new endoscopic suturing device: the Double-arm-bar Suturing System (with video). Surg Endosc 2014;28:683–90.
30. Hiki N, Yamamoto Y, Fukunaga T, et al. Laparoscopic and endoscopic cooperative surgery for gastrointestinal stromal tumor dissection. Surg Endosc 2008;22: 1729–35.
31. Abe N, Takeuchi H, Yanagida O, et al. Endoscopic full-thickness resection with laparoscopic assistance as hybrid NOTES for gastric submucosal tumor. Surg Endosc 2009;23:1908–13.
32. Han TS, Kong SH, Lee HJ, et al. Dissemination of free cancer cells from the gastric lumen and from perigastric lymphovascular pedicles during radical gastric cancer surgery. Ann Surg Oncol 2011;18:2818–25.
33. Nunobe S, Hiki N, Gotoda T, et al. Successful application of laparoscopic and endoscopic cooperative surgery (LECS) for a lateral-spreading mucosal gastric cancer. Gastric Cancer 2012;15:338–42.
34. Inoue H, Ikeda H, Hosoya T, et al. Endoscopic mucosal resection, endoscopic submucosal dissection, and beyond: full-layer resection for gastric cancer with nonexposure technique (CLEAN-NET). Surg Oncol Clin N Am 2012;21:129–40.
35. Goto O, Mitsui T, Fujishiro M, et al. New method of endoscopic full-thickness resection: a pilot study of non-exposed endoscopic wall-inversion surgery in an ex vivo porcine model. Gastric Cancer 2011;14:183–7.
36. Mitsui T, Goto O, Shimizu N, et al. Novel technique for full-thickness resection of gastric malignancy: feasibility of nonexposed endoscopic wall-inversion surgery (NEWS) in porcine models. Surg Laparosc Endosc Percutan Tech 2013;23: e217–21.
37. Mitsui T, Niimi K, Yamashita H, et al. Non-exposed endoscopic wall-inversion surgery as a novel partial gastrectomy technique. Gastric Cancer 2014;17: 594–9.
38. Kim CG, Yoon HM, Lee JY, et al. Nonexposure endolaparoscopic full-thickness resection with simple suturing technique. Endoscopy 2015;47(12):1171–4.
39. Takizawa K, Knipschield MA, Gostout CJ. Submucosal endoscopy as an aid to full-thickness resection: pilot study in the porcine stomach. Gastrointest Endosc 2015;81:450–4.
40. Schmidt A, Bauder M, Riecken B, et al. Endoscopic full-thickness resection of gastric subepithelial tumors: a single-center series. Endoscopy 2015;47:154–8.
41. Seto Y, Nagawa H, Muto Y, et al. Preliminary report on local resection with lymphadenectomy for early gastric cancer. Br J Surg 1999;86:526–8.
42. Abe N, Mori T, Takeuchi H, et al. Successful treatment of early stage gastric cancer by laparoscopy-assisted endoscopic full-thickness resection with lymphadenectomy. Gastrointest Endosc 2008;68:1220–4.
43. Cho WY, Kim YJ, Cho JY, et al. Hybrid natural orifice transluminal endoscopic surgery: endoscopic full-thickness resection of early gastric cancer and laparoscopic regional lymph node dissection - 14 human cases. Endoscopy 2011;43: 134–9.
44. Takeuchi H, Kitagawa Y. New sentinel node mapping technologies for early gastric cancer. Ann Surg Oncol 2013;20:522–32.
45. Kitagawa Y, Takeuchi H, Takagi Y, et al. Sentinel node mapping for gastric cancer: a prospective multicenter trial in Japan. J Clin Oncol 2013;31:3704–10.
46. Goto O, Takeuchi H, Kawakubo H, et al. Feasibility of non-exposed endoscopic wall-inversion surgery with sentinel node basin dissection as a new surgical

method for early gastric cancer: a porcine survival study. Gastric Cancer 2015; 18:440–5.

47. Goto O, Takeuchi H, Kawakubo H, et al. First case of non-exposed endoscopic wall-inversion surgery with sentinel node basin dissection for early gastric cancer. Gastric Cancer 2015;18:434–9.

48. Goto O, Fujimoto A, Shimoda M, et al. Estimation of subepithelial lateral extent in submucosal early gastric cancer: retrospective histological analysis. Gastric Cancer 2015;18:810–6.

Novel NOTES Techniques and Experimental Devices for Endoscopic Full-thickness Resection (EFTR)

Hirohito Mori, MD, PhD[a,b,*], Hideki Kobara, MD, PhD[a], Tsutomu Masaki, MD, PhD[a]

KEYWORDS

- Natural orifice transluminal endoscopic surgery • Ultraminimally invasive
- Exposed EFTR • Nonexposed EFTR • Feasible surgical procedure

KEY POINTS

- Endoscopic full-thickness resection (EFTR) is an ultraminimally invasive endoscopic surgery for radical tumor resection.
- There are 2 types of EFTR: exposed EFTR and nonexposed EFTR.
- Nonexposed EFTR is ideal.

INTRODUCTION

EFTR is an ultraminimally invasive procedure in which a flexible endoscope alone is used, and endoscopic submucosal dissection (ESD), is used for full-thickness local excision of a gastrointestinal epithelial malignancy, such as gastric or colon cancer, or a gastrointestinal submucosal tumor, such as a gastrointestinal stromal tumor (GIST).[1–5]

From improvements in diagnostic performance to therapeutics, flexible endoscopes have progressively been developed; these include development of the various peripheral devices and accessories to the endoscope, including those used to perform polypectomies and endoscopic mucosal resection. With the evolution of incision devices from snares to electrosurgical knives, flexible endoscopes have been used for ESD as an ultraminimally invasive treatment of gastrointestinal

Conflict of Interest: None.
[a] Department of Gastroenterology and Neurology, Kagawa University, Kita, Kagawa, Japan;
[b] Department of Gastroenterological Surgery, Ehime Rosai Hospital, Niihama, Ehime, Japan
* Corresponding author. Department of Gastroenterology and Neurology, Kagawa University, 1750-1 Ikenobe, Miki, Kita, Kagawa 761-0793, Japan.
E-mail address: hiro4884@med.kagawa-u.ac.jp

tract malignancies and currently as the standard treatment of early-stage gastrointestinal cancer.[6–8]

Although an excellent therapeutic technique, ESD is still limited to intraluminal treatments, and robust full-thickness closure devices and countertraction devices need to be developed to perform full-thickness excision.

Although full-thickness closure devices have been developed, only the OverStitch Endoscopic Suturing System (Apollo Endosurgery, Austin, Texas)[9] and the Over-The-Scope Clip (Ovesco, Tübingen, Germany) have been commercialized,[10] and the development of full-thickness suturing devices is difficult. The authors have been working toward commercialization of inexpensive suturing devices that have a simple configuration, have highly reliable suturing strength, are simple to operate, and can be used in clinical practice.[5]

Ensuring an appropriate endoscopic surgical field for full-thickness excision and suturing is also a major challenge, but there have been few reports on devices for expanding the field of view.[11] Suturing is impossible if an adequate field of view cannot be achieved. Other than insufflation, there are no means of increasing the field of view of flexible endoscopes in diagnosis and treatment. Thus, if the gastrointestinal tract walls are punctured, the insufflated air flows out from the lumen into the abdominal cavity, and collapse of the gastrointestinal tract makes it difficult to secure the field of view. There are 2 different methods for securing the operative field of view. One is to extend/expand an enclosed cavity by insufflation of CO_2 or a similar gas to increase the field of view for laparoscopy, and another is to mechanically expand the tissue with instruments, such as a surgical retractor, without insufflation. Because the insufflation method is hampered by loss of CO_2 during full-thickness procedures, developing mechanical devices that maintain an adequate field of view is important.

In clinical practice, a pathway of development of NOTES for many of these procedures has been to start with hybrid NOTES procedures, which include collaboration of endoscopists and surgeons.[12]

Laparoscopy and endoscopy cooperative surgery (LECS) was proposed in 2006[13]; this superior procedure, which incorporates both safety of laparoscopy and the diagnostic accuracy of endoscopy, has been recognized as safe by both surgeons and endoscopists and has expanded the potential for new minimally invasive surgeries, with various new surgical procedures developed and reported. LECS and hybrid NOTES are similar.

Among NOTES-related procedures, specifically EFTR, it is beneficial to have an endoscopist who is skilled in advanced flexible endoscope treatments, such as ESD. With further development of devices and surgical procedures in the future, an increasing number of gastrointestinal endoscopists may operate in this field. This article describes the authors' efforts as one of the pioneering EFTR groups to study and address challenges of EFTR, including 2 endoscope techniques to facilitate pure EFTR, prevention of peritoneal contamination, minimization of the risk of tense capnoperitoneum, achieving secure closure with a suturing device that can be operated via a single-channel regular gastroscope, and countertraction devices to maintain visibility during loss of luminal insufflation.

EXPOSED ENDOSCOPIC FULL-THICKNESS RESECTION AND NONEXPOSED ENDOSCOPIC FULL-THICKNESS RESECTION

EFTR includes what the authors term, *exposed EFTR* (**Fig. 1**), in which an endoscope inserted from the mouth or anus is used to intentionally perforate the muscle layer and then perform a full-thickness excision, followed by full-thickness suturing, and also

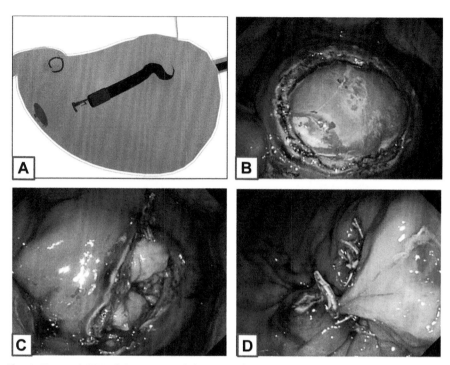

Fig. 1. Exposed EFTR. (*A*) Conceptual diagram of exposed EFTR, in which an endoscope is inserted from the mouth to intentionally perforate the muscle layer and then a full-thickness excision is performed and followed by full-thickness suturing. (*B*) An incision reaching as far as the muscle layer is made around the entire circumference using ESD. (*C*) The DBSS, which is a full-thickness suturing device prototype, is used to suture the full-thickness excision wound. (*D*) Full-thickness suture is performed using a 3-mm bite and a 3-mm pitch.

includes what is termed, *non-exposed EFTR* (**Fig. 2**), in which the lesion is inverted, and the full-thickness excision is performed only after full-thickness suturing has been performed. In clinical practice, the device development has been in pace with pure EFTR, in which a flexible endoscope alone is used, and the field of view and full-thickness suturing are secured laparoscopically as hybrid-exposed EFTR (so-called LECS).

Nonexposed EFTR involves nonexposed endoscopic wall-inversion surgery (NEWS), a procedure in which hand-sewn sutures are made laparoscopically, followed by full-thickness excision under endoscopy and a combination of laparoscopic and endoscopic approaches for neoplasia using a nonexposure technique, where the mucosa forms a barrier to exposing the peritoneum to luminal contents (see elsewhere in this issue).[14]

Although still in an ex vivo experimental setting, nonexposure EFTR has been achieved as a proof of principle using 2 flexible endoscopes—one inserted through the mouth into the lumen of the stomach and another inserted via an 10-mm umbilical laparoscopic port created by open technique and allowing access to the gastric wall from the peritoneal side (see **Fig. 2**A).[15] Using the gastroscope inserted through the mouth, ESD technique is used to perform a circumferential mucosal and submucosal incision around the tumor, leaving the muscular layer intact. The flexible endoscope

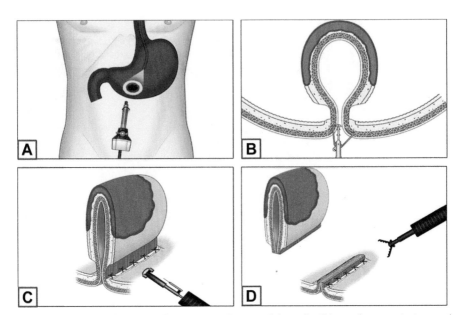

Fig. 2. Conceptual diagram of nonexposed EFTR. (*A*) A flexible endoscope is inserted through a 10-mm umbilical laparoscopic port, which is created by open technique. This endoscope allows access to the peritoneal side of the gastric wall. Transillumination is seen from the orally inserted gastroscope. Light filters through the circumferential submucosal incision created by the intraluminal gastroscope and through the intact muscular layer. This ring of transillumination clearly marks the desired EFTR borders on the peritoneal side. (*B*) The borders of the planned excision region (demarcated by the transillumination ring) are grasped with the Twin Grasper (Ovesco Endoscopy) and the gastric wall is inverted. (*C*) The inverted full-thickness plication of the stomach is sutured from the luminal side using an endoscope fitted with the DBSS, a full-thickness suturing device. (*D*) After suturing, full-thickness excision is performed with an endoscope from the inside of the stomach without any risk of exposure of luminal contents.

inserted via the 10-mm umbilical laparoscopic port allows visualization of transmitted light from the orally inserted endoscope as it filters through the circumferential submucosal incision and ring of intact muscularis propria around the lesion. This ring of transmitted light defines the proper resection border on the peritoneal side. Thus, the endoscope on the peritoneal side can grasp the muscularis along this ring using the Twin Grasper (Ovesco Endoscopy) and thus invert the gastric wall (**Fig. 3**A, B). This inverted full-thickness plication of the stomach is sutured with an endoscope equipped with the double-armed bar suturing system (DBSS), a full-thickness suturing device (see **Fig. 3**C). After suturing, the resection is completed from the luminal side by full-thickness excision seromuscular excision with a DualKnife (KD-650L; Olympus, Tokyo, Japan) (see **Fig. 3**D).

RATIONALE AND INDICATIONS OF ENDOSCOPIC FULL-THICKNESS RESECTION

There is no need for lymph node dissection in GIST cases, and EFTR is regarded as safe for use in such cases clinically. Pure EFTR, which is completed entirely using flexible endoscopes, allows for removal of the excised lesions, which are usually approximately 3 cm in size, through the mouth. During laparoscopic partial gastrectomy,

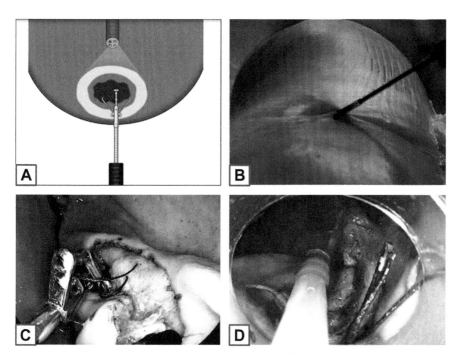

Fig. 3. Ex vivo study on nonexposed EFTR. (*A*) Conceptual illustration of gastric inversion using Twin Grasper. (*B*) Gastric inversion using Twin Grasper. (*C*) Full-thickness suturing from the luminal side of the stomach using the DBSS. (*D*) Full-thickness excision of the lesion is completed from the luminal side using a flexible endoscope.

ports are placed in the abdominal wall, and a full-thickness excision of a significant portion of the stomach wall is performed because usually laparoscopic staplers are used. Therefore, a laparoscopic approach is invasive in 2 ways: (1) violation of the abdominal wall and peritoneal paragastric structures to access the stomach and (2) when wedge resection/partial gastrectomy is used, removal of a larger portion of the stomach wall than is the case with simple circumferential excision of a GIST. EFTR is minimally invasive because full-thickness excision of the lesion is performed without violating the abdomen and without removing any excess gastric tissue. Thus, EFTR seems a desirable minimally invasive approach for gastric GISTs that do not require lymph node dissection.[16]

Nonexposed EFTR is also indicated for epithelial tumors in certain clinical scenarios, including early gastric cancers, for which ESD is impossible because of extensive submucosal fibrosis, or early gastrointestinal cancers in locations where ESD has a high risk of perforation and thus possible peritoneal dissemination of cancer cells (locations such as the gastric fornix or duodenum with reported perforation rates as high as 20%–25% with ESD).[17–19] Nonexposed EFTR is ideal when the risk of peritoneal infection or peritoneal dissemination of the tumor is considered increased.

PREOPERATIVE LUMINAL LAVAGE

Particularly with exposed EFTR, because the endoscope is inserted into the stomach through the oral cavity, the endoscope is exposed to the oral flora, which it can then translocate into the peritoneal cavity. There are no established guidelines, however, regarding systematic methods of disinfection or cleaning. Because exposed EFTR is a new procedure that goes beyond what constitutes familiar boundaries for endoscopists and surgeons, it is important to consider the utility of disinfection or cleaning methods.

A report on porcine animal experimentation with NOTES stated that irrigation with 500 mL of saline and 200 mL of 5% povidone iodine (Betadine) obtained by diluting Betadine with purified water reduced the bacterial content from culturing gastric juice before gastric cleaning, from 15 to 17 $\times 10^3$ colony-forming units/mL to 0 to 3 colony-forming units/mL, and made it possible to suppress intra-abdominal adhesion and abscesses formation after NOTES.[20] Gastric cleaning with povidone iodine solution in the transgastric route in humans is valid, but incidence of systemic bacteremia has not been studied. In the transgastric route, gastric cleaning with either povidone iodine solution or 500 mL of saline has been reported to eliminate clearly evident adhesions or formation of abscesses; it is not known whether either has a reliable bacteria-reducing effect.[21,22]

The authors recently completed a study comparing the effect of hybrid EFTR for gastric GISTs on white blood cell count and C-reactive protein in the earlier patients in a series who did not receive systematic lavage of the stomach versus the later patients who did receive systematic lavage of the stomach with saline. In the group who received systematic lavage, bacterial counts in the gastric juice before the systematic lavage were compared with counts in gastric juice and in peritoneal lavage fluid at completion of the procedure. In the patients who did not have preoperative systematic cleaning, a proton-pump inhibitor was administered once a day from the day prior using an endoscope that was disinfected using 2.4% glutaraldehyde (Cidex; Johnson & Johnson, Irvine, California); the endoscopist, without prior scrubbing, performed the procedure from the patient's cranial side away from the surgeon's sterile field. Gastric irrigation was performed only as dictated by the procedure. At the completion of the EFTR, intraperitoneal lavage was performed with 1000 mL by the laparoscopic surgeon prior to procedure termination.

The group with systematic cleaning received once-daily administration of a proton-pump inhibitor from the day prior. Before surgery, 20 mL of distilled water was uniformly sprayed inside the stomach, and 20 mL of gastric juice was collected with a sterile tube and submitted to culturing. The inside of the stomach was the cleaned with 2000 mL of saline. The face, mouthpiece, and area around the mouth were also disinfected with iodine, and an endoscope sterilized with ethylene oxide gas was used. The endoscopist and assistant scrubbed and maintained sterility where possible. At completion of the hybrid EFTR, 20 mL of distilled water was sprayed on the stomach wall and 20 mL of gastric juice was collected with a sterile tube and submitted for culturing. In addition, 20 mL of peritoneal fluid was collected laparoscopically and submitted for culturing. The authors' study showed significantly lower white blood cell count, C-reactive protein, and body temperature at postoperative days 1 and 3 in the patients who received systematic gastric cleaning. Furthermore, systematic stomach cleaning dramatically suppressed the bacterial load in the gastric juice. Preoperative gastric cleaning with saline exhibited a bacteria-reducing effect that was equivalent to reductions seen in other studies using disinfection with iodine solution.[23]

ADAPTING ENDOSCOPIC SUBMUCOSAL DISSECTION TECHNIQUE FOR FULL-THICKNESS RESECTION: THE AUTHORS' TECHNIQUE

Cases of GISTs in the stomach that are difficult to accurately localize laparoscopically can be marginated by ESD technique from the luminal side. Using ESD for incision and hemostasis extending through the mucosal and submucosal layers reduces bleeding during the full-thickness laparoscopic excision, through the serous membrane/muscular layers, and allows precise localization of the lesion from the peritoneal side by means of transillumination; if the laparoscopic light intensity is reduced, then transmission of the light of the endoscope through the endoscopic marginal incision precisely defines the area to be resected to ensure complete en bloc excision of the lesion.

Margination of the lesion is performed as follows: a shallow mucosal incision is made first using ESD to prevent vascular damage or bleeding, and gradually the incision is deepened; the penetrating vessels passing through the muscle and supplying the mucosa and submucosa are completely cauterized with hemostatic forceps under direct visual guidance. A ring-shaped incision and vascular treatments are performed up to an adequate submucosal depth, and the muscle layer incision is prepared. The seromuscular incision can be performed by laparoscopic means or endoscopically to achieve a purely endoscopic resection. The authors' reported approach for endoscopic seromuscular incision consists of making small perforations through the seromuscular layers measuring approximately 1.5 mm in diameter and located at intervals of approximately 10 mm around the circumference of the marginal incision to ensure a reliable connect-the-dots excision pathway that can be followed even after visibility becomes limited due to stomach collapse from loss of insufflation once the wall of the gastrointestinal tract is breeched. These perforation holes serve as landmarks for full-thickness excision with the ITknife2 (KD-611L, Olympus), which is taken through an excision path that joins these small perforations.[24]

DEVELOPMENT OF FLEXIBLE ENDOSCOPE FULL-THICKNESS SUTURING DEVICES

EFTR requires secure closure of the full-thickness defect in the gastrointestinal wall to avoid risk of life-threatening complications from leakage of luminal contents. It is well appreciated by surgeons that suturing is one of the most secure closure methods. It is essential to develop full-thickness suturing devices that possess a suturing strength equivalent to that of surgical hand-sewn sutures. Currently, the world's only marketed flexible endoscope full-thickness suturing device that use suture thread is the OverStitch. The Over-The-Scope Clip devices (eg, the bear-claw device from Ovesco Endoscopy and the Padlock Clip device from Aponos Medical [Kingston, New Hampshire]) have been marketed as clip-type full-thickness suturing devices but are large tissue apposing clips with teeth that obtain deep tissue bites but are not true suturing devices and are restricted on the size of defects they can close and the depth of tissue penetration. These 2 different suturing devices have advantages and disadvantages, but both represent innovations in suture layer devices for flexible endoscopes. Nonetheless, there currently is no full-thickness suturing device that is inexpensive and simple and can be easily fitted onto a general-purpose endoscope and operated. Mori and colleagues[25] developed a flexible endoscope full-thickness suturing device that has suturing strength comparable to surgical hand-sewn sutures. This DBSS consists of a hood portion that fits onto the tip of a single-channel general-purpose endoscope. The accessory channel of the endoscope is not used by the device and, therefore, it remains available for use by other accessories (**Fig. 4**A). The arms have various sizes in accordance with the size of the perforation opening; after 1 suture, the first arm is removed, and, from the second suture, replacing the tip makes rapid suturing possible, as with endoscopic variceal ligation (see **Fig. 4**B).[25] A DBSS prototype has been used in various studies on

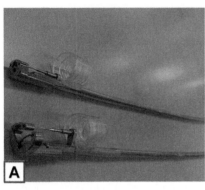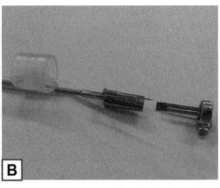

Fig. 4. The DBSS, a full-thickness suturing device. (*A*) Various sizes of the DBSS. It can be easily used by simply inserting the flexible endoscope into the hood portion. (*B*) The first arm is removable, allowing for quick suturing.

full-thickness suturing with resected pig stomachs. One of these basic experiments assessed whether the suturing strength is equivalent to surgical hand-sewn sutures, using an air leak test. The defect after EFTR in 10 pig stomachs was closed and air leak test was performed. No significant difference was observed in the pressure values between surgical hand-sewn sutures and DBSS (median of 3350 Pa [G] [95% CI, 2470–4250 Pa (G)] for hand-sewn sutures versus median of 3665 Pa [G] [95% CI, 1600–4400 Pa (G)] for DBSS; $P = .542$).[5] After full-thickness excision of a 40-mm simulated gastric lesion in dogs, closure was performed using this full-thickness suturing device and suturing was performed with a 4-mm bite and 4-mm pitch; 1-year survival confirmed safety and efficacy of the closure with the DBSS device.

MEASURING AND CONTROLLING PNEUMOPERITONEUM DURING ENDOSCOPIC FULL-THICKNESS RESECTION

In gastrointestinal endoscopy, the endoscopist manually operates suction and insufflation, and the internal pressure of the gastrointestinal tract is ascertained by the endoscopist subjectively. Pneumoperitoneum, however, is inevitable with EFTR, as it is with laparoscopic surgery, and safe EFTR necessitates carefully controlling abdominal pressure to avoid a compartment syndrome that could compromise ventilation and cardiovascular function. The authors have developed a hood that is equipped with a simple, semiautomatic constant-pressure device that can be fitted onto general-purpose endoscopes and is inexpensive with a simple structure (**Fig. 5**A). The efficacy of the microelectromechanical system (MEMS) hood equipped with a MEMS pressure sensor was verified in animal experiments (see **Fig. 5**B). Using an endoscope fitted with the MEMS hood inserted into the stomach, pressures were measured through a gastric fistula and true measured pressure values were compared with the values measured with the MEMS hood. While testing the increase/decrease in internal pressure over time, the signal intensity (V) of the MEMS hood showed good correlation with the pressure measurement sensor (mm Hg), with a signal intensity from −0.01 V to 0.138 V, and the true measured internal pressure from the sensor was favorable, from 0 mm Hg to 22 mm Hg. Simply fitting an endoscope with the MEMS hood makes it possible to measure the pressure at the endoscope tip in real time (**Fig. 6**).[26]

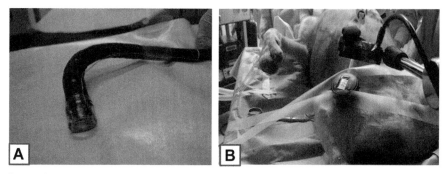

Fig. 5. The pressure-measuring MEMS hood. (*A*) Hood with built-in MEMS. (*B*) In animal experiments, true pressure values were measured from a gastric fistula. The internal gastric pressure was measured by inserting into the stomach an endoscope fitted with an MEMS hood.

IMPROVING ENDOSCOPIC VISUALIZATION DURING INSUFFLATION LOSS AT ENDOSCOPIC FULL-THICKNESS RESECTION

Exposed EFTR necessarily entails collapse of the gastrointestinal tract, because the gastrointestinal tract is perforated. No study has addressed securing surgical field visualization during exposed EFTR. In EFTR at the lesser and greater curvatures, the lesser or greater omentum limits outflow of CO_2 from the gastrointestinal tract, and thus it may be possible to maintain sufficient endoscopic visualization to complete the full-thickness excision and suturing. When the EFTR involves the anterior or posterior wall, however, the gastrointestinal tract collapses, making it difficult to operate

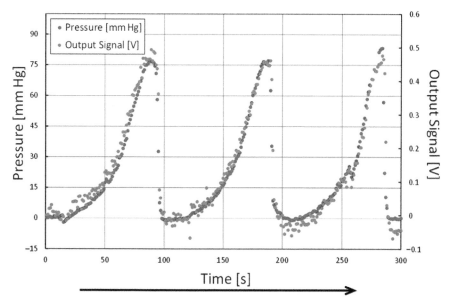

Fig. 6. Results of internal gastric pressure in an insufflation-deflation test. Simply fitting an endoscope with the MEMS hood enables measurement of the pressure at the endoscope tip in real time.

the endoscope. This is one of the limitations of pure EFTR performed solely with an endoscope. The authors are developing a countertraction device that maintains an expanded view within the operative field at the tip of the endoscope by mechanical traction obviating continued insufflation (**Fig. 7**). This device has been developed to ensure good endoscopic visualization while minimizing CO_2 insufflation and thus avoiding excessive pneumoperitoneum.[11]

Several animal experiments have shown favorable results of the countertraction device in ex vivo animal models. In animal experimentation in vivo, however, the authors concluded that the surgical field cannot be expanded in a manner similar to ex vivo, in light of the multiorgan load and compression of the abdominal wall onto the gastric wall. Therefore, the authors have narrowed the focus to develop nonexposed EFTR techniques, where conventional insufflation is effective because loss of CO_2 to the peritoneal cavity is prevented. Pure nonexposed EFTR involves the use of a flexible endoscope throughout the surgical process, and a dedicated full-thickness suturing device needs to be developed, but no countertraction device is required, so it would be feasible. There also would be no intraoperative exposure of the peritoneum to epithelial malignancies, and no exposure to luminal bacteria, thus making it safe in terms of infection. In the authors' opinion, nonexposed EFTR is the most feasible procedure for next-generation EFTR.[15]

SUMMARY

EFTR, both exposed and nonexposed, is a new endoscopic technique that is becoming popular in the expanding fields of endoscopic diagnostics, endoscopic therapeutics, and endoscopic surgery. Gastrointestinal tumors can be approached via natural orifices using a flexible endoscope more directly and less invasively than with laparoscopic surgery. Despite the minimal invasiveness of EFTR, however, there is an urgent need to establish EFTR guidelines for its safe implementation and to continue efforts to develop safer and more efficient instrumentation for this highly challenging procedure. The authors' group has been one of the pioneering groups extensively invested in the development of devices and techniques that can help solve EFTR challenges. This article reviews the authors' efforts in this regard, including a technique that uses 2 endoscopes to address the need for visualization and

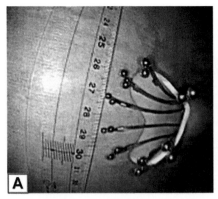 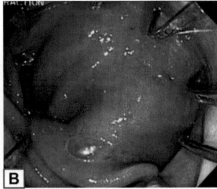

Fig. 7. Mechanical countertraction device. (*A*) Eight countertraction prongs protruding from a specially designed overtube. (*B*) In animal experimentation, a favorable surgical field was ensured.

instrumentation from the peritoneal side of the gastrointestinal lumen and several devices that the authors developed, including a device that can measure pressures at the tip of the endoscope to help avoid tense pneumoperitoneum, a suturing device that utilizes a diagnostic endoscope and still allows use of the accessory channel of the scope for other accessories, and a device that also fits on a diagnostic endoscope without blocking its accessory channel and achieves countertraction to maintain a field of view even in the setting of lost insufflation. The ability to safely use existing general-purpose flexible endoscopes for EFTR would reduce medical expenses and patients' economic, physical, and mental burdens, as noted for ultraminimally invasive surgeries.

REFERENCES

1. Abe N, Takeuchi H, Ooki A, et al. Recent developments in gastric endoscopic submucosal dissection: towards the era of endoscopic resection of layers deeper than the submucosa. Dig Endosc 2013;25(Suppl 1):64–70.

2. von Renteln D, Rösch T, Kratt T, et al. Endoscopic full-thickness resection of submucosal gastric tumors. Dig Dis Sci 2012;57:1298–303.

3. Elmunzer BJ, Trunzo JA, Marks JM, et al. Endoscopic full-thickness resection of gastric tumors using a novel grasp-and-snare technique: feasibility in ex vivo and in vivo porcine models. Endoscopy 2008;40:931–5.

4. von Renteln D, Riecken B, Walz B, et al. Endoscopic GIST resection using Flush-Knife ESD and subsequent perforation closure by means of endoscopic full-thickness suturing. Endoscopy 2008;40(Suppl 2):E224–5.

5. Mori H, Kobara H, Fujihara S, et al. Feasibility of pure EFTR using an innovative new endoscopic suturing device: the double-arm-bar suturing system (with video). Surg Endosc 2014;28:683–90.

6. Fujishiro M, Yahagi N, Kakushima N, et al. Endoscopic submucosal dissection of esophageal squamous cell neoplasm. Clin Gastroenterol Hepatol 2006;4:688–94.

7. Ono H, Kondo H, Gotoda T, et al. Endoscopic mucosal resection for treatment of early gastric cancer. Gut 2001;48:225–9.

8. Yamamoto H, Kawata H, Sunada K, et al. Successful en bloc resection of large superficial tumor in the stomach and colon using sodium hyaluronate and small-caliber-tip transparent hood. Endoscopy 2003;35:690–4.

9. Kantsevoy SV, Thuluvath PJ. Successful closure of a chronic refractory gastrocutaneous fistula with a new endoscopic suturing device (with video). Gastrointest Endosc 2012;75:688–90.

10. von Renteln D, Vassiliou MC, Rothstein RI. Randomized controlled trial comparing endoscopic clips and over-the-scope clips for closure of natural orifice transluminal endoscopic surgery gastrotomies. Endoscopy 2009;41: 1056–61.

11. Mori H, Rafiq K, Kobara H, et al. Innovative non insufflation EFTR: sufficient endoscopic operative field by mechanical counter traction device. Surg Endosc 2013; 27:3028–34.

12. Mori H, Kobara H, Fujihara S, et al. Establishment of the hybrid endoscopic full-thickness resection of gastric gastrointestinal stromal tumors. Mol Clin Oncol 2015;3:18–22.

13. Hiki N, Nunobe S, Matsuda T, et al. Laparoscopic endoscopic cooperative surgery. Dig Endosc 2015;27:197–204.

14. Goto O, Mitsui T, Fujishiro M, et al. New method of endoscopic full-thickness resection: a pilot study of non-exposed endoscopic wall-inversion surgery in an ex vivo porcine model. Gastric Cancer 2011;14:183–7.

15. Mori H, Kobara H, Nishiyama N, et al. Non exposure endoscopic full-thickness resection (Neo-EFTR) with two flexible endoscopes equipped with a suturing device (ex vivo study). Endoscopy 2015;47(Suppl 1):E501–2.

16. Warsi AA, Peyser PM. Laparoscopic resection of gastric GIST and benign gastric tumours: evolution of a new technique. Surg Endosc 2010;24:72–8.

17. Inoue T, Uedo N, Yamashina T, et al. Delayed perforation: a hazardous complication of endoscopic resection for non-ampullary duodenal neoplasm. Dig Endosc 2014;26:220–7.

18. Basford PJ, George R, Nixon E, et al. Endoscopic resection of sporadic duodenal adenomas: comparison of endoscopic mucosal resection (EMR) with hybrid endoscopic submucosal dissection (ESD) techniques and the risks of late delayed bleeding. Surg Endosc 2014;28:1594–600.

19. Mori H, Shintaro F, Kobara H, et al. Successful closing of duodenal ulcer after endoscopic submucosal dissection with over-the-scope clip to prevent delayed perforation. Dig Endosc 2013;25:459–61.

20. Zheng YZ, Wang D, Gu JJ, et al. An experimental study of betadine irrigation for preventing infection during the natural orifice transluminal endoscopic surgery (NOTES) procedure. J Dig Dis 2011;12:217–22.

21. Rao GV, Reddy DN, Banerjee R. NOTES: human experience. Gastrointest Endosc Clin N Am 2008;18:361–70.

22. Steele K, Schweitzer MA, Lyn-Sue J, et al. Flexible transgastric peritoneoscopy and liver biopsy: a feasibility study in human beings (with videos). Gastrointest Endosc 2008;68:61–6.

23. Mori H, Kobara H, Tsushimi T, et al. Reduction effect of bacterial counts by preoperative saline lavage of the stomach in performing laparoscopic and endoscopic cooperative surgery. World J Gastroenterol 2014;20:15763–70.

24. Mori H, Kobara H, Kobayashi M, et al. Establishment of pure NOTES procedure using a conventional flexible endoscope: review of six cases of gastric gastrointestinal stromal tumors. Endoscopy 2011;43:631–4.

25. Mori H, Kobara H, Kazi R, et al. Balloon-armed mechanical counter traction and double-armed bar suturing systems for pure endoscopic full-thickness resection. Gastroenterology 2014;147:278–80.

26. Mori H, Takao H, Kobara H, et al. Precise tumor size measurement under constant pressure by novel real-time micro-electro-mechanical-system hood for proper treatment (with videos). Surg Endosc 2015;29:212–9.

Hybrid NOTES
Combined Laparo-endoscopic Full-thickness Resection Techniques

Hyung Hun Kim, MD[a],*, Noriya Uedo, MD[b]

KEYWORDS

- Full-thickness resection • Laparoscopic and endoscopic cooperative surgery
- Laparoscopy-assisted endoscopic full-thickness resection
- Combination of laparoscopic and endoscopic approaches for neoplasia with a nonexposure technique • Nonexposed endoscopic wall-inversion surgery
- Laparoscopic transgastric surgery • Laparoscopy-assisted endoscopic resection
- Gastrointestinal stromal tumor

KEY POINTS

- The combination of laparoscopy and endoscopic submucosal dissection represents a new minimally destructive surgical method.
- Laparoscopic and endoscopic cooperative surgery and laparoscopy-assisted endoscopic full-thickness resection are effective methods of removing gastric subepithelial tumors (SETs), but they are not appropriate for gastric cancer because of the possibility of peritoneal seeding.
- Nonexposure techniques, such as combination of laparoscopic and endoscopic approaches to the treatment of neoplasia with a nonexposure technique (CLEAN-NET), nonexposed endoscopic wall-inversion surgery (NEWS), and laparoscopy transgastric surgery, are appropriate for SETs with mucosal defects.
- CLEAN-NET and NEWS have the potential for use in gastric cancer resection because these techniques can prevent peritoneal seeding.
- Laparoscopy-assisted endoscopic resection is an effective method that facilitates efficient therapeutic endoscopic procedures for colorectal neoplasm.

Disclosure Statement: The authors have no conflicts of interest to disclose.
Company Relationship: There is no conflict of interest.
[a] Department of Gastroenterology, Endoscopy Center for Gastrointestinal Oncology, Hansol Hospital, 138-844, Songpadasero 445, Songpa-gu, Seoul, Korea; [b] Department of Gastrointestinal Oncology, Osaka Medical Center for Cancer and Cardiovascular Diseases, 1-3-3 Nakamichi, Tosei-ku, Osaka 537-8511, Japan
* Corresponding author.
E-mail address: drhhkim@gmail.com

Gastrointest Endoscopy Clin N Am 26 (2016) 335–373
http://dx.doi.org/10.1016/j.giec.2015.12.011
1052-5157/16/$ – see front matter © 2016 Elsevier Inc. All rights reserved.

giendo.theclinics.com

INTRODUCTION

In the era of minimally destructive surgery, 2 important points must be considered: removal of the target lesion without removing normal tissue and obtaining a sufficient resection margin. These 2 aims seem to be contradictory, but advances in surgical procedures and therapeutic endoscopic technology allow operators to accomplish these difficult tasks in a stepwise manner. The development of laparoscopy paved the way for minimally invasive surgery. Laparoscopic wedge resection of the stomach is used to remove stomach tumors, such as gastrointestinal stromal tumors (GISTs),[1] neuroendocrine tumors, and adenocarcinoma. However, it is difficult to determine the appropriate incision line from the outside of the stomach when these lesions are intraluminal. Excessive gastric resection might result in transformation of the stomach, with consequent gastric stasis during food uptake. Furthermore, the open approach was used for large tumors and tumors located at specific locations, such as the posterior gastric wall, esophagogastric junction, and the area near the pylorus, to ensure negative margins. Surgeons have used various methods to determine the appropriate incision line for local resection of the stomach, such as lesion-lifting gastrectomy,[2] hand-assisted laparoscopic surgery,[3] the tumor eversion method,[4] and laparoscopic-endoscopic rendezvous resection.[5,6] In addition to these methods, endoscopic submucosal dissection (ESD) has been used to transform organ-saving treatment into a minimally destructive surgical procedure.[7] Currently, these 2 techniques are being merged with the aim of developing less invasive and less destructive treatments in the future.

Laparoscopic and endoscopic cooperative surgery (LECS) was developed as a less invasive and less destructive surgical technique that overcomes the disadvantages of laparoscopy-only procedures. Currently, LECS is evolving such that endoscopy has a more significant role (ie, it is not used to simply guide laparoscopic resection; rather, it has an active role in the resection itself).[8] Following the development of the original LECS procedure, many researchers investigated several modified LECS procedures. Laparoscopy-assisted endoscopic full-thickness resection (LAEFR) was developed to manipulate lesions that cannot be easily approached via LECS. Several nonexposure techniques, such as inverted LECS,[9] a combination of laparoscopic and endoscopic approaches to the treatment of neoplasia with a nonexposure technique (CLEAN-NET),[10] nonexposed endoscopic wall-inversion surgery (NEWS),[11–13] and laparoscopic transgastric surgery (LTGS),[14] have been developed to avoid creating an opening in the gastric wall leading to the peritoneal cavity. Use of LECS and its variants has resulted in minimal resection of the normal gastric wall, with minimal gastric transformation.

As techniques have advanced, several attempts have been made to achieve local removal of gastric cancer (GC) or colorectal cancer (CRC) with laparoendoscopic full-thickness resection. Evaluating lymph node metastasis is another important issue that must be considered when laparoendoscopic full-thickness resection is used to remove GC and CRC rather than subepithelial tumors (SETs) such as GISTs, because laparoendoscopic full-thickness resection is essentially predicated on limited lymph node dissection based on sentinel lymph node (SN) mapping. SN navigation of GC and CRC has not been performed universally because of the complicated lymphatic flow from the stomach and colon and skip metastases, which sometimes occur in GC and CRC.[15–22] However, laparoscopy-assisted endoscopic resection (LAER) and other techniques have been consistently used for colon polyp removal.[19,23–25] Use of the colon collaborative technique eventually allowed the achievement of full-thickness laparoendoscopic excision (FLEX) and eversion full-thickness laparoendoscopic excision (eFLEX) using a new thread device.[23,26]

Currently, laparoendoscopic full-thickness resection procedures are being combined with natural orifice transluminal endoscopic surgery (NOTES). These combined procedures are commonly referred to as "hybrid NOTES" because additional laparoscopic or thoracoscopic surgical instruments are used to assist with the endoscopic surgical procedure. Laparoendoscopic full-thickness resection performed with LECS and LECS variants nearly achieved the goals of removing a smaller specimen and obtaining a sufficient resection margin. Furthermore, a simultaneous laparoscopic approach has the potential to concomitantly remove SNs or SN basins. It is thought that these collaborative procedures satisfy the concept of minimally destructive surgery. In this article, we investigate the theoretic basis and technical feasibility of laparoendoscopic full-thickness resection for muscular propria (MP)-origin SETs, GC, and CRC. Furthermore, we analyze the advantages and limitations of laparoendoscopic full-thickness resection compared with endoscopic full-thickness resection (EFTR), as well as the role of laparoendoscopic full-thickness resection as a bridge technique for pure NOTES.

THEORETICAL INDICATIONS FOR LAPAROENDOSCOPIC FULL-THICKNESS RESECTION
Local Resection of Gastrointestinal Stromal Tumors and Principles of Surgery

SETs consist of many different histologic entities, such as leiomyoma, GIST, lipoma, neuroma, and others. However, it is important to note that GISTs account for most cases.[27] Thus, investigations of the theoretic basis for local resection of GISTs should be prioritized. Most GISTs are regarded to have malignant potential to some degree; roughly 20% to 25% of gastric GISTs show malignant behavior.[28] One of the most prominent features of GISTs is their unpredictable and variable behavior. Risk can be estimated preoperatively based on size and location; however, there are currently no reliable criteria for surgery. Unlike GC, regional lymph node metastasis of GISTs reportedly ranges from 1.1% to 3.4%.[29–31] Due to the unpredictable malignant behavior of GISTs and rare lymph node metastasis, local resection without primary lymph node dissection is recommended. The goal of surgery is complete resection without capsule injury because rupture is associated with intra-abdominal dissemination and poor prognosis.[32] It has been demonstrated that laparoscopic wedge resection, less invasive than laparotomy, provides comparable results in terms of efficacy, safety, and length of hospitalization.[1,33–39] Although some researchers showed that a microscopically positive margin does not cause recurrence,[40,41] one study reported that it was an adverse factor for survival.[42] Therefore, it is obvious that achieving R0 resection and preventing capsule rupture should be the goals of laparoendoscopic full-thickness resection.

Local Resection of Gastric Cancer and Colorectal Cancer: the Sentinel Lymph Node Concept

Surgical therapy for gastrointestinal cancer involves removal of the cancer lesion and complete lymph node dissection. This approach stems from the belief that removal of all lymph nodes potentially containing metastases should contribute not only to successful extraction of the surgical specimen and reconstruction of the alimentary tract, which is technically difficult even for experienced surgeons, but also to patient survival. In addition, these resected lymph nodes provide important information that can be used to predict recurrence and survival and to guide decision-making regarding adjuvant therapy. This principle has also been applied to laparoscopic techniques for early-stage GC and CRC. Minimally destructive surgical techniques have been previously attempted, and lymphatic mapping and SN biopsy are progressing toward clinical applicability for early-stage GC and CRC, extending the criteria for minimally invasive resection beyond the current ESD criteria. More favorable clinical outcomes have been obtained with laparoscopic surgery compared with conventional surgery.[43–45] Laparoendoscopic full-thickness resection with SN biopsy or SN basin dissection could be feasible and could fulfill the concept of minimally destructive surgery for GC and CRC if the SN concept is successfully established.[46] Preliminary data reported in 2002 have shown a high degree of sensitivity and diagnostic accuracy for a technique using radiotracer to mark SNs that are detected intraoperatively with a gamma probe.[47] However, despite the large number of studies that have attempted to validate the feasibility and accuracy of SN in GC, the results are still conflicting, likely because of different protocols and surgical techniques.[17,48–56] The outcomes of SN in CRC are similar.[57,58] Considering these experimental data, the active clinical use of laparoendoscopic full-thickness resection with SN biopsy or SN basin dissection is not yet supported.

LAPAROENDOSCOPIC FULL-THICKNESS RESECTION TECHNIQUES FOR THE UPPER GASTROINTESTINAL TRACT
Procedure Setup

a. The surgeon is on the patient's right side, and the first assistant stands on the patient's left side. The laparoscopist stands between the patient's legs[59] (**Fig. 1**).
b. The endoscopic operator stands at the top of the patient's head.
c. A camera port is inserted into the inferior umbilical area.
d. Four additional ports are inserted into the points as follows: left upper, left lower, right upper, and right lower quadrants, respectively.

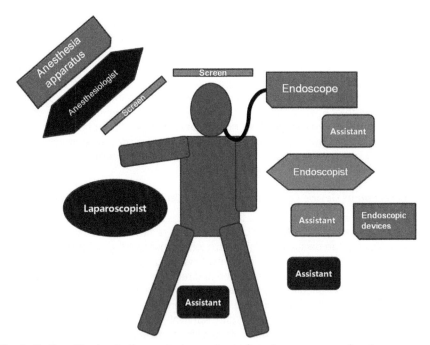

Fig. 1. Staff positioning in the surgical room to perform laparoscopy and endoscopy cooperative surgery.

Laparoscopic and Endoscopic Cooperative Surgery

For the first time, Izumi and colleagues[60] reported the use of a combination of gastrointestinal endoscopy and laparoscopy for the removal of an esophageal SET.[10] Using this technique, the SET was pushed out by a balloon on an endoscope, and thoracoscopic enucleation was performed to remove the protruded tumor.[10,60] Hiki and colleagues[8] reported the successful use of ESD for aiding local laparoscopic gastric GIST resection. In their technique, named LECS, laparoscopic staplers were used for resection after an approximately three-fourths cutline was completed. Tsujimoto and colleagues[61] also reported satisfactory surgical outcomes after LECS for gastric SETs. LECS has the important advantage of reducing the volume of the resected gastric wall compared with conventional laparoscopic wedge resection performed solely by using a linear stapler (**Fig. 2**).[62,63]

Laparoscopic and endoscopic cooperative surgery procedure

a. Preparation of blood vessels in the excision area (**Fig. 3**).
   Blood vessels in the excision area are treated using an ultrasonically activated device. Minimal blood vessel harvesting is recommended because excessive blood vessel manipulation can cause postoperative reduced gastric mobility.
b. ESD around the tumor.
   The mucosal incision technique is performed using a needle knife. First, the periphery of the tumor is marked as close as possible to the tumor edge. After injecting fluid into the submucosal layer, a small initial incision is made with a needle knife, and the tip of an insulated tip (IT) knife is inserted into the submucosal layer. Then, three-fourths of the marked area is cut circumferentially using the IT knife in usual ESD technique.
c. Laparoscopic seromuscular incision.
   The tip of the needle knife is apparent beyond the seromuscular layer, and artificial perforation is performed. The tip of the ultrasonically activated device is inserted into the perforation hole to make a seromuscular incision. After seromuscular incision of three-quarters of the circumference of the tumor, the tumor is delivered into the abdominal cavity attached only by the pedicle of tissue in the quarter of the circumference that was left intact. The tumor and the edge of the incision line are then lifted up by the laparoscopic assistant using forceps, and a laparoscopic stapler is used to simultaneously close the incision and complete the tumor resection.

Laparoscopic and endoscopic cooperative surgery advantages

The use of LECS avoids excessive resection of the gastric wall. This technique is relatively simple and typically takes 2 to 3 hours to perform. Moreover, the LECS procedure is not affected by challenging tumor locations, such as those in the vicinity of the esophagogastric junction (EGJ) or pyloric ring.[8] Hoteya and colleagues[64] demonstrated the feasibility and safety of the LECS procedure in 25 cases of gastric SET, including lesions adjacent to the EGJ.

Laparoscopic and endoscopic cooperative surgery limitations

LECS can be used to remove lesions at the EGJ, but dissection of the esophageal wall must be confined to less than one-third of the esophageal circumference to reduce the possibility of complications. Luminal stenosis or obstruction and leaks can be caused by difficult esophageal suturing. For gastric resections, opening of the gastric wall might result in spillage of gastric contents, including bacteria and tumor cells, into the abdominal cavity. Consequently, intra-abdominal infection and/or peritoneal

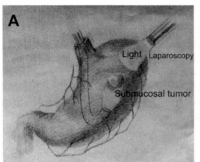

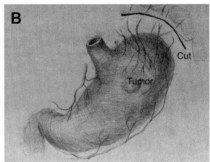

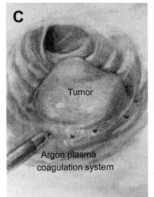

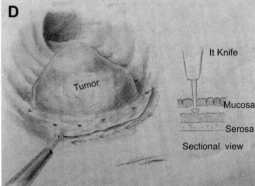

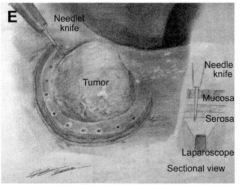

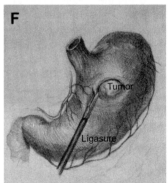

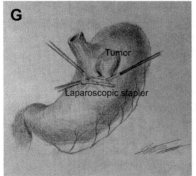

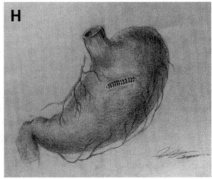

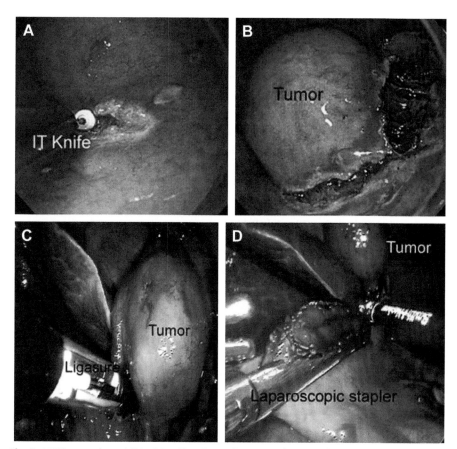

Fig. 3. LCES procedure. (*A*) Incision line for endoscopic submucosal resection around the tumor is guided by argon plasma markings. (*B*) Incision and submucosal layer trimming is completed around the tumor. (*C*) Laparoscopic seromuscular dissection is performed with ultrasonically activated device inserted to the hole after active perforation is caused by a needle knife. (*D*) The tumor (nonresected part) and the edge of the incision line are lifted into a laparoscopic stapler that is used to complete the resection and perform stapled closure of the resection defect (Endo-GIA laparoscopic stapler; Tyco Autosuture, Tokyo, Japan). (*Data from* Hiki N, Yamamoto Y, Fukunaga T, et al. Laparoscopic and endoscopic cooperative surgery for gastrointestinal stromal tumor dissection. Surg Endosc 2008;22:1731–2; with permission.)

Fig. 2. LECS schematic illustration. (*A*) Identifying a lesion by both endoscopy and laparoscopy. (*B*) Preparing vessels before the procedure. (*C*) Marking with APC around the lesion. (*D*) Incision with IT knife around the markers. (*E*) Seromuscular puncture with a needle knife after three-fourth mucosal/submucosal incision is completed. (*F*) Laparoscopic scissors are inserted into the hole and full seromuscular dissection is performed. (*G*) The tumor (nonresected part) and the edge of the incision line are lifted up by the assistant using forceps, and completion of the resection along with closure of the incision line is achieved using laparoscopic stapling devices. (*H*) Image of the stapled closure site.

dissemination of tumor cells could occur during procedure. Thus, LECS currently cannot be used for local dissection of SETs with mucosal defects or GC.[61,63]

Laparoscopic and endoscopic cooperative surgery outcomes

All studies have demonstrated 100% complete resection without complications in LECS procedures (**Table 1**).[8,61,64–66] The mean operative time is less than 3 hours.

Laparoscopy-Assisted Endoscopic Full-Thickness Resection

Abe and colleagues[62,67] described EFTR with laparoscopic assistance (LAEFR) as an alternative to LECS for the treatment of gastric SETs. Contrary to LECS, LAEFR involves an endoscopic full-thickness incision and a hand-sewn suture for artificial gastric perforation, instead of linear staples.[62,64,67] Although the full-thickness incision is performed endoscopically, countertraction was applied to stretch the gastric wall by laparoscopic manipulation (**Fig. 4**).[62,64,67]

Laparoscopy-assisted endoscopic full-thickness resection procedure

a. Endoscopic deep submucosal incision is performed using ESD[62] (**Fig. 5**).
b. Endoscopic full-thickness incision (three-fourths or two-thirds of the circumference of the lesion) is performed. Countertraction was made by laparoscopic assistance.
c. Laparoscopic full-thickness resection of the remaining circumference of the lesion is performed.
d. Hand sewing closure was done.

Laparoscopy-assisted endoscopic full-thickness resection advantages

LAEFR results in minimal resection, whereas LECS affords easier and faster resection.[62,64]

Laparoscopy-assisted endoscopic full-thickness resection limitations

LAEFR and LECS have the same limitations; they cannot be used for GC or SETs with mucosal ulceration.

Laparoscopy-assisted endoscopic full-thickness resection outcomes

Abe and colleagues[67] performed 4 LAEFR procedures; the mean tumor diameter was 30 mm, and the mean operation time was 201 minutes. All tumors were completely removed without complications.

Table 1
Publications reporting laparoscopy and endoscopy cooperative surgery for subepithelial tumors in the upper gastrointestinal tract

Reference	No.	Mean Operation Time, min	Mean Tumor Diameter, mm	Complete Resection Rate, %	Complications
Hoteya et al,[64] 2014	25	156	32	100[a]	0
Kawahira et al,[66] 2012	16	172	—	100	0
Tsujimoto et al,[61] 2012	20	157	38	100[a]	0
Hiki,[100] 2011	38	—	—	100	0
Hiki et al,[8] 2008	7	169	46	100	0

[a] Pathologically evaluated.

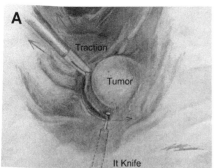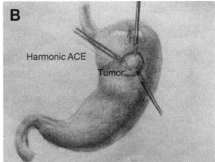

Fig. 4. Schematic illustration of the differences of LAEFR compared with LECS. (*A*) Unlike LECS, full-thickness endoscopic incision is conducted with the IT knife over three-quarters of the circumference around the lesion. (*B*) Harmonic ACE is then inserted in the incision and to complete resection of the remaining undissected part, followed by hand-sewn suture laparoscopically to close the defect.

Inverted Laparoscopic and Endoscopic Cooperative Surgery

LECS can be used to treat early GC when ESD is difficult, and it is essential that tumor cells are not seeded into the peritoneal cavity during LECS procedures for epithelial neoplasms. To prevent contact between the tumor and visceral tissue, the tumor was turned toward the intragastric cavity using traction on the stitches at the edge of the resected specimen, and the resection line of the stomach was pulled up like a bowl with several stitches.[9,65,68]

Inverted laparoscopic and endoscopic cooperative surgery procedure

a. After setup for laparoscopic surgery, the tumor location was confirmed by intraluminal endoscopy (**Fig. 6**).
b. Blood vessels in the excision area around the tumor were prepared using an ultrasonically activated device.
c. The periphery of the tumor was marked to the tumor edge with a 1-cm margin.
d. The incision and submucosal dissection was performed using the IT knife.
e. The seromuscular layer was perforated by the needle knife for inserting the ultrasonically activated device.
f. The seromuscular layer was dissected along the incision line, created by the IT knife, using the ultrasonically activated device.
g. To prevent contact between the tumor and the visceral tissue, the tumor was inverted to face the intragastric cavity using the traction of the stitch at the edge of the resected specimen, and the resection line of the stomach was pulled up like a bowl by several stitches.
h. The tumor was resected into the gastric cavity and collected via the per-oral route.
i. The edge of the incision line was closed temporarily using hand-sewn sutures.
j. The incision line was properly closed using a laparoscopic stapling device.

Inverted laparoscopic and endoscopic cooperative surgery advantages and limitations

This technique may prevent the gastric contents from leaking into the peritoneal cavity and the tumor from contacting any intra-abdominal tissue; however, there can still

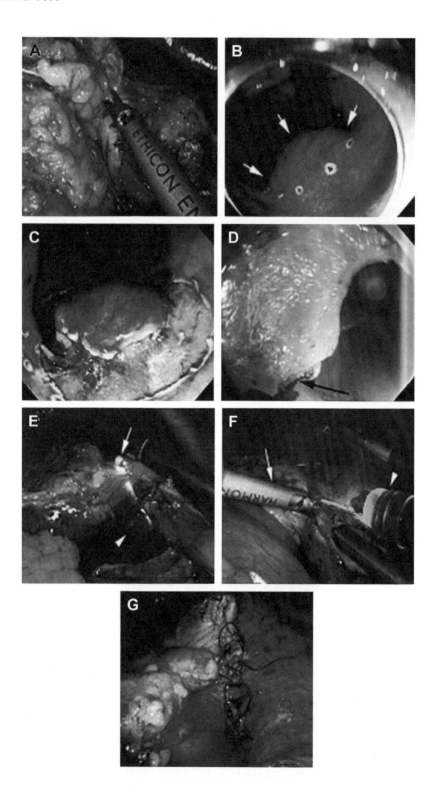

be a risk of gastric content contamination, as the gastric lumen is exposed to the peritoneal cavity for portions of the procedure with leakage being prevented by simple traction to keep the luminal contents on a dependent position away from the resection orifice.

Inverted laparoscopic and endoscopic cooperative surgery outcomes
Nunobe and colleagues[9] removed lateral-spreading intramucosal gastric tumors measuring 60 × 47 mm in diameter through inverted LECS. The operation time was 152 minutes, and the estimated blood loss was 0 mL during the operation. The postoperative course was mostly uneventful.

Combination of Laparoscopic and Endoscopic Approaches for Treatment of Neoplasia with a Nonexposure Technique

CLEAN-NET is one type of nonexposure full-thickness gastric wall resection technique.[10,65] CLEAN-NET involves a seromuscular incision with a laparoscopic instrument to maintain the continuity of the mucosa, which functions as a barrier of "CLEAN-NET." The mucosal tissue is pulled out toward the outside of the stomach, and the stretched mucosa is dissected together with a minimal amount of full-thickness stomach wall (**Fig. 7**).

Combination of laparoscopic and endoscopic approaches to the treatment of neoplasia with a nonexposure technique procedure

a. After endoscopic marking for the location of the lesion with indocyanine green, the mucosal layer is fixed to the seromuscular layer with 4 full-layer stay sutures (**Fig. 8**).
b. After submucosal injection of solution, the seromuscular layer is dissected along the outside of the 4 stay sutures using a laparoscopic electrocautery knife.
c. The full-layer specimen is lifted with the 4 stay sutures, and the mucosa surrounding the full-layer specimen is also pulled up.
d. Using a laparoscopic stapling device, the full-layer specimen is dissected with a sufficient margin.

Combination of laparoscopic and endoscopic approaches to the treatment of neoplasia with a nonexposure technique advantages
In addition to nonexposed removal of GC, CLEAN-NET can be used for GIST with ulceration, which has a high likelihood of peritoneal seeding when LECS and LAEFR are used.[68]

Fig. 5. LAEFR procedure. (*A*) Laparoscopic view of the lesser omentum around the tumor site being dissected. (*B*) Endoscopic view after marking around the gastric subepithelial tumor (*white arrows*) located on the lesser curvature side of the gastric body. (*C*) Endoscopic view after incision as deep as the submucosal layer around the lesion. (*D*) Endoscopic view of the full-thickness incision from inside the stomach using the IT knife (*black arrow*). (*E*) Laparoscopic view of the full-thickness incision from inside the stomach using the IT knife (*arrow*, the tip of the IT knife; *arrowhead*, the gastroscope). (*F*) Laparoscopic view of the remaining full-thickness incision from outside the stomach using a Harmonic ACE (*arrow*). *Arrowhead*, the gastroscope. (*G*) Laparoscopic view after laparoscopic hand-sewn closure of the gastric-wall defect. (*Data from* Abe N, Takeuchi H, Yanagida O, et al. Endoscopic full-thickness resection with laparoscopic assistance as hybrid NOTES for gastric submucosal tumor. Surg Endosc 2009;23:1910; with permission.)

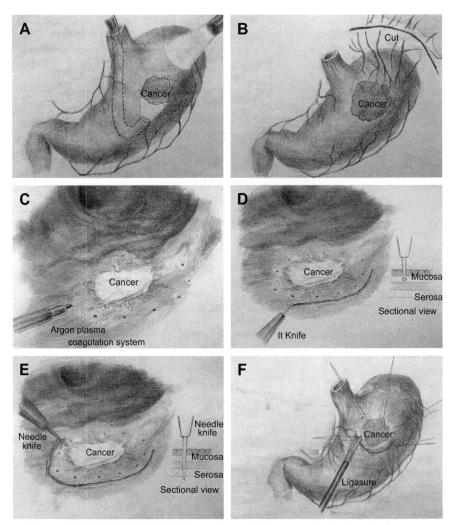

Fig. 6. Illustration of the important points of inverted LECS. (*A*) After setup for laparoscopic surgery, the tumor location is confirmed by intraluminal endoscopy. (*B*) Blood vessels in the excision area around the tumor are prepared using an ultrasonically activated device. (*C*) The periphery of the tumor is marked to the tumor edge with a 1-cm margin. (*D*) The mucosal circumferential incision and submucosal dissection is completed using the IT knife. (*E*) The seromuscular layer is perforated by the needle knife to allow insertion of a laparoscopic ultrasonic scalpel. (*F*) The seromuscular layer is dissected along the incision line, created by the IT knife, using the ultrasonic scalpel. (*G*) To prevent contact between the tumor and the visceral tissue or escape of luminal contents into the peritoneal cavity, the tumor is inverted to face the intragastric cavity using traction on sutures placed just outside of the planned resection area, which allows the resection line of the stomach to be pulled up like the rim of a bowl by these sutures. (*H*) The tumor is kept intraluminally and collected via the per-oral route. (*I*) The edge of the incision line is closed temporarily using hand-sewn sutures. (*J*) The incision line is then more securely closed using a laparoscopic stapling device. (*K*) Image of the closed incision line from the laparoscopic view.

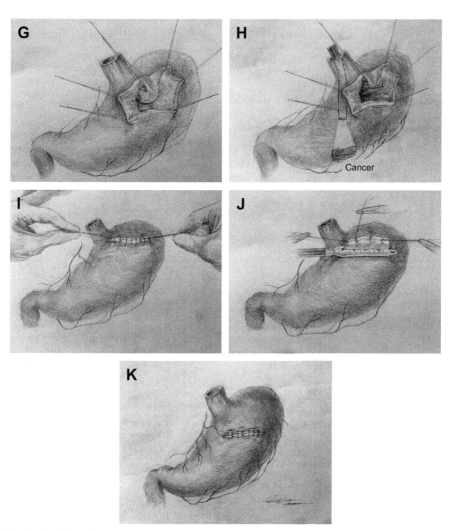

Fig. 6. (*continued*).

Combination of laparoscopic and endoscopic approaches to the treatment of neoplasia with a nonexposure technique limitations

There are some limitations associated with CLEAN-NET in the case of SET. First, the mucosal tissue is pulled out toward the outside of the stomach, and the stretched mucosa functions as a barrier to prevent the spillage of gastric contents; thus, the specimen size is limited to less than 3 cm to avoid mucosal laceration. However, if CLEAN-NET is used for epithelial neoplasms, such as GC, the size limit can be increased because deformation of the specimen is possible. Second, in this procedure, the incision line is determined from the serosal side; thus, the appropriate mucosal incision might be difficult to determine, particularly for intraluminal protruding SETs and mucosal lesions, such as GC. Additionally, location can sometimes be a limiting factor for this procedure, and it may not be useful in areas near the EGJ or the pyloric ring.

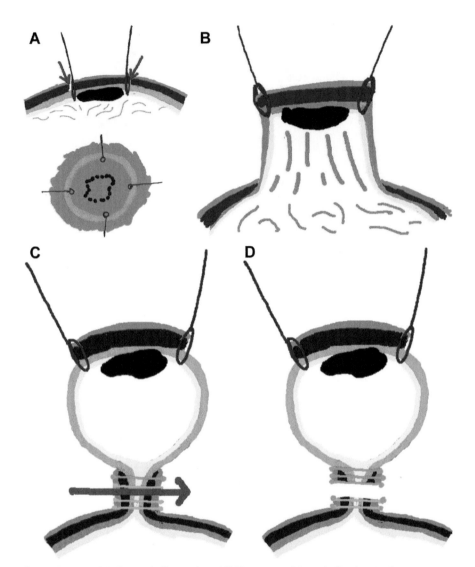

Fig. 7. CLEAN-NET schematic illustration. (*A*) The mucosal layer is fixed onto the seromuscular layer using 4 stay sutures, and selective seromuscular dissection outside the 4 stitches (*red arrows*) is performed laparoscopically. (*B*) The full-thickness specimen is lifted by 4 stay sutures. (*C*) Laparoscopic resection (*red arrows*) is performed. (*D*) The lesion is thus removed without risk of exposure of the peritoneal cavity to the surface of the lesion or luminal contents.

Combination of laparoscopic and endoscopic approaches to the treatment of neoplasia with a nonexposure technique outcomes

CLEAN-NET was used for 24 consecutive cases: 16 GC cases and 8 GIST cases. In 22 cases, the procedure was completed successfully with good clinical results. In 1 case, surgical repair was necessary because of incomplete closure of the resected line by the linear stapling device. In another case, additional surgery was necessary to correct gastric deformity. No clinical signs of recurrence were identified in any of the cases.[10]

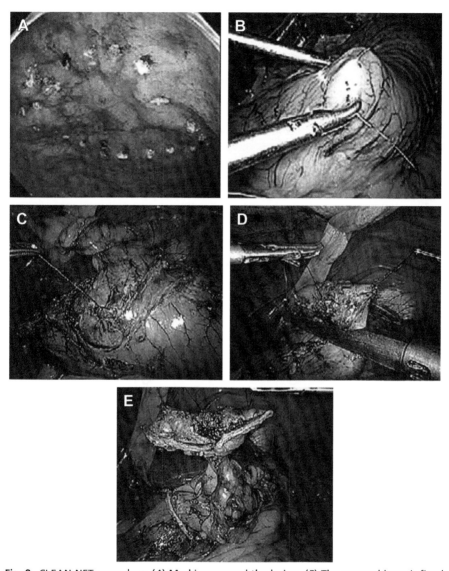

Fig. 8. CLEAN-NET procedure. (*A*) Marking around the lesion. (*B*) The mucosal layer is fixed onto the seromuscular layer using 4 stay sutures, which are introduced using laparoscopic vision and controlled by endoscopic vision from inside the stomach. (*C*) By pulling the 4 sutures with laparoscopic forceps, selective seromuscular dissection outside the 4 stitches is performed using a laparoscopic electrocautery knife. The continuity of the mucosal layer remains intact, preventing the gastric contents from flowing out into the peritoneal cavity. The mucosal layer works as a "clean net," which potentially avoids peritoneal seeding of cancer cells. (*D*) The full-thickness specimen is lifted by 4 stay sutures and laparoscopic resection is performed. (*E*) The lesion is thus resected without exposing its mucosal surface or luminal contents to the peritoneal cavity. (*Data from* Inoue H, Ikeda H, Hosoya T, et al. Endoscopic mucosal resection, endoscopic submucosal dissection, and beyond: full-layer resection for gastric cancer with nonexposure technique (CLEAN-NET). Surg Oncol Clin N Am 2012;21:137; with permission.)

Adding to this series, 2 GISTs with mucosal ulceration (3.5 cm and 4.0 cm in size) were successfully removed using CLEAN-NET.[68] There were no postoperative complications.

Nonexposed Endoscopic Wall-Inversion Surgery

NEWS is a newly developed nonexposure technique that minimizes the resected tissue volume and prevents peritoneal contamination.[69] It differs from CLEAN-NET in that NEWS involves suturing the serosal side to move the lesion to the intra-luminal side, and the procedure is completed through endoscopic resection (**Fig. 9**).[12,69]

Nonexposed endoscopic wall-inversion surgery procedure

a. The mucosa around a lesion is marked (**Fig. 10**).
b. Serosal marking is performed using laparoscopy at the sites of the mucosal markings.
c. Submucosal injection is performed.
d. Laparoscopic circumferential seromuscular layer incision is performed.
e. The seromuscular layer is sutured.
f. Seromuscular sutures achieve inversion of the lesion.
g. A circumferential endoscopic incision is made in the mucosal and submucosal layer.

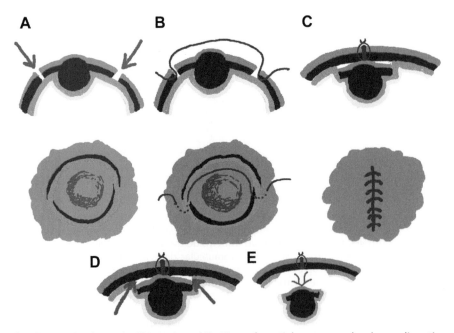

Fig. 9. NEWS schematic illustration. (*A*) Circumferential seromuscular layer dissection outside markings around the lesion (*red arrows*). (*B*) Seromuscular sutures are placed to achieve lesion inversion. (*C*) The lesion is now "sealed" inside the stomach by the seromuscular layer apposition. (*D*) Purely endoscopic resection is completed by ESD technique (*red arrows*). (*E*) The lesion falls into the stomach.

Nonexposed endoscopic wall-inversion surgery advantages
Theoretically, NEWS is an optimal method for the prevention of peritoneal seeding and contamination during surgery.

Nonexposed endoscopic wall-inversion surgery limitations
NEWS and CLEAN-NET share most of the same limitations in terms of size (≤ 3 cm), location (not useful near the EGJ or the pyloric ring), and delineation of lesion difficulty.

Nonexposed endoscopic wall-inversion surgery outcomes
Mitsui and colleagues[69] reported 2 perforations in 6 cases: 1 laparoscopic mucosal injury during the seromuscular incision and musculoserosal tearing during ESD. Two of 6 cases also converted due to poor recognition of the tumor margin.[69] The selection of appropriate lesions and advancements in the technique are necessary for the wider application of NEWS in ordinary clinical fields.

Laparoscopic Transgastric Surgery

LTGS is a procedure for the removal of gastric SETs primarily using a laparoscopic technique with the aid of endoscopy.[14,70] Laparoscopy is used to remove a SET in the gastric luminal side, and endoscopy is used to perorally extract the specimen (**Fig. 11**).

Laparoscopic transgastric surgery setup
Under general anesthesia, the patient is placed in a supine lithotomy position; the surgeon is positioned between the patient's legs, and the assistant is positioned to the right of the patient (**Fig. 12**). The assistant endoscopist is positioned at the patient's head. The first 5-mm trocar is inserted 10 cm below the xiphoid, left of the midline, using a trocar insertion and visualization technique. CO_2 is used to create pneumoperitoneum to a pressure of 15 mm Hg. A 5-mm laparoscope is then inserted into the abdominal cavity. After exploration of the abdominal cavity, an assistant performs endoscopy and insufflates the stomach with CO_2. Using both laparoscopic and endoscopic views, 2 balloon-tipped trocars (5-mm and 12-mm in diameter) are placed transabdominally and into the stomach via small gastrotomies. The balloons on the trocars are inflated and the pneumoperitoneum is partially released to a pressure of 10 mm Hg, allowing the stomach to be retracted against the anterior abdominal wall.

Laparoscopic transgastric surgery procedure

a. The tumor is grasped, and resection is achieved using a linear cutting stapler that is placed through the 12-mm transgastric trocar (**Fig. 13**).[70]
b. After being resected, the tumor is placed in a retrieval bag (see **Fig 13**B), and an endoscopic grasper is then used to retrieve the specimen through the mouth.
c. Last, a linear cutting stapler is used from within the peritoneal cavity to close the gastrostomies.

Laparoscopic transgastric surgery advantages
Using a gastroscope for visualization in the gastric cavity, the operators can reduce the need for an additional gastrotomy for insertion of a laparoscopic camera and the added complexity and risk of a fourth laparoscopic instrument into the gastric cavity. Furthermore, the endoscopist can use endoscopic closure devices such as clips to close the gastrotomies used to insert the laparoscopic instruments into the stomach. Compared with normal laparoscopic suturing, this technique is minimally invasive. Tumors measuring less than 3 cm in size can be removed through the mouth to reduce trauma to the abdominal wall. The exterior and interior of the gastric cavity can be

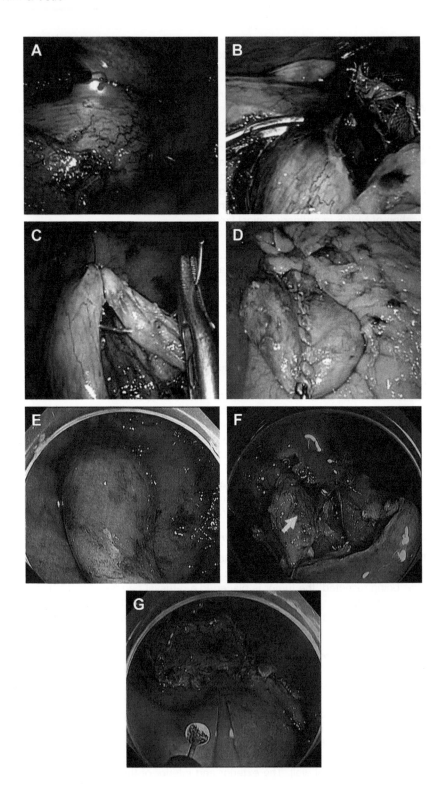

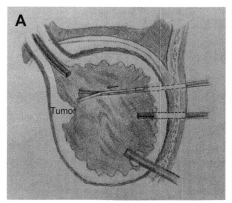 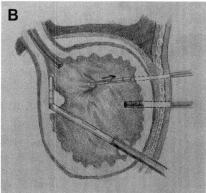

Fig. 11. LTGS schematic illustration. (*A*) Laparoscope and endoscope inserted into the stomach, and a laparoscopic grasper grasp the stomach wall (*arrow*). (*B*) With endoscopic guidance, a laparoscopic stapler is inserted into the stomach and used to resect the lesion from the luminal side with the assistance of laparoscopic graspers (*arrow*).

observed with laparoscopy and gastroscopy, respectively, to reduce the incidence of postoperative complications. Finally, this technique can prevent peritoneal contamination and, therefore, can be used for GIST with ulceration.

Laparoscopic transgastric surgery limitations
This technique has 2 limitations: (1) a size limitation of less than 3 cm for SETs due to the per-oral extraction route, and (2) difficulty in removing SETs growing in an extraluminal direction due to inaccurate delineation from the gastric side.

Laparoscopic transgastric surgery outcomes
Recent studies have reported 100% complete resection with minor postoperative complications, such as postoperative bleeding controlled through endoscopic management and medication (**Table 2**).[70–72]

Therapeutic Options Depending on Lesion Characteristics (Size, Location, and Histology)

When choosing therapeutic options for local resection, SETs originating from the MP must be classified into several types according to their locations in the gastric wall (**Fig. 14**).[73] Type I is an SET that has a narrow connection with the MP and protrudes into the luminal side, similar to polyps (see **Fig. 14**A). Type II has a wider connection with the MP and protrudes into the luminal side at an obtuse angle (see **Fig. 14**B). Type III is centered in the gastric wall (see **Fig. 14**C). Type IV has a significant extraluminal, "exophytic" protrusion on the serosal side of the gastric wall (see **Fig. 14**D). Of the 4 types, type I is the best candidate for endoscopic enucleation due to its

---

Fig. 10. NEWS procedure. (*A*) Laparoscopic markings on the serosal surface guided by transmitted light from the endoscope located in the gastric lumen. (*B*) Circumferential seromuscular layer dissection outside the serosal markings. (*C*) Seromuscular layer sutured closure. (*D*) Laparoscopic view of inversion of the dissected area. (*E*) Endoscopic view of massive protrusion of the inverted tissue. (*F*) Serosal surface (*arrow*) identified during endoscopic dissection. (*G*) Resected lesion to be retrieved. (*Data from* Mitsui T, Niimi K, Yamashita H, et al. Non-exposed endoscopic wall-inversion surgery as a novel partial gastrectomy technique. Gastric Cancer 2014;17:596; with permission.)

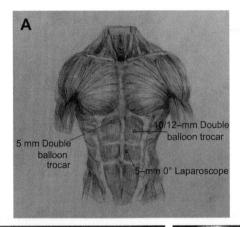

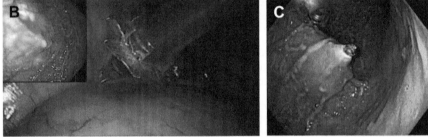

Fig. 12. LTGS setup. (*A*) Trocar placement. (*B*) Trocar placement, laparoscopic view. (*C*) Trocar placement, endoscopic view. (*Data from* Barajas-Gamboa JS, Acosta G, Savides TJ, et al. Laparo-endoscopic transgastric resection of gastric submucosal tumors. Surg Endosc 2015;29:2151; with permission.)

narrow connection with the MP layer, and it appears to be possible to remove type II lesions through endoscopic enucleation or EFTR. Type III can be managed by EFTR, but laparoendoscopic full-thickness resection may provide a more invasive but possibly technically easier option for safe R0 resection. Achieving complete resection

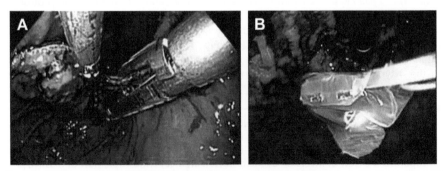

Fig. 13. LTGS procedure. (*A*) Tumor resection and stapling. (*B*) Tumor extraction using an endobag. (*Data from* Barajas-Gamboa JS, Acosta G, Savides TJ, et al. Laparo-endoscopic transgastric resection of gastric submucosal tumors. Surg Endosc 2015;29:2152; with permission.)

Table 2
Publications reporting laparoscopic transgastric surgery for subepithelial tumors in the upper gastrointestinal tract

Reference	No.	Mean Operation Time, min	Mean Tumor Diameter, mm	Complete Resection Rate, %	Complications
Barajas-Gamboa et al,[70] 2015	8[a]	84	33	100[b]	2 postoperative bleedings
Wilhelm et al,[71] 2008	34	114	28.5	100[b]	[c]
Privette et al,[72] 2008	4	236	46	100[b]	1 postoperative bleeding[d]

[a] Five of 14 patients had conversions to traditional laparoscopic surgery, and in 1 of 14 patients the resection was aborted.
[b] Pathologically evaluated.
[c] Cannot be assessed due to heterogeneous data.
[d] Patient with von Willebrand disease.

of type IV SETs through EFTR is technically challenging and requires extensive experience and skill in endoscopic resection. Laparoendoscopic full-thickness resection may be a technically less challenging option for type IV tumors and thus provide a more controlled and potentially safer resection but at the cost of higher invasiveness (laparoscopic surgery). Until now, LECS and LAEFR have shown excellent outcomes. The best indication for LECS and LAEFR may be the presence of gastric SETs growing in an intraluminal direction (types I and II) originating from the MP layer. Such lesions cannot be easily identified from the serosal side of the stomach; therefore, there is a high probability that conventional laparoscopic wedge resection will lead to the resection of more tissue than expected and cause gastric deformity or stenosis or, conversely, produce a positive surgical margin.[62] LECS or LAEFR can be used to avoid such problems, as a relatively larger specimen and a pathologically acceptable resection margin can be more easily obtained while minimizing the amount of tissue resected.[62,66,67,74] Inverted LECS was devised for GC, but this technique can cause spillage of tumor cells into the peritoneal cavity, and, thus, it cannot be implemented without more clinical data.[9,68] CLEAN-NET and NEWS were developed to use the mucosal barrier to prevent tumor seeding.[10,65,69] These 2 techniques are promising for type III and IV SETs with ulceration and resection of GC. However, the size limitation of a target SET lesion is thought to be 3 cm, and the EGJ and pyloric ring are difficult areas in which to work. LTGS also can be categorized as a nonexposure technique and might be the most feasible procedure for type I and II lesions along the posterior wall of the stomach that are 3 cm or smaller. The recommended lesions for each technique are summarized in **Table 3**.

LAPAROENDOSCOPIC COLLABORATIVE PROCEDURES FOR TREATMENT OF COLON NEOPLASMS

As early as 1993, laparoendoscopic procedures for the excision of large colonic polyps were described as alternatives to colectomy.[75] These procedures involve laparoscopic mobilization and external visualization of the colonic wall to permit the use of more aggressive colonoscopic polypectomy techniques, and they include LAER, endoscopy-assisted laparoscopic wedge resection (EAWR), endoscopy-assisted laparoscopic transluminal resection (EATR), and endoscopy-assisted laparoscopic

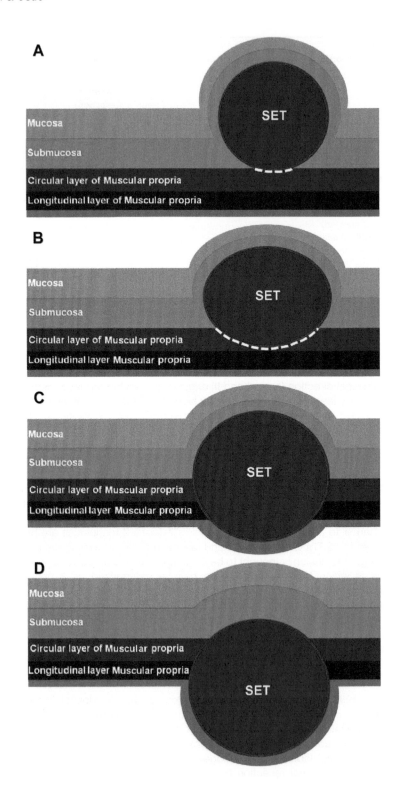

Table 3
Recommended lesions for laparoendoscopic full-thickness resection procedures

Characteristics of SETs	LECS	LAEFR	Inverted LECS	CLEAN-NET	NEWS	LTGS
Appropriate SET type	I, II	I, II	I, II	III, IV	III, IV	I, II
SET with mucosal ulceration	No	No	Equivocal	Yes	Yes	Yes
Tumor location	Any location	Any location	Any location	Except EGJ or pyloric ring	Except EGJ or pyloric ring	Except pyloric ring
Tumor size	≤5 cm	≤5 cm	≤5 cm	≤3 cm	≤3 cm	≤3 cm
Indication for early gastric cancer	No	No	Equivocal	Yes	Yes	No

Abbreviations: CLEAN-NET, combination of laparoscopic and endoscopic approaches to neoplasia with a nonexposure technique; EGJ, esophagogastric junction; LAEFR, laparoscopy-assisted endoscopic full-thickness resection; LECS, laparoscopic and endoscopic cooperative surgery; LTGS; laparoscopic transgastric surgery; NEWS, nonexposed endoscopic wall-inversion surgery.

segment resection (EASR).[76–80] In EAWR, EATR, and EASR, endoscopy was used to identify laparoscopic resection points.[78–80] ESD, of course, is an excellent organ-saving technique in cases of colon polyps and early CRC,[81,82] but it is time-consuming, and there is a greater risk of perforation and bleeding.[83,84] With new technologies, laparoendoscopic full-thickness resection may be another option for safer, faster, and more secure R0 resection for colonic neoplasia. We describe the LAER procedures that are currently performed and introduce FLEX and eFLEX procedures as new options for difficult colon polyps and early CRC resection.[23,26]

Procedure Setup

a. Under general anesthesia and after placing a nasogastric tube and urethral catheter, the patients are placed in a modified lithotomy position to allow for anal access[59] (**Fig. 15**).
b. Laparoscopy and colonoscopy monitors are placed in the room, depending on the colonic segment involved, to provide a good view for the surgeon and colonoscopist.
c. The patient is draped in the abdomen and anal regions, and the procedure begins with the establishment of pneumoperitoneum with carbon dioxide.
d. A camera port is inserted into the inferior umbilical position using an open technique.
e. A 5-mm cannula with a trocar is introduced in the contralateral flank or an area in which there has been no previous surgery, followed by a 5-mm laparoscope and

Fig. 14. Classification of SETs according to their location in the gastric wall. (*A*) Type I is a SET that has a very narrow connection with the proper muscle layer and protrudes into the luminal side like a polyp. (*B*) Type II has a wider connection with the proper muscle layer and protrudes into the luminal side at an obtuse angle. (*C*) Type III is located in the middle of the gastric wall. (*D*) Type IV protrudes mainly into the serosal side of the gastric wall. White dotted lines indicate the area dissected from the proper muscle layer.

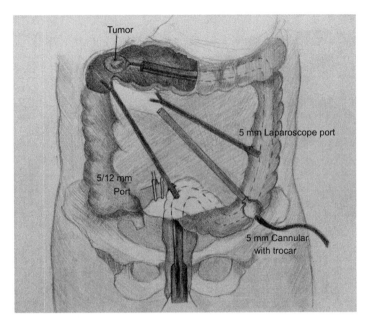

Fig. 15. LAER for colon neoplasms. Operative setup: 5-mm cannula with a trocar is introduced in the contralateral flank or where there has been no previous surgery, followed by a 5-mm laparoscope and additional ports (5/12 mm) distributed according to lesion location.

additional ports (5 or 5/12 mm under direct vision) distributed according to the lesion site.

Laparoscopy-Assisted Endoscopic Resection

Laparoscopically assisted procedures can serve as alternatives to colonic resection for extensive or inaccessible polyps. Franklin and colleagues[76] reported on a series of 110 patients undergoing colonoscopic polypectomy following laparoscopic mobilization of the colon. Other reports have described the utility of this technique.[24,25,77,85,86] Laparoscopic colonic mobilization has the potential to orient the colon to a more favorable and stable position and to facilitate intraoperative endoscopic mucosal resection (EMR) using a colonoscope. It also allows the identification of sites of potential iatrogenic bowel injury, with the option of immediate laparoscopic repair.

Laparoscopically assisted endoscopic resection procedure

a. After the procedure setup, abdominal exploration and lysis of adhesions are performed, as needed (**Fig. 16**).
b. The affected segment or segments are identified, and mobilization of the area is performed, similar to resection.
c. The vascular structures are isolated and preserved.
d. The bowel is clamped proximally with 2 laparoscopic bulldog clamps to prevent distension of the proximal bowel as colonoscopy is instituted. This step is crucial because loss of domain makes it difficult to perform resection if needed.

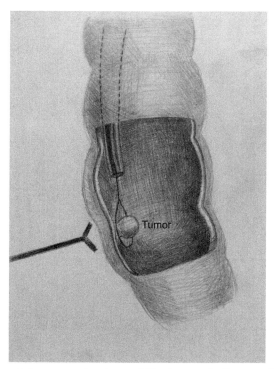

Fig. 16. LAER concept. Laparoscopic colon mobilization can facilitate endoscopic resection.

e. Colonoscopy is performed, frequently aided by laparoscopic manipulation of the sigmoid colon.
f. The polyp is located with the colonoscope, and its position is noted through laparoscopic visualization, often with the use of transillumination. The colon segment is mobilized by laparoscopic maneuvering. Consistent efforts are made to expose the base of the polyp.
g. Polypectomy, EMR, or ESD is performed with the aid of laparoscopic manipulation.
h. The specimen is extracted transanally, and seromuscular sutures are placed when an obvious perforation or full-thickness burn is present or when it is considered necessary to avoid partial-thickness injuries manifested at a later time.
i. If an invasive neoplasm is suspected during the resection, intraoperative pathology assessment of frozen sections can be obtained and, depending on the findings, the procedure is concluded or converted to laparoscopic resection if needed.

Laparoscopically assisted endoscopic resection advantages
LAER represents an alternative that may obviate the need for colonic resection in a select group of patients. Complete colonoscopic excision of these types of polyps can be safely undertaken using laparoscopic assistance, which enables prompt diagnosis and treatment of any perforation or full-thickness injury as well as manipulation of the polyp to allow resection.

Laparoscopically assisted endoscopic resection limitations
Several types of laparoscopic surgery–associated complications can occur after LAER, including atelectasis due to general anesthesia (**Table 4**).[78,87–90]

Table 4
Outcomes of laparoendoscopic collaborative procedures for colon polyps

Reference	Method	No.	Mean Operation Time, min	Mean Polyp Size, mm	Successful Removal, %	Complications
Lee et al,[91] 2013	LAER	5	159	23	100	0
Goh et al,[87] 2014	LAER	30	105	—	73[a]	3 postoperative bleeding, 1 ileus, and 3 urinary tract infection
Wilhelm et al,[78] 2009	LAER	8	75	—	95[b]	25%[c]
	EAWR	72	92			
	EATR	40	93			
	EASR	26	123			
Yan et al,[92] 2011	LAER or EAWR	23	—	30	87[e]	0
Cruz et al,[88] 2011	LAER	25	92.7	24	76[d]	1 ileus and 1 abdominal abscess
Franklin & Portillo,[90] 2009	LAER	176	96.5	36.9	87.5[f]	9 atelectasis, 3 seroma, and 4 ileus
Franklin et al,[89] 2000	LAER	47	—	28	89.4[g]	1 seroma

Abbreviations: EASR, endoscopic-assisted segmental resection; EATR, endoscopy-assisted transluminal resection; EAWR, endoscopic-assisted wedge resection; LAER, laparoscopic-assisted endoscopic resection.

[a] Eight (26.6%) of 30 procedures were converted to colotomy or laparoscopic colectomy due to the following: 2 patients, large polyps; 3 patients, polyps in difficult locations; 2 failed polypectomies; 1 ulcer.

[b] Conversion to open surgery was required in 5% (7/146) of patients due to the following: 3 lesions suspected of being malignant, 1 bowel perforation during colonoscopy in a patient with severe adhesions, 2 difficult closures of the colostomy site, 1 incomplete resection of a polyp.

[c] Complications were reported in 25% (36/146); wound infections, 9.6% (14/146); urinary tract infections, 3.4% (5/146); intra-abdominal abscesses, 2.7% (4/146); delayed bleeding,1.4% (2/146); phlegmon, 1 patient; and cardiac arrhythmias in 1 patient during surgery. Reoperation was necessary in 11% (16/146) of patients due to the following: 7 postoperative complications and 9 patients with pathologic confirmation of malignant disease.

[d] Operative failure was due to failed elevation of the polyp by submucosal saline injected. Conversion to laparoscopic colectomy was required in 4% (1/25) of patients treated by LAER due to intraoperative diagnosis of adenocarcinoma.

[e] Three (13%) of 23 patients were converted to laparoscopic resection after laparoendoscopic evaluations: 2 patients, failed elevation of the polyp: 1 patient, identification of a polyp larger than 5 cm in diameter.

[f] Four (2.3%) of 176 patients were converted to a "formal resection" due to failure of the combined approach; 10.2% (18/176) of patients were converted to a "formal resection" due to histopathological evidence of cancer.

[g] Conversion to other types of surgical procedures was required in 10.6% (5/47) of patients: 3 patients, laparoscopic segmental resection for malignancy that had not been diagnosed preoperatively; 2 patients with benign disease, laparoscopic segmental resection due to circumferential involvement; 2 patients with benign to pathologic diagnosis, colotomy due to large polyps (>6 cm).

Outcomes of laparoscopically assisted endoscopic resection and other collaborative
procedures for treatment of colon neoplasms

Although ESD is frequently practiced in the Eastern world to resect large colonic polyps, the procedure is technically demanding and time-consuming, even for experts.[83,84] Hence, for large colonic polyps occupying more than one-third of the bowel circumference or spanning more than 2 haustral folds, the laparoendoscopic collaborative procedure is a viable treatment option. The laparoendoscopic collaborative procedure can be performed using several techniques, including LAER, EAWR, EATR, and EASR.[91] The overall success rate of polyp resection is between 74% and 100% (see **Table 4**).[76,78,87–92] The morbidity rate is 3% to 10%, with a short hospital stay of 1 to 2 days. The polyp recurrence rate at the same location is between 2% and 5%. Therefore, this approach appears to be feasible, safe, and associated with a high success rate.

Full-Thickness Laparoendoscopic Excision and Eversion Full-Thickness Laparoendoscopic Excision

The FLEX and eFLEX techniques involve the use of BraceBars (Olympus Medical Systems, Olympus KeyMed, Southend-on-Sea, UK) to create an artificial polyplike structure for easy removal via endoscopic resection (FLEX) and laparoscopic resection (eFLEX) (**Fig. 17**). The major difference between FLEX and eFLEX is the direction in which the lesion and surrounding colonic wall is plicated.[23,26] FLEX involves the

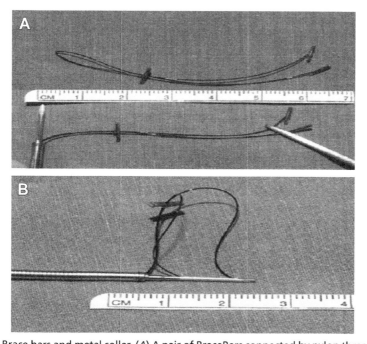

Fig. 17. Brace bars and metal collar. (*A*) A pair of BraceBars connected by nylon thread and a metal collar used to approximate the BraceBars when deployed is shown alone and secured in a needle catheter. (*B*) Brace bars are preloaded into the needle before the needle and the metal collar are retracted into the catheter. (*Data from* Brigic A, Southgate A, Sibbons P, et al. Full-thickness laparoendoscopic colonic excision in an experimental model. Br J Surg 2013;100:1650; with permission.)

inversion of a lesion toward the luminal side of the colon, and the procedure is finalized with endoscopic resection. In contrast, eFLEX involves the eversion of a lesion toward the extraluminal side of the colon, and laparoscopic resection is the final step.

Full-thickness laparoendoscopic excision procedure

a. Argon plasma coagulation marks are placed 1 cm lateral to the polyp to mark the excision line (**Fig. 18**).
b. Hook diathermy of the serosa 1 cm outside the argon mark identifies the BraceBar placement sites, guided by endoscopic counter pressure.
c. The BraceBar is placed laparoscopically, and the collar is tightened down to plicate the colon; after 3 BraceBars are placed, all are cinched together to achieve inversion of a fold containing the "pseudopolyp" into the colonic lumen.
d. The BraceBars are oversewn laparoscopically with 2 layers of continuous sutures.
e. The prior steps essentially achieve "pre-closure" of the anticipated full-thickness defect before proceeding with EFTR. EFTR of the polyp can then be efficiently and safely performed via the colonoscope. If necessary, a second endoscope can be used to apply traction on the lesion and ensure complete resection of the inverted lesion.

Eversion full-thickness laparoendoscopic excision procedure

a. Argon plasma coagulation (APC) marks 1 cm away from the edge of the polyp delineate the proximal and distal resection margins. A single APC mark is placed at 3 o'clock and 9 o'clock (**Fig. 19**).
b. Endoscopic placement of BraceBars is performed guided by the APC marks, and eversion of the bowel area is achieved by tightening the BraceBars.
c. The everted polypoid protuberance is resected using a laparoscopic linear stapler; the stapler is placed below the BraceBars to ensure an adequate clearance margin, and the colonic defect is closed simultaneously by the stapler.

Full-thickness laparoendoscopic excision and eversion full-thickness laparoendoscopic excision advantages

FLEX and eFLEX are effective and safe methods of achieving full-thickness resection of colon polyps with diameters exceeding 2 cm without any risk of spillage of intraluminal contents or cells into the peritoneal cavity.[23,26] The possible benefits of the technique over conventional segmental colectomy likely include enhanced postoperative recovery along with preservation of the bowel length (and, therefore, function). Because the excision avoids pan-circumferential resection, impairment of the blood supply is avoided; thus, the likelihood of anastomotic leakage may be reduced.

Full-thickness laparoendoscopic excision and eversion full-thickness laparoendoscopic excision limitations

When considering the favorable data reported from animal studies, differences between porcine and human anatomy should be considered. For example, the mesentery and marginal vessels could impede the procedure in humans. Retroperitoneal locations are likely to require colonic mobilization to allow access, as suggested by Wilhelm and colleagues[78] and Franklin and colleagues[76] Computed tomographic colonography would clarify the locations of the polyps in relation to the mesentery and retroperitoneum, facilitating surgical planning. It is likely that a proportion of polyps will not be suitable for this procedure, particularly those located on the mesenteric border.

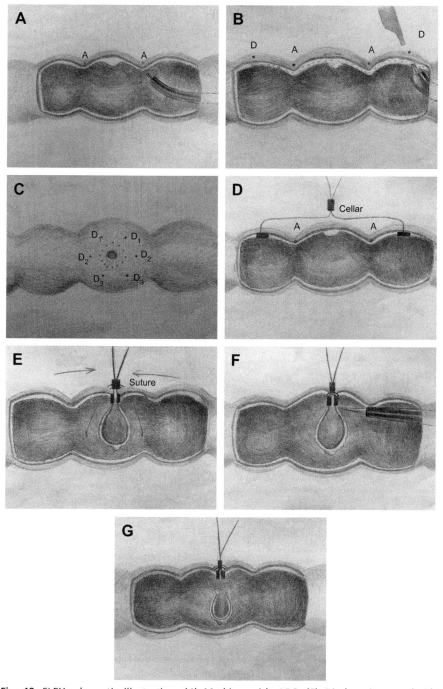

Fig. 18. FLEX schematic illustration. (*A*) Marking with APC. (*B*) Diathermic serosal side marking by laparoscope with endoscopic guidance and aid. (*C*) Serosal side markings for brace bars. (*D*) Brace bars placed by laparoscopy. (*E*) The collar is tightened (*arrows* outside the colon) and the tissue encircling the lesion is inverted to the luminal side forming a pseudopolyp (*arrows* inside the colon). This is followed by a 2-layer suture at the serosal side. (*F*) Endoscopic resection is performed with the aid of a grasper (*arrows*). (*G*) Full-thickness resection is completed.

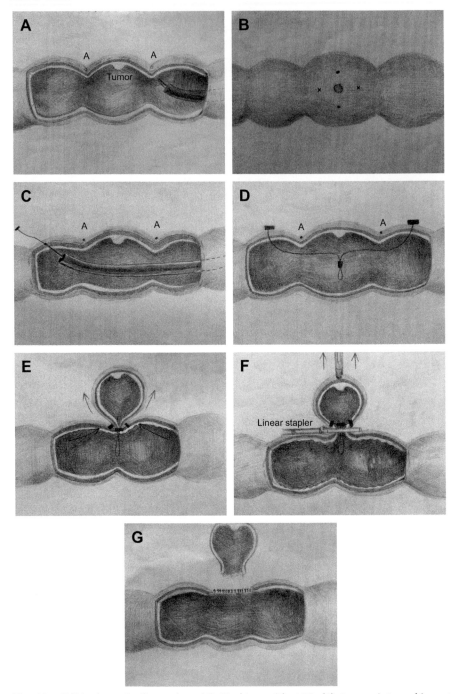

Fig. 19. eFLEX schematic illustration. (*A*) Marking with APC. (*B*) Four-point marking at luminal side. (*C*) Brace bars placed by endoscopy. (*D*) Deployed BraceBars. (*E*) Tightening of the collar of the BraceBars (*arrows* inside the colon) results in eversion of the tissue around the lesion and the lesion itself toward the peritoneal side forming a pseudopolyp (*arrows* outside the colon). (*F*) Laparoscopic resection of this pseudopolyp containing the lesion is performed with the aid of a grasper (*arrows*). (*G*) Full-thickness resection is completed.

*Full-thickness laparoendoscopic excision and eversion full-thickness
laparoendoscopic excision outcomes*

FLEX and eFLEX are still being tested in animal studies; therefore, only porcine study results can be described. All procedures were completed without complications. The FLEX procedure required a long operative time (201–245 minutes for specimens 2–3 cm in size), but eFLEX required only a short procedure time (20–31 minutes from marking to specimen excision for specimens 4.5–6.3 cm in size) (**Fig. 20**). Therefore, eFLEX was much faster and could be used to remove larger specimens.

ADVANTAGES OF LAPAROENDOSCOPIC COOPERATIVE SURGERY OVER ENDOSCOPY ALONE

Although endoscopy-only procedures, such as endoscopic enucleation and EFTR, appear to be more attractive as minimally invasive operations, laparoendoscopic hybrid techniques have important advantages. The most important advantage is obviously possibly an increased likelihood of an R0 resection. Although careful pure EFTR should achieve R0 resection by completely removing the tumor along with the full thickness of the gastrointestinal wall from which it arises, in cases of endoscopic enucleation, there may be remnant GIST tissue at the deep margin resulting in an R1 resection. Most studies have only assessed en bloc resection.[93–96] The dissection surface is ablated with an electrical knife or snare; therefore, there may be no remnant GIST cells even when R1 resection is achieved (**Fig. 21**). Although this assertion seems logical, no data supporting this hypothesis have been reported. Moreover, a recent study reported that a 5.8% local recurrence rate was observed even when complete endoscopic resection was achieved in all cases.[97] Another advantage is a higher likelihood that the capsule remains intact during the entire local resection when laparoendoscopic full-thickness resection is performed, whereas endoscopic enucleation and EFTR may be more likely to cause capsule injury and perforation simultaneously. In particular, in the case of endoscopic enucleation, perforation is usually accompanied by pseudocapsule injury. Therefore, the possibility of peritoneal seeding increases.

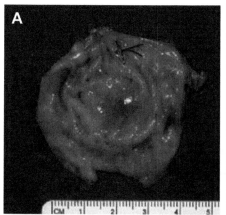 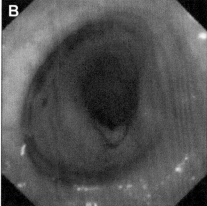

Fig. 20. Outcome of eFLEX. (*A*) An opened excision specimen 5 cm in diameter with APC markings delineating a tumor-free margin. (*B*) Endoscopic view of a partially circumferential stapled anastomosis after resection demonstrating a patent lumen in a surviving animal. (*Data from* Brigic A, Southgate A, Sibbons P, et al. Full-thickness laparoendoscopic colonic excision in an experimental model. Br J Surg 2013;100:1652; with permission.)

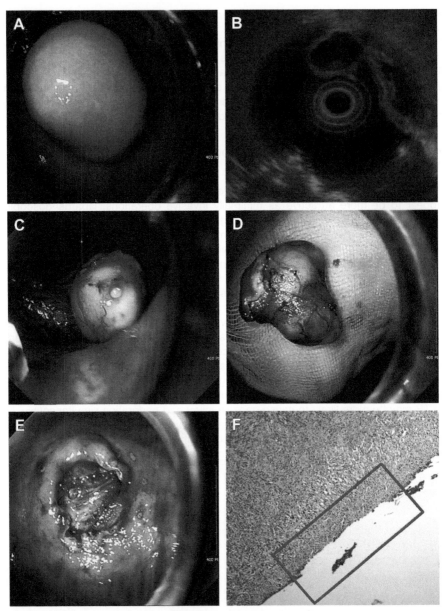

Fig. 21. R1 resection after en block endoscopic enucleation. (*A*) An approximately 2.5-cm SET is identified at the greater curvature side of the upper body of the stomach. (*B*) Endoscopic ultrasound image demonstrating 2.6-cm mixed echogenic tumor with a slightly irregular border arising from the proper muscle layer. (*C*) Endoscopic enucleation using ESD technique is performed. (*D*) En bloc resection is achieved. (*E*) There is no perforation at the operation site. (*F*) On pathologic examination, a vertical resection margin is apparently involved with tumor cells (*red boxed area*) (hematoxylin eosin stain, magnification × 10); R1 resection is confirmed. (*Courtesy of* Kyung Oh Kim, MD, PhD, Gil Hospital, Incheon, Korea.)

Peritoneal seeding is accompanied by a high recurrence rate and can result in a poor prognosis. If MP layer dissection does not cause perforation, capsule injury may not be a serious problem; the tumor cells will shed into the lumen of the gut and will be destroyed. However, there is some likelihood of concomitant perforation and capsule rupture or injury during the procedure, particularly in cases in which there is difficulty performing the procedure. In such situations, shedding of tumor cells into the peritoneal cavity may occur. A third advantage is that laparoendoscopic full-thickness resection allows closure of the artificial perforation by laparoscopic means, which may be easier and more secure than what can be achieved by some of the endoscopic methods (such as clips and endoloops) used during EFTR.[98,99] In EFTR, the surgeon performing the resection must have advanced skills to close the sizable 2-cm to 3-cm iatrogenic perforation that results from EFTR. EFTR is also limited by tumor size (ie, <4 cm for SETs) and location.[73] Finally, laparoendoscopic full-thickness resection can be used to perform SN biopsy or SN basin dissection in a minimally destructive way in patients with GC or CRC. Nevertheless, a pure endoscopic approach, such as EFTR, is significantly less invasive than hybrid approaches that involve laparoscopic surgery. Therefore, more comparative data are needed, particularly in light of recent EFTR technique improvements, such as the use of endoscopic suturing for closure of the iatrogenic perforation, a technique that may be more efficient and secure than closure with endoscopic clips and endoloops.

THE POTENTIAL TO BE A BRIDGE TO ENDOSCOPIC FULL-THICKNESS RESECTION

It should be noted that although EFTR is currently being performed in clinical settings, the performance of this technique requires great skill. Note that endoscopists can perform more aggressive procedures with the aid of laparoscopists, and unexpected complications can be readily managed through laparoscopic treatment. Thus, accumulating laparoendoscopic full-thickness resection experience and developing surgical skill would be preferable compared with relying on endoscopy alone. After developing a skillful technique, endoscopists can be less dependent on laparoscopic assistance and can eventually initiate and complete the procedure independently.

SUMMARY

Due to advances in modern medical technology, various endoscopic procedures have emerged that have challenged conventional surgical techniques. In terms of its theoretic efficacy and technical feasibility, laparoendoscopic full thickness resection is considered to be an appropriate option for removal of upper gastrointestinal SETs, particularly GISTs, and it is superior to procedures involving endoscopy alone. However, it is too early to use laparoendoscopic full thickness resection for GC or CRC with only SN biopsy or SN basin dissection because the SN concept has not yet been fully developed. In managing difficult colon polyps, laparoendoscopic collaborative procedures appear to be feasible and safe. Moreover, new techniques are being developed, although ESD is a powerful tool in this field. If the clinical outcomes of FLEX and eFLEX are similar to those of ESD, faster, safer, and easier surgical procedures can be performed. Complete EFTR would be an attractive operation for both endoscopists and patients. However, we know that there are many hurdles to overcome. Improving operator technique is the most important factor related to successful EFTR. We are certain that endoscopists can easily become more active and more comfortable with laparoscopic techniques. Completion of LEFR procedures can provide valuable experience for endoscopists, who can use their EFTR skill in a safe environment.

REFERENCES

1. Choi SM, Kim MC, Jung GJ, et al. Laparoscopic wedge resection for gastric GIST: long-term follow-up results. Eur J Surg Oncol 2007;33:444–7.
2. Ohgami M, Otani Y, Kumai K, et al. Curative laparoscopic surgery for early gastric cancer: five years experience. World J Surg 1999;23:187–92 [discussion: 92–3].
3. Yano H, Kimura Y, Iwazawa T, et al. Hand-assisted laparoscopic surgery for a large gastrointestinal stromal tumor of the stomach. Gastric Cancer 2005;8: 186–92.
4. Hyung WJ, Lim JS, Cheong JH, et al. Laparoscopic resection of a huge intraluminal gastric submucosal tumor located in the anterior wall: eversion method. J Surg Oncol 2005;89:95–8.
5. Ludwig K, Wilhelm L, Scharlau U, et al. Laparoscopic-endoscopic rendezvous resection of gastric tumors. Surg Endosc 2002;16:1561–5.
6. Ridwelski K, Pross M, Schubert S, et al. Combined endoscopic intragastral resection of a posterior stromal gastric tumor using an original technique. Surg Endosc 2002;16:537.
7. Gotoda T, Yanagisawa A, Sasako M, et al. Incidence of lymph node metastasis from early gastric cancer: estimation with a large number of cases at two large centers. Gastric Cancer 2000;3:219–25.
8. Hiki N, Yamamoto Y, Fukunaga T, et al. Laparoscopic and endoscopic cooperative surgery for gastrointestinal stromal tumor dissection. Surg Endosc 2008; 22:1729–35.
9. Nunobe S, Hiki N, Gotoda T, et al. Successful application of laparoscopic and endoscopic cooperative surgery (LECS) for a lateral-spreading mucosal gastric cancer. Gastric Cancer 2012;15:338–42.
10. Inoue H, Ikeda H, Hosoya T, et al. Endoscopic mucosal resection, endoscopic submucosal dissection, and beyond: full-layer resection for gastric cancer with nonexposure technique (CLEAN-NET). Surg Oncol Clin N Am 2012;21:129–40.
11. Mitsui T, Goto O, Shimizu N, et al. Novel technique for full-thickness resection of gastric malignancy: feasibility of nonexposed endoscopic wall-inversion surgery (news) in porcine models. Surg Laparosc Endosc Percutan Tech 2013;23: e217–21.
12. Goto O, Mitsui T, Fujishiro M, et al. New method of endoscopic full-thickness resection: a pilot study of non-exposed endoscopic wall-inversion surgery in an ex vivo porcine model. Gastric Cancer 2011;14:183–7.
13. Goto O, Takeuchi H, Kawakubo H, et al. Feasibility of non-exposed endoscopic wall-inversion surgery with sentinel node basin dissection as a new surgical method for early gastric cancer: a porcine survival study. Gastric Cancer 2015;18:440–5.
14. Dong HY, Wang YL, Li J, et al. New-style laparoscopic and endoscopic cooperative surgery for gastric stromal tumors. World J Gastroenterol 2013;19:2550–4.
15. Lips DJ, Schutte HW, van der Linden RL, et al. Sentinel lymph node biopsy to direct treatment in gastric cancer. A systematic review of the literature. Eur J Surg Oncol 2011;37:655–61.
16. Ryu KW. The future of sentinel node oriented tailored approach in patients with early gastric cancer. J Gastric Cancer 2012;12:1–2.
17. Wang Z, Dong ZY, Chen JQ, et al. Diagnostic value of sentinel lymph node biopsy in gastric cancer: a meta-analysis. Ann Surg Oncol 2012;19:1541–50.

18. Tsioulias GJ, Wood TF, Spirt M, et al. A novel lymphatic mapping technique to improve localization and staging of early colon cancer during laparoscopic colectomy. Am Surg 2002;68:561–5.

19. Bilchik AJ, Trocha SD. Lymphatic mapping and sentinel node analysis to optimize laparoscopic resection and staging of colorectal cancer: an update. Cancer Control 2003;10:219–23.

20. Nagata K, Endo S, Hidaka E, et al. Laparoscopic sentinel node mapping for colorectal cancer using infrared ray laparoscopy. Anticancer Res 2006;26:2307–11.

21. Bianchi PP, Ceriani C, Rottoli M, et al. Laparoscopic lymphatic mapping and sentinel lymph node detection in colon cancer: technical aspects and preliminary results. Surg Endosc 2007;21:1567–71.

22. Rivet EB, Mutch MG, Ritter JH, et al. Ex vivo sentinel lymph node mapping in laparoscopic resection of colon cancer. Colorectal Dis 2011;13:1249–55.

23. Brigic A, Southgate A, Sibbons P, et al. Full-thickness laparoendoscopic colonic excision in an experimental model. Br J Surg 2013;100:1649–54.

24. Smedh K, Skullman S, Kald A, et al. Laparoscopic bowel mobilization combined with intraoperative colonoscopic polypectomy in patients with an inaccessible polyp of the colon. Surg Endosc 1997;11:643–4.

25. Hensman C, Luck AJ, Hewett PJ. Laparoscopic-assisted colonoscopic polypectomy: technique and preliminary experience. Surg Endosc 1999;13:231–2.

26. Kennedy RH, Cahill RA, Sibbons P, et al. The "FLEX" procedure: a new technique for full-thickness laparo-endoscopic excision in the colon. Endoscopy 2011;43:223–9.

27. Kang HC, Menias CO, Gaballah AH, et al. Beyond the GIST: mesenchymal tumors of the stomach. Radiographics 2013;33:1673–90.

28. Miettinen M, Lasota J. Gastrointestinal stromal tumors: review on morphology, molecular pathology, prognosis, and differential diagnosis. Arch Pathol Lab Med 2006;130:1466–78.

29. Arber DA, Tamayo R, Weiss LM. Paraffin section detection of the c-kit gene product (CD117) in human tissues: value in the diagnosis of mast cell disorders. Hum Pathol 1998;29:498–504.

30. Aparicio T, Boige V, Sabourin JC, et al. Prognostic factors after surgery of primary resectable gastrointestinal stromal tumours. Eur J Surg Oncol 2004;30:1098–103.

31. Tashiro T, Hasegawa T, Omatsu M, et al. Gastrointestinal stromal tumour of the stomach showing lymph node metastases. Histopathology 2005;47:438–9.

32. Demetri GD, von Mehren M, Antonescu CR, et al. NCCN Task Force report: update on the management of patients with gastrointestinal stromal tumors. J Natl Compr Canc Netw 2010;8(Suppl 2):S1–41 [quiz: S2–4].

33. Catena F, Di Battista M, Fusaroli P, et al. Laparoscopic treatment of gastric GIST: report of 21 cases and literature's review. J Gastrointest Surg 2008;12:561–8.

34. Bedard EL, Mamazza J, Schlachta CM, et al. Laparoscopic resection of gastrointestinal stromal tumors: not all tumors are created equal. Surg Endosc 2006;20:500–3.

35. Huguet KL, Rush RM Jr, Tessier DJ, et al. Laparoscopic gastric gastrointestinal stromal tumor resection: the Mayo Clinic experience. Arch Surg 2008;143:587–90 [discussion: 91].

36. Lai IR, Lee WJ, Yu SC. Minimally invasive surgery for gastric stromal cell tumors: intermediate follow-up results. J Gastrointest Surg 2006;10:563–6.

37. Nguyen SQ, Divino CM, Wang JL, et al. Laparoscopic management of gastrointestinal stromal tumors. Surg Endosc 2006;20:713–6.

38. Novitsky YW, Kercher KW, Sing RF, et al. Long-term outcomes of laparoscopic resection of gastric gastrointestinal stromal tumors. Ann Surg 2006;243: 738–45 [discussion: 45–7].

39. Rivera RE, Eagon JC, Soper NJ, et al. Experience with laparoscopic gastric resection: results and outcomes for 37 cases. Surg Endosc 2005;19:1622–6.

40. McCarter MD, Antonescu CR, Ballman KV, et al. Microscopically positive margins for primary gastrointestinal stromal tumors: analysis of risk factors and tumor recurrence. J Am Coll Surg 2012;215:53–9 [discussion: 9–60].

41. DeMatteo RP, Lewis JJ, Leung D, et al. Two hundred gastrointestinal stromal tumors: recurrence patterns and prognostic factors for survival. Ann Surg 2000; 231:51–8.

42. Catena F, Di Battista M, Ansaloni L, et al. Microscopic margins of resection influence primary gastrointestinal stromal tumor survival. Onkologie 2012;35: 645–8.

43. Lacy AM, Ibarzabal A. Gastric surgery and notes. Curr Gastroenterol Rep 2012; 14:460–6.

44. Guillou PJ, Quirke P, Thorpe H, et al. Short-term endpoints of conventional versus laparoscopic-assisted surgery in patients with colorectal cancer (MRC CLASICC trial): multicentre, randomised controlled trial. Lancet 2005;365: 1718–26.

45. Arezzo A, Passera R, Scozzari G, et al. Laparoscopy for rectal cancer reduces short-term mortality and morbidity: results of a systematic review and meta-analysis. Surg Endosc 2013;27:1485–502.

46. Cho WY, Kim YJ, Cho JY, et al. Hybrid natural orifice transluminal endoscopic surgery: endoscopic full-thickness resection of early gastric cancer and laparoscopic regional lymph node dissection–14 human cases. Endoscopy 2011;43: 134–9.

47. Kitagawa Y, Fujii H, Mukai M, et al. Radio-guided sentinel node detection for gastric cancer. Br J Surg 2002;89:604–8.

48. Becher RD, Shen P, Stewart JH, et al. Sentinel lymph node mapping for gastric adenocarcinoma. Am Surg 2009;75:710–4.

49. Tajima Y, Yamazaki K, Masuda Y, et al. Sentinel node mapping guided by indocyanine green fluorescence imaging in gastric cancer. Ann Surg 2009;249: 58–62.

50. Kelder W, Nimura H, Takahashi N, et al. Sentinel node mapping with indocyanine green (ICG) and infrared ray detection in early gastric cancer: an accurate method that enables a limited lymphadenectomy. Eur J Surg Oncol 2010;36: 552–8.

51. Miyashiro I, Hiratsuka M, Sasako M, et al. High false-negative proportion of intraoperative histological examination as a serious problem for clinical application of sentinel node biopsy for early gastric cancer: final results of the Japan Clinical Oncology Group multicenter trial JCOG0302. Gastric Cancer 2014;17:316–23.

52. Ryu KW, Eom BW, Nam BH, et al. Is the sentinel node biopsy clinically applicable for limited lymphadenectomy and modified gastric resection in gastric cancer? A meta-analysis of feasibility studies. J Surg Oncol 2011;104:578–84.

53. Stojanovic D, Milenkovic SM, Mitrovic N, et al. The feasibility of sentinel lymph node biopsy for gastric cancer: the experience from Serbia. J BUON 2013;18: 162–8.

54. Dong LF, Wang LB, Shen JG, et al. Sentinel lymph node biopsy predicts lymph node metastasis in early gastric cancer: a retrospective analysis. Dig Surg 2012;29:124–9.

55. Tonouchi H, Mohri Y, Tanaka K, et al. Laparoscopic lymphatic mapping and sentinel node biopsies for early-stage gastric cancer: the cause of false negativity. World J Surg 2005;29:418–21.

56. Ichikura T, Chochi K, Sugasawa H, et al. Individualized surgery for early gastric cancer guided by sentinel node biopsy. Surgery 2006;139:501–7.

57. Pedrazzani C, Moro M, Ghezzi G, et al. What should we intend for minimally invasive treatment of colorectal cancer? Surg Oncol 2014;23:147–54.

58. van der Zaag ES, Bouma WH, Tanis PJ, et al. Systematic review of sentinel lymph node mapping procedure in colorectal cancer. Ann Surg Oncol 2012; 19:3449–59.

59. Mori H, Kobara H, Fujihara S, et al. Establishment of the hybrid endoscopic full-thickness resection of gastric gastrointestinal stromal tumors. Mol Clin Oncol 2015;3:18–22.

60. Izumi Y, Inoue H, Endo M. Combined endoluminal-intracavitary thoracoscopic enucleation of leiomyoma of the esophagus. A new method. Surg Endosc 1996;10:457–8.

61. Tsujimoto H, Yaguchi Y, Kumano I, et al. Successful gastric submucosal tumor resection using laparoscopic and endoscopic cooperative surgery. World J Surg 2012;36:327–30.

62. Abe N, Takeuchi H, Ooki A, et al. Recent developments in gastric endoscopic submucosal dissection: towards the era of endoscopic resection of layers deeper than the submucosa. Dig Endosc 2013;25(Suppl 1):64–70.

63. Qiu WQ, Zhuang J, Wang M, et al. Minimally invasive treatment of laparoscopic and endoscopic cooperative surgery for patients with gastric gastrointestinal stromal tumors. J Dig Dis 2013;14:469–73.

64. Hoteya S, Haruta S, Shinohara H, et al. Feasibility and safety of laparoscopic and endoscopic cooperative surgery for gastric submucosal tumors, including esophagogastric junction tumors. Dig Endosc 2014;26:538–44.

65. Hiki N, Nunobe S, Matsuda T, et al. Laparoscopic endoscopic cooperative surgery. Dig Endosc 2015;27:197–204.

66. Kawahira H, Hayashi H, Natsume T, et al. Surgical advantages of gastric SMTs by laparoscopy and endoscopy cooperative surgery. Hepatogastroenterology 2012;59:415–7.

67. Abe N, Takeuchi H, Yanagida O, et al. Endoscopic full-thickness resection with laparoscopic assistance as hybrid NOTES for gastric submucosal tumor. Surg Endosc 2009;23:1908–13.

68. Nabeshima K, Tomioku M, Nakamura K, et al. Combination of laparoscopic and endoscopic approaches to neoplasia with non-exposure technique (CLEAN-NET) for GIST with ulceration. Tokai J Exp Clin Med 2015;40:115–9.

69. Mitsui T, Niimi K, Yamashita H, et al. Non-exposed endoscopic wall-inversion surgery as a novel partial gastrectomy technique. Gastric Cancer 2014;17:594–9.

70. Barajas-Gamboa JS, Acosta G, Savides TJ, et al. Laparo-endoscopic transgastric resection of gastric submucosal tumors. Surg Endosc 2015;29:2149–57.

71. Wilhelm D, von Delius S, Burian M, et al. Simultaneous use of laparoscopy and endoscopy for minimally invasive resection of gastric subepithelial masses—analysis of 93 interventions. World J Surg 2008;32:1021–8.

72. Privette A, McCahill L, Borrazzo E, et al. Laparoscopic approaches to resection of suspected gastric gastrointestinal stromal tumors based on tumor location. Surg Endosc 2008;22:487–94.

73. Kim HH. Endoscopic treatment for gastrointestinal stromal tumor: advantages and hurdles. World J Gastrointest Endosc 2015;7:192–205.

74. Sakon M, Takata M, Seki H, et al. A novel combined laparoscopic-endoscopic cooperative approach for duodenal lesions. J Laparoendosc Adv Surg Tech A 2010;20:555–8.

75. Beck DE, Karulf RE. Laparoscopic-assisted full-thickness endoscopic polypectomy. Dis Colon Rectum 1993;36:693–5.

76. Franklin ME Jr, Leyva-Alvizo A, Abrego-Medina D, et al. Laparoscopically monitored colonoscopic polypectomy: an established form of endoluminal therapy for colorectal polyps. Surg Endosc 2007;21:1650–3.

77. Winter H, Lang RA, Spelsberg FW, et al. Laparoscopic colonoscopic rendezvous procedures for the treatment of polyps and early stage carcinomas of the colon. Int J Colorectal Dis 2007;22:1377–81.

78. Wilhelm D, von Delius S, Weber L, et al. Combined laparoscopic-endoscopic resections of colorectal polyps: 10-year experience and follow-up. Surg Endosc 2009;23:688–93.

79. Monkemuller K, Neumann H, Fry LC, et al. Polypectomy techniques for difficult colon polyps. Dig Dis 2008;26:342–6.

80. Benedix F, Kockerling F, Lippert H, et al. Laparoscopic resection for endoscopically unresectable colorectal polyps: analysis of 525 patients. Surg Endosc 2008;22:2576–82.

81. Currie AC, Cahill R, Delaney CP, et al. International expert consensus on endpoints for full-thickness laparoendoscopic colonic excision. Surg Endosc 2015. [Epub ahead of print].

82. Kaimakliotis PZ, Chandrasekhara V. Endoscopic mucosal resection and endoscopic submucosal dissection of epithelial neoplasia of the colon. Expert Rev Gastroenterol Hepatol 2014;8:521–31.

83. Saito Y, Uraoka T, Yamaguchi Y, et al. A prospective, multicenter study of 1111 colorectal endoscopic submucosal dissections (with video). Gastrointest Endosc 2010;72:1217–25.

84. Farhat S, Chaussade S, Ponchon T, et al. Endoscopic submucosal dissection in a European setting. A multi-institutional report of a technique in development. Endoscopy 2011;43:664–70.

85. Prohm P, Weber J, Bonner C. Laparoscopic-assisted coloscopic polypectomy. Dis Colon Rectum 2001;44:746–8.

86. Mal F, Perniceni T, Levard H, et al. Colonic polyps considered unresectable by endoscopy. Removal by combinations of laparoscopy and endoscopy in 65 patients. Gastroenterol Clin Biol 1998;22:425–30 [in French].

87. Goh C, Burke JP, McNamara DA, et al. Endolaparoscopic removal of colonic polyps. Colorectal Dis 2014;16:271–5.

88. Cruz RA, Ragupathi M, Pedraza R, et al. Minimally invasive approaches for the management of "difficult" colonic polyps. Diagn Ther Endosc 2011;2011:682793.

89. Franklin ME Jr, Diaz EJ, Abrego D, et al. Laparoscopic-assisted colonoscopic polypectomy: the Texas Endosurgery Institute experience. Dis Colon Rectum 2000;43:1246–9.

90. Franklin ME Jr, Portillo G. Laparoscopic monitored colonoscopic polypectomy: long-term follow-up. World J Surg 2009;33:1306–9.

91. Lee MK, Chen F, Esrailian E, et al. Combined endoscopic and laparoscopic surgery may be an alternative to bowel resection for the management of colon polyps not removable by standard colonoscopy. Surg Endosc 2013;27:2082–6.

92. Yan J, Trencheva K, Lee SW, et al. Treatment for right colon polyps not removable using standard colonoscopy: combined laparoscopic-colonoscopic approach. Dis Colon Rectum 2011;54:753–8.

93. Liu BR, Song JT, Qu B, et al. Endoscopic muscularis dissection for upper gastrointestinal subepithelial tumors originating from the muscularis propria. Surg Endosc 2012;26:3141–8.

94. Gong W, Xiong Y, Zhi F, et al. Preliminary experience of endoscopic submucosal tunnel dissection for upper gastrointestinal submucosal tumors. Endoscopy 2012;44:231–5.

95. Hwang JC, Kim JH, Shin SJ, et al. Endoscopic resection for the treatment of gastric subepithelial tumors originated from the muscularis propria layer. Hepatogastroenterology 2009;56:1281–6.

96. Lee IL, Lin PY, Tung SY, et al. Endoscopic submucosal dissection for the treatment of intraluminal gastric subepithelial tumors originating from the muscularis propria layer. Endoscopy 2006;38:1024–8.

97. Wang Y, Li Y, Luo H, et al. Efficacy analysis of endoscopic submucosal excavation for gastric gastrointestinal stromal tumors. Zhonghua Wei Chang Wai Ke Za Zhi 2014;17:352–5 [in Chinese].

98. Zhou PH, Yao LQ, Qin XY, et al. Endoscopic full-thickness resection without laparoscopic assistance for gastric submucosal tumors originated from the muscularis propria. Surg Endosc 2011;25:2926–31.

99. Feng Y, Yu L, Yang S, et al. Endolumenal endoscopic full-thickness resection of muscularis propria-originating gastric submucosal tumors. J Laparoendosc Adv Surg Tech A 2014;24:171–6.

100. Hiki N. Feasible technique for laparoscopic wedge resection for gastric submucosal tumor-laparoscopy endoscopy cooperative surgery (LECS) [in Japanese]. Gan To Kagaku Ryoho 2011;38:728–32.

Endoscopic Suturing, an Essential Enabling Technology for New NOTES Interventions

Sergey V. Kantsevoy, MD, PhD[a,b,c],*,
Joseph Ramon Armengol-Miro, MD[c,d]

KEYWORDS

- Natural orifice transluminal endoscopic surgery (NOTES) • Full-thickness resection
- Gastrointestinal tract

KEY POINTS

- Reliable closure of the transluminal entrance site is paramount to prevent postoperative leakages and infectious complications.
- The Overstitch (Apollo Endosurgery Inc, Austin, TX) endoscopic suturing device creates a reliable, full-thickness, surgical-quality, airtight closure of transmural gastrointestinal tract defects.
- Endoscopic suturing is an essential enabling technology for new natural orifice transluminal endoscopic surgery interventions.

Peroral transluminal endoscopic surgery was started with a series of animal experiments, which demonstrated the ability to enter the peritoneal cavity through the gastric wall without any damage to organs surrounding the stomach.[1] During the first reported transluminal interventions in animal models, a full-thickness gastric wall incision was made, a flexible endoscope was introduced into the peritoneal cavity to perform liver biopsy, and then the endoscope was withdrawn back to the stomach and the gastric wall defect was completely closed with endoscopic clips.[1] After this report of feasibility of transluminal endoscopic intraperitoneal interventions, numerous abstracts and full-length articles have described in acute and survival

[a] University of Maryland School of Medicine, Baltimore, MD, USA; [b] Institute for Digestive Health and Liver Diseases, Mercy Medical Center, 301 St. Paul Place, POB 7th Floor, Suite 718, Baltimore, MD 21202, USA; [c] World Institute for Digestive Endoscopy (WIDER), Barcelona, Spain; [d] Digestive Endoscopy, Vall D'Hebron University Hospital, Barcelona, Spain
* Corresponding author. Institute for Digestive Health and Liver Diseases, Mercy Medical Center, 301 St. Paul Place, POB 7th Floor, Suite 718, Baltimore, MD 21202.
E-mail address: skan51@hotmail.com

Gastrointest Endoscopy Clin N Am 26 (2016) 375–384
http://dx.doi.org/10.1016/j.giec.2015.12.005
1052-5157/16/$ – see front matter © 2016 Elsevier Inc. All rights reserved.

animal studies transgastric peritoneoscopy, gastro-jejunostomy, tubal ligation, cholecystectomy, splenectomy, and other intraperitoneal interventions on live animal models.[2–6] In 2006, the Natural Orifice Consortium for Assessment and Research was formed and the term *natural orifice transluminal endoscopic surgery* (NOTES) was invented.[7,8]

Since that time numerous NOTES procedures in humans were performed, including transgastric peritoneoscopy and liver biopsy, transgastric and transvaginal cholecystectomies and appendectomies, NOTES percutaneous endoscopic gastrostomy rescue procedures, and other interventions.[9–12]

However, peroral and transvaginal interventions on intraperitoneal organs have not demonstrated convincing advantages over traditional laparoscopic surgery.[13]

The authors think that the real potential of NOTES has not yet been explored. The unique advantages of a NOTES approach over traditional and laparoscopic surgery are in procedures such as purely endoscopic full-thickness resection of gastrointestinal (GI) tract lesions. These new NOTES procedures are not possible without reliable, surgical-quality closure of transmural GI tract wall defects.

Table 1 summarizes accessories and endoscopic suturing devices previously used for closure of NOTES entrance sites into the peritoneal cavity.

Through-the-scope endoscopic clips are commercially available devices, which were widely used during initial NOTES animal experiments. Unfortunately, these clips were created for endoscopic hemostasis and not for tissue approximation. Through-the scope clips only provided mucosa-to-mucosa apposition. Endoscopic hemostatic

Table 1
Accessories and devices for closure of the NOTES incision

Type	Name	Manufacturer	Available for Clinical Use
Through-the-scope endoscopic clips	QuickClip2 and QuickClip Pro	Olympus Optical Ltd, Tokyo, Japan	Yes
	Resolution	Boston Scientific, Natick, MA	Yes
	Instinct	Cook Medical, Bloomington, IN	Yes
Over-the-scope clip	Over-The-Scope Clip (OTSC) System	*Ovesco*, Tübingen, Germany	Yes
	Padlock Clip	Aponos, Kingston, NH	Yes
Suction based	EndoCinch	Bard, Murray Hill, NJ	Yes
	LSI Solution	Victor, NY	No
	Spiderman	Ethicon Endo Surgery, Cincinnati, OH	No
Working overtube delivering preloaded stitch	NDO plicator	NDO Surgical, Mansfield, MA	No
T-bars deployment with subsequent cinching	TAS system	Ethicon Endo Surgery, Cincinnati, OH	No
	T-bars	Cook Endoscopy, Winston-Salem, NC	No
	T-bars	Olympus Optical LTD, Tokyo, Japan	No
Flexible stapler	PowerMedical	Acquired by Medtronic, Minneapolis, MN	No
Use of curved needle	G-Prox	USGI Medical, San Clemente, CA	Yes
	Eagle Claw	Olympus Optical LTD, Tokyo, Japan	No
	Overstitch	Apollo Endosurgery Inc, Austin, TX	Yes

clips could not achieve reliable closure of NOTES incisions and were far inferior to surgical suturing closure as demonstrated in animal experiments comparing burst pressures between various types of endoscopic closure techniques.[14,15]

Compared with the small through-the-scope clips, the over-the-scope clips (OTSC [Ovesco Endoscopy, Tübingen, Germany], Padlock Clip [Aponos, Kingston, NH]) are very robust devices allowing even a full-thickness closure of GI tract defects. Over-the-scope clips are preloaded on the distal end of the flexible endoscope for delivery to the site of their application. However, the size of defect amenable to closure with these devices is limited by the space inside the over-the-scope clip; in case of suboptimal placement, these clips are very difficult to remove and cannot be repositioned after initial deployment.[16]

The first endoscopic suturing devices, which were used in animal experiments for closure of NOTES entrances into the peritoneal cavity (EndoCinch [Bard, Murray Hill, NJ], LSI Solution [Victor, NY], Spiderman [Ethicon Endo Surgery, Cincinnati, OH]), were based on suctioning of tissue into a suction chamber mounted on the distal tip of the flexible endoscope. Then a needle with suture was passed through the suctioned tissue to deliver a stitch.[17] After advancement of the needle through both edges of the NOTES incision, the suture was finished with extracorporeal knot tying or intracorporeal cinching. Unfortunately, use of suction could not provide predictable and adequate depth of the suture delivery and most sutures were too superficial, located only in the mucosal and submucosal layers.[18]

NDO plicator (NDO Surgical, Mansfield, MA) used a specially created overtube with preloaded stitches.[17,19] Although this device was created specifically for correction of gastroesophageal reflux disease, it was successfully used for endoscopic full-thickness suturing and potentially could be used for closure of NOTES entrance into peritoneal cavity.[20] However, this device could only deliver a single stitch of predetermined length and after each application needed removal from patients for reloading. Manufacturing of this suturing device was discontinued, and it is no longer commercially available for clinical use in humans.

Several companies (Ethicon Endo Surgery, Cincinnati, OH; Cook Endoscopy, Winston-Salem, NC; Olympus Optical LTD, Tokyo, Japan) developed suturing devices based on hollow needles delivering T-bars.[21–23] Unfortunately, T-bars were delivered into the edges of the NOTES incision through a blind puncture of the GI tract wall, which could potentially cause damage to adjacent intraperitoneal organs and blood vessels.[24] None of these devices is currently commercially available for clinical use in humans.

A flexible endoscopic stapler was originally developed by PowerMedical and later acquired by Medtronic (Minneapolis, MN). Numerous acute and survival animal experiments demonstrated effectiveness of this device for closure of full-thickness defects in the GI tract wall.[25–28] However, this device was very difficult to navigate and required removal from patients for reloading. It is no longer available for clinical use.

Endoscopic suturing devices using a curved needle (G-Prox [USGI Medical, San Clemente, CA], Eagle Claw [Olympus Optical LTD, Tokyo, Japan], and Overstitch [Apollo Endosurgery Inc, Austin, TX]) most closely resemble surgical suturing. The G-Prox tissue approximation system uses a curved needle to deliver specially designed suture material with baskets on both ends.[29] The outer diameter of the G-Prox device is bigger than the biopsy channel of existing flexible endoscopes and requires the use of the special TransPort system (USGI Medical, San Clemente, CA).[29]

Eagle Claw was specifically created for endoscopic suturing including closure of NOTES entrance into the peritoneal cavity, creation of anastomosis, and other interventions inside the peritoneal cavity and GI tract.[30–32] However, Eagle Claw could only create separate stitches of limited length and required removal from patients after completion of each stitch for reloading. Although several consecutive prototypes of Eagle Claw have been made, it is still not available for human use.

The only commercially available endoscopic suturing device now (currently available in Europe and the United States) is Overstitch made by Apollo Endosurgery Inc, (Austin, TX).[33,34] The current version of Overstitch is front-loaded on a double-channel endoscope (GiF-2T160 or GiF-2T180, Olympus Optical Ltd, Tokyo, Japan) fitted inside the endoscope's larger channel with a special spring-loaded mechanism and actuated by a handle that clips onto the endoscope (**Fig. 1**).

Endoscopic closure of full-thickness GI tract wall defects with Overstitch requires several consecutive steps (**Fig. 2**)[16,35]:

1. The suturing arm is closed driving the needle and suture through one of the edges of the GI tract wall defect (see **Fig. 2**A).
2. The needle holder is advanced forward to take hold of the needle. Then the needle holder is pulled back removing the needle from the spike at the end of the suturing arm. The empty suturing arm is opened releasing the edge of GI tract wall defect (see **Fig. 2**B). Then the suturing arm is closed, and the needle holder is advanced forward returning the needle back onto the suturing arm (see **Fig. 2**C). The needle is released from the needle holder, and it is again is mounted on the suturing arm.
3. The endoscope is advanced toward the opposite edge of the GI tract wall defect. The suturing arm is opened (see **Fig. 2**D) and then closed driving the needle and the suture through the tissue (see **Fig. 2**E). The needle holder is again pushed forward to take hold of the needle and then pulled back to remove the needle from the suturing arm. The empty suturing arm is opened again releasing the edge of GI tract wall defect (see **Fig. 2**F).
4. At this point, both edges of the full-thickness GI tract wall defect are connected by the suture. Now the needle can be released from the needle holder to become a T-bar. The free end of the suture is loaded into a specially designed cinching

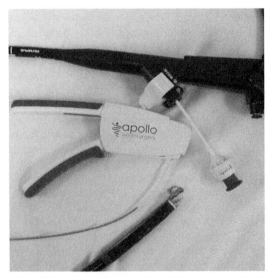

Fig. 1. Overstitch endoscopic suturing device is assembled on a double-channel Olympus upper endoscope.

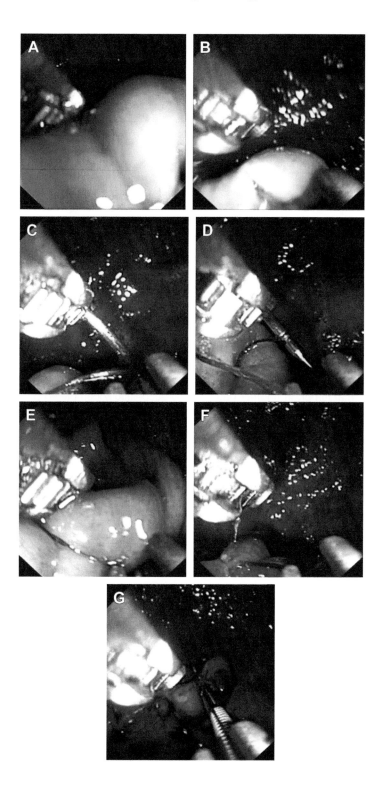

mechanism. Deployment of the cinching mechanism will complete a separate stitch connecting both edges of the full-thickness defect in the GI tract wall together (see **Fig. 2**G).[16,35]

After completion of the first stitch, a new needle with a suture can be loaded into the Overstitch an unlimited number of times to create additional separate stitches until the full-thickness GI tract wall defect is closed completely. Alternatively, for closure of large full-thickness defects, the aforementioned steps (1–3) can be repeated as necessary to create a continuous suturing line completely closing a NOTES entrance into the peritoneal cavity.[16,35]

Previous small case reports demonstrated successful use of the Overstitch for endoscopic closure of full-thickness GI tract iatrogenic perforations.[36–39] A recent larger study (21 patients) confirmed that the Overstitch suturing device provided adequate and reliable endoscopic repair of full-thickness colonic perforations, which was more effective than endoscopic clips closure and eliminated the need for rescue surgery (**Fig. 3**).[40]

The authors have previously reported their preliminary results demonstrating safety and feasibility of a new NOTES procedure: full-thickness, purely endoscopic resection of GI tract lesions.[13,41,42] In 9 survival experiments on a live porcine model, the authors successfully performed endoscopic full-thickness resection of the GI tract wall. The colonic and gastric wall defects were successfully closed with the Overstitch endoscopic suturing device. There were no problems or complications in the postoperative period. The follow-up postmortem examination revealed good full-thickness healing of the GI tract wall at all sites of resection.[13,41,42] After completion of animal experiments, the authors performed purely endoscopic full-thickness resection of a 2 × 5-cm gastric stromal tumor; in another patient, they successfully completed purely endoscopic full-thickness resection (**Fig. 4**) of an actively bleeding 2 × 4-cm colon cancer located at the hepatic flexure.[41,42] The patients tolerated these NOTES procedures very well and had no pain in the postoperative period. Follow-up endoscopy revealed good healing of the resection sites without any residual lesions or strictures. Both patients are tumor free 4 years after the procedure.

Stavropoulos and colleagues[43] reported 25 successful full-thickness purely endoscopic resections of GI tract subepithelial tumors. Transmural defects after resection were initially closed with omental patch attached to the gastric wall with endoscopic clips. In subsequent cases, the Overstitch endoscopic suturing device was successfully used to achieve reliable closure of the NOTES full-thickness GI tract wall defects.

In conclusion, the Overstitch endoscopic suturing device creates reliable, full-thickness, surgical-quality airtight closure of transmural GI tract defects. Endoscopic suturing with Overstitch has become an essential enabling technology for clinical introduction of new NOTES procedures: purely endoscopic full-thickness resection of GI tract lesions.

Fig. 2. Suturing with the Overstitch endoscopic suturing device. (*A*) The suturing arm is closed driving the needle and suture through one of the edges of the GI tract wall defect. (*B*) The needle is removed from the suturing arm, and the empty suturing arm is opened releasing the edge of GI tract wall defect. (*C*) The needle is mounted again onto the suturing arm. (*D*) The endoscope is advanced toward the opposite edge of the GI tract wall defect, and the suturing arm is opened. (*E*) The suturing arm is closed driving the needle and the suture through the second edge of the GI tract defect. (*F*) The needle is again removed from the suturing arm, and the empty suturing arm is opened releasing the second edge of the GI tract wall defect. (*G*) Deployment of the cinching mechanism completes a separate stitch connecting both edges of the full-thickness defect in the GI tract wall together.

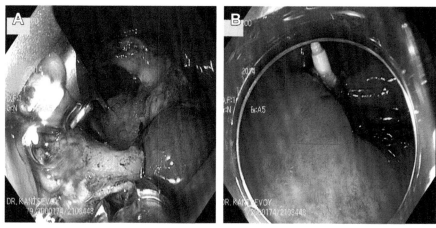

Fig. 3. Endoscopic suturing closure of full-thickness colonic perforation. (*A*) Suturing arm of the Overstitch is closed driving the needle through the distal (anal) edge of the large colonic full-thickness perforation. (*B*) Endoscopic suturing is completed. The cinch is deployed completely closing the large full-thickness colonic perforation.

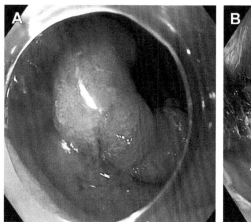

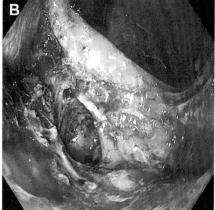

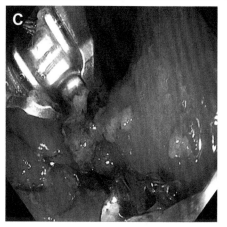

Fig. 4. NOTES for endoscopic full-thickness removal of colon cancer. (*A*) Endoscopic view of a large colon cancer. (*B*) Endoscopic en bloc full-thickness resection of the colon cancer is completed. (*C*) Full-thickness colonic defect after resection of colon cancer is completely closed with a continuous suturing line using the Overstitch endoscopic suturing device.

REFERENCES

1. Kalloo AN, Singh VK, Jagannath SB, et al. Flexible transgastric peritoneoscopy: a novel approach to diagnostic and therapeutic interventions in the peritoneal cavity. Gastrointest Endosc 2004;60:114–7.
2. Park PO, Bergstrom M, Ikeda K, et al. Experimental studies of transgastric gallbladder surgery: cholecystectomy and cholecystogastric anastomosis (videos). Gastrointest Endosc 2005;61:601–6.
3. Jagannath SB, Kantsevoy SV, Vaughn CA, et al. Peroral transgastric endoscopic ligation of fallopian tubes with long-term survival in a porcine model. Gastrointest Endosc 2005;61:449–53.
4. Merrifield BF, Wagh MS, Thompson CC. Peroral transgastric organ resection: a feasibility study in pigs. Gastrointest Endosc 2006;63:693–7.
5. Kantsevoy SV, Jagannath SB, Niiyama H, et al. Endoscopic gastrojejunostomy with survival in a porcine model. Gastrointest Endosc 2005;62:287–92.
6. Kantsevoy SV, Hu B, Jagannath SB, et al. Transgastric endoscopic splenectomy: is it possible? Surg Endosc 2006;20:522–5.
7. Rattner D, Kalloo A. ASGE/SAGES working group on natural orifice translumenal endoscopic surgery. Surg Endosc 2005;2006(20):329–33.
8. Rattner D, Hawes RH. NOTES: gathering momentum. Surg Endosc 2006;20:711–2.
9. Marks JM, Ponsky JL, Pearl JP, et al. PEG "rescue": a practical NOTES technique. Surg Endosc 2007;21:816–9.
10. Palanivelu C, Rajan PS, Rangarajan M, et al. Transvaginal endoscopic appendectomy in humans: a unique approach to NOTES-world's first report. Surg Endosc 2008;22(5):1343–7.
11. Steele K, Schweitzer MA, Lyn-Sue J, et al. Flexible transgastric peritoneoscopy and liver biopsy: a feasibility study in human beings (with videos). Gastrointest Endosc 2008;68:61–6.
12. Lehmann KS, Ritz JP, Wibmer A, et al. The German registry for natural orifice translumenal endoscopic surgery: report of the first 551 patients. Ann Surg 2010;252:263–70.
13. Armengol-Miro JR, Dot Bach J, Suboh Abadia MA, et al. Natural orifice translumenal endoscopic surgery (NOTES) for G.I. tract neoplasia. In: Testoni PA, Arcidiacono PG, Mariani A, editors. Endoscopic management of gastrointestinal cancer and precancerous conditions. Turin (Italy): Edizoni Minerva Medica; 2015. p. 277–83.
14. Ryou M, Pai RD, Sauer JS, et al. Evaluating an optimal gastric closure method for transgastric surgery. Surg Endosc 2007;21:677–80.
15. Ryou M, Fong DG, Pai RD, et al. Transluminal closure for NOTES: an ex vivo study comparing leak pressures of various gastrotomy and colotomy closure modalities. Endoscopy 2008;40:432–6.
16. Kantsevoy SV. Endoscopic suturing devices. In: Testoni PA, Arcidiacono PG, Mariani A, editors. Endoscopic management of gastrointestinal cancer and precancerous conditions. Turin (Italy): Edizoni Minerva Medica; 2015. p. 249–55.
17. Chen YK. Endoscopic suturing devices for treatment of GERD: too little, too late? Gastrointest Endosc 2005;62:44–7.
18. Schwartz MP, Schreinemakers JR, Smout AJ. Four-year follow-up of endoscopic gastroplication for the treatment of gastroesophageal reflux disease. World J Gastrointest Pharmacol Ther 2013;4:120–6.
19. Yew KC, Chuah SK. Antireflux endoluminal therapies: past and present. Gastroenterol Res Pract 2013;2013:481417.

20. von Renteln D, Schmidt A, Riecken B, et al. Gastric full-thickness suturing during EMR and for treatment of gastric-wall defects (with video). Gastrointest Endosc 2008;67:738–44.
21. Raju GS, Shibukawa G, Ahmed I, et al. Endoluminal suturing may overcome the limitations of clip closure of a gaping wide colon perforation (with videos). Gastrointest Endosc 2007;65:906–11.
22. Ikeda K, Fritscher-Ravens A, Mosse CA, et al. Endoscopic full-thickness resection with sutured closure in a porcine model. Gastrointest Endosc 2005;62:122–9.
23. Dray X, Krishnamurty DM, Donatelli G, et al. Gastric wall healing after NOTES procedures: closure with endoscopic clips provides superior histological outcome compared with threaded tags closure. Gastrointest Endosc 2010;72:343–50.
24. Kantsevoy SV. Endoscopic full-thickness resection: new minimally invasive therapeutic alternative for GI-tract lesions. Gastrointest Endosc 2006;64:90–1.
25. Kaehler GF, Langner C, Suchan KL, et al. Endoscopic full-thickness resection of the stomach: an experimental approach. Surg Endosc 2006;20:519–21.
26. Kaehler G, Grobholz R, Langner C, et al. A new technique of endoscopic full-thickness resection using a flexible stapler. Endoscopy 2006;38:86–9.
27. Meireles OR, Kantsevoy SV, Assumpcao LR, et al. Reliable gastric closure after natural orifice translumenal endoscopic surgery (NOTES) using a novel automated flexible stapling device. Surg Endosc 2008;22:1609–13.
28. Magno P, Giday SA, Dray X, et al. A new stapler-based full-thickness transgastric access closure: results from an animal pilot trial. Endoscopy 2007;39:876–80.
29. Swanstrom LL. Current technology development for natural orifice transluminal endoscopic surgery. Cir Esp 2006;80:283–8 [in Spanish].
30. Hu B, Chung SC, Sun LC, et al. Eagle claw II: a novel endosuture device that uses a curved needle for major arterial bleeding: a bench study. Gastrointest Endosc 2005;62:266–70.
31. Hu B, Chung SC, Sun LC, et al. Endoscopic suturing without extracorporeal knots: a laboratory study. Gastrointest Endosc 2005;62:230–3.
32. Kantsevoy SV, Hu B, Jagannath SB, et al. Technical feasibility of endoscopic gastric reduction: a pilot study in a porcine model. Gastrointest Endosc 2007;65:510–3.
33. Kantsevoy SV, Thuluvath PJ. Successful closure of a chronic refractory gastrocutaneous fistula with a new endoscopic suturing device (with video). Gastrointest Endosc 2012;75:688–90.
34. Armengol-Miro JR, Dot J, Abu-Suboh Abadia M, et al. New endoscopic suturing device for closure of chronic gastrocutaneous fistula in an immunocompromised patient. Endoscopy 2011;43(Suppl 2 UCTN):E403–4.
35. Kantsevoy SV. Endoscopic suturing for closure of transmural defects. Tech Gastrointest Endosc 2015;17:136–40.
36. Kumar N, Thompson CC. A novel method for endoscopic perforation management by using abdominal exploration and full-thickness sutured closure. Gastrointest Endosc 2014;80:156–61.
37. Stavropoulos SN, Modayil R, Friedel D. Current applications of endoscopic suturing. World J Gastrointest Endosc 2015;7:777–89.
38. Henderson JB, Sorser SA, Atia AN, et al. Repair of esophageal perforations using a novel endoscopic suturing system. Gastrointest Endosc 2014;80:535–7.
39. Kantsevoy SV, Bitner M, Davis JM, et al. Endoscopic suturing closure of large iatrogenic colonic perforation. Gastrointest Endosc 2015;82:754–5.
40. Kantsevoy SV, Bitner M, Hajiyeva G, et al. Endoscopic management of colonic perforations: clips versus suturing closure (with videos). Gastrointest Endosc 2015. [Epub ahead of print].

41. Armengol-Miro JR, Dot J, Abu-Suboh Abadia M, et al. Full-thickness purely endoscopic resection of colon cancer. Gastrointest Endosc 2012;75:AB114–5.

42. Armengol-Miro JR, Abu-Suboh Abadia M, Dot J, et al. Full-thickness endoscopic resection of gastrointestinal cancer: from animal experiments to humans. Gastrointest Endosc 2013;77:AB458.

43. Stavropoulos SN, Modayil R, Friedel D, et al. Endoscopic full-thickness resection for GI stromal tumors. Gastrointest Endosc 2014;80:334–5.

New NOTES Clinical Training and Program Development

Payal Saxena, MBBS, FRACP[a,b], Mouen A. Khashab, MD[b,c],*

KEYWORDS

- NOTES • POEM • Endoscopy • STER • Fellowship • Pyloromyotomy • Training
- Peroral endoscopic myotomy

KEY POINTS

- Natural orifice translumenal endoscopic surgery (NOTES) is an intense area of research, and is arguably the most significant endoscopic innovation of this decade.
- After initial enthusiasm of ideas, there was some early disappointment owing to the limitations of instruments and accessories to facilitate intraabdominal surgery via flexible endoscopes.
- "New NOTES" procedures have been performed by both gastroenterologists and GI surgeons worldwide.
- This paper outlines the current status of new NOTES procedures and the skills and training required for the new generation of trainees to become proficient in new NOTES.

INTRODUCTION

The concept of natural orifice translumenal endoscopic surgery (NOTES) has been a radical and innovative idea that changed the way we think about the field of endoscopy and minimally invasive surgery. In 2004, Kalloo and colleagues[1] performed the first transgastric peritoneoscopy in a porcine model. Next, Rao and Reddy[2] demonstrated the first human transgastric natural orifice translumenal endoscopic surgery (NOTES) appendectomy. In 2005, the American Society of Gastrointestinal

Conflicts of Interest: P. Saxena is a consultant for Boston Scientific, Cook Medical, Pentax, Apollo Endosurgery, and scientific advisory board member for Oncosil Medical. M.A. Khashab is a consultant for Boston Scientific.

^a Division of Gastroenterology and Hepatology, Department of Medicine, Royal Prince Alfred Hospital, Missenden Rd, Camperdown, NSW 2050, Australia; ^b Division of Gastroenterology and Hepatology, Department of Medicine, The Johns Hopkins Medical Institutions, 1800 Orleans St, Baltimore, MD 21205, USA; ^c Department of Medicine, Johns Hopkins Hospital, 1800 Orleans Street, Suite 7125B, Baltimore, MD 21205, USA
* Corresponding author. Johns Hopkins Hospital, 1800 Orleans Street, Suite 7125B, Baltimore, MD 21205.
E-mail address: mkhasha1@jhmi.edu

Gastrointest Endoscopy Clin N Am 26 (2016) 385–400
http://dx.doi.org/10.1016/j.giec.2015.12.009
1052-5157/16/$ – see front matter © 2016 Elsevier Inc. All rights reserved.

Endoscopy and Society of American Gastrointestinal Endoscopic Surgeons formed a working party of gastroenterologists and surgeons, namely the Natural Orifice Surgery Consortium for Assessment and Research, with the aim of safely developing and introducing NOTES techniques.[3]

After initial enthusiasm of ideas, there was some early disappointment owing to the limitations of instruments and accessories to facilitate intraabdominal surgery via flexible endoscopes. Nevertheless, 10 years later, the concept of NOTES has become a clinical reality. After extensive investigation carried out in animal models and cadavers, we have seen an eruption of various NOTES procedures, including the initial human transgastric cholecystectomy,[4] transvaginal cholecystectomy,[5] transvaginal nephrectomy,[6] and transanal mesorectal resection.[7] However, such procedures have not been adopted widely in clinical practice and some would argue that NOTES is "dead" because the hype has not generated a revolution as was seen with laparoscopic surgery in the 1990s.[8] This argument is likely misguided.

It is best to consider that NOTES is not a technique, but a concept of accessing organs or tissue beyond the lumen of the gastrointestinal (GI) tract. As the skill set of NOTES pioneers and interventional endoscopists became more sophisticated, they began pushing the limits of what could be accomplished endoluminally, eventually exiting the confines of the GI lumen. Along the way, the "third space" that lies within the wall of the gut became apparent.[9]

There has been extensive dialogue with regard to who is best suited to carry out NOTES procedures. With regard to traditional NOTES, opinion over time has largely favored a multidisciplinary team combing the skill sets from both gastroenterologists and GI laparoscopic surgeons. However, "new NOTES" procedures have been performed by both gastroenterologists and GI surgeons worldwide. This paper outlines the current status of new NOTES procedures in addition to the skills and training required for the new generation of trainees to become proficient in new NOTES.

LONG-RANGE AND SHORT-RANGE (NEW) NATURAL ORIFICE TRANSLUMENAL ENDOSCOPIC SURGERY

It is important to recognize that not all NOTES procedures are the same. NOTES can broadly be divided into 2 categories: long-range and short-range NOTES. Long-range NOTES refers to procedures where access through a healthy visceral organ is gained to target another, distant organ (eg, transgastric appendectomy). Short-range NOTES refers to procedures whereby the organ of interest is accessed directly, without disrupting another organ (eg, peroral endoscopic myotomy [POEM]). Other examples are listed in **Table 1**.

Table 1 Examples of short-range and long-range NOTES procedures	
Short-Range NOTES	**Long-Range NOTES**
POEM	Transgastric cholecystectomy
EFTR	Transgastric appendectomy
STER	Transvaginal cholecystectomy
G-POEM	Transvaginal appendectomy

Abbreviations: EFTR, endoscopic full-thickness resection of tumors; G-POEM, peroral pyloromyotomy; NOTES, natural orifice translumenal endoscopic surgery; POEM, peroral endosipic myotomy; STER, submucosal tunneling and endoscopic resection.

It has become clear to operators that long-range NOTES requires not only advanced endoscopic skills, but also knowledge of intraabdominal anatomy and the ability to manage complications such as bleeding. For patient safety, conversion to laparoscopic or open surgery remains a possibility and therefore surgical skills are paramount. It has been well-accepted that, for safe and successful application of long-range NOTES, a multidisciplinary team of practitioners including surgeons and gastroenterologists is required.[10]

On the other hand, short-range or "new NOTES" procedures are largely performed in the third space. Hence, advanced endoscopic skills including submucosal dissection are the vital skill constituents for the operator.

SKILL SET FOR NEW NATURAL ORIFICE TRANSLUMENAL ENDOSCOPIC SURGERY

The ongoing challenges of traditional NOTES procedures do not apply to new NOTES. For instance, transvisceral access to the peritoneal cavity for resection of intraabdominal organs (eg, cholecystectomy, appendectomy) requires triangulation of instruments and detailed knowledge of intraabdominal anatomy. Laparoscopic surgical skills are also mandatory to ensure safety of the procedure as well as potential conversion in the event of inability to complete the resection via NOTES techniques or occurrence of complications.

In contrast, the skill set pertinent to new NOTES are those of an advanced endoscopist (**Box 1**). Advanced techniques such as endoscopic mucosal resection (EMR) or endoscopic submucosal dissection (ESD) are well-investigated methods for endoscopic resection of superficial GI neoplasms.[11,12] ESD operators have developed expertise in recognizing and working within the layers of the GI tract. Appreciation of the planes is essential for performing submucosal endoscopy, the most successful off-shoot of NOTES procedures. New NOTES procedures include POEM, submucosal tunneling and endoscopic resection (STER), endoscopic full-thickness resection of tumors (EFTR), and peroral endoscopic pyloromyotomy (G-POEM). These procedures offer minimally invasive therapeutic options for motility disorders (achalasia, spastic esophageal disorders, gastroparesis) and subepithelial masses of the upper GI tract (eg, GI stromal tumors, leiomyomas). Mastery of endoscopic dexterity within the narrow submucosal or "third space" with an in-depth understanding of the tissue planes is essential for technical expertise.

Box 1
Recommended skill set of new NOTES operators

Essential

Endoscopy

Colonoscopy

EMR

ESD

Desirable

EUS

Abbreviations: EMR, endoscopic mucosal resection; ESD, endoscopic submucosal dissection; EUS, endoscopic ultrasound; NOTES, natural orifice translumenal endoscopic surgery.

To manage motility disorders, the operator should either have an in-depth understanding of the disorders and ability to interpret manometry studies, or have a close collaboration and working relationship with a gastroenterologist with a special expertise in motility disorders. With regard to subepithelial lesions, the appropriate resection technique depends the layer of origin of the mass. Endoscopic ultrasonography plays a very important role in not only identifying the origin of the lesion, but also proximity of associated structures, such as the great mediastinal vessels. Hence, the operator should either be proficient in performing endoscopic ultrasonography or work closely with an endosonographer who can communicate the findings of the examination relevant to endoscopic resection. The new NOTES procedures are reliant on the endoscopists' familiarity and knowledge of submucosal dissection, therefore ESD experience is an advantage. In particular, the operator should be familiar with ESD principles, techniques, equipment, and cautery settings. Last, and most important, to achieve complete success of these procedures, the new NOTES operator should also have mastery in the management of potential endoscopic complications such as bleeding, mucosal perforation, or full-thickness perforation. Hence, use of endoscopic hemostasis devices and proficiency of closure techniques using through-the-scope (TTS) clips, over the scope clips (OTSC, Ovesco Endoscopy AG, Tübingen, Germany), endoscopic suturing (Overstitch, Apollo Endosurgery, Austin, TX, USA; **Boxes 2** and **3**).

WHO CURRENTLY PERFORMS NEW NATURAL ORIFICE TRANSLUMENAL ENDOSCOPIC SURGERY?
Peroral Endoscopic Myotomy

POEM is an incisionless therapeutic procedure that shows great efficacy for the treatment of achalasia and spastic esophageal disorders. The technique was developed in 2007 by Pasricha and colleagues[13] in a porcine model and subsequently translated to clinical practice by Inoue and associates in 2008.[14,15] The 4 steps are (1) mucosal incision, (2) submucosal tunneling, (3) myotomy, and (4) closure of mucosal incision.[16] Maintaining an intact mucosa prevents leakage of esophageal contents and is the key to the safety of the procedure. Seven years later the technique has been adopted world-wide. More than 10,000 procedures have been performed with technical and clinical success rates ranging from 71% to 100%.[17] An international survey performed in 2012 identified 25 POEM operators.[18] Of these, 14 were surgeons and 11 gastroenterologists. The majority (84%) of all operators had prior ESD experience. Interestingly, only 66% of operators had experience of long-range NOTES procedures and 25% of operators performed POEM in the endoscopy suite (as opposed to operating room).

Box 2
Devices used during new NOTES procedures

ESD knives

Coagraspers

TTS clips

Endoscopic suturing device

OTSC

Abbreviations: ESD, endoscopic submucosal dissection; NOTES, natural orifice translumenal endoscopic surgery; OTSC, over the scope clip; TTS, through the scope.

Box 3
Rescue kit for managing potential adverse events during new NOTES procedures

Spare ESD knives

Fully covered and partially covered enteral stents

Veress needle

Cyanoacrylate glue

OTSC

Injector needles/catheters

Abbreviations: ESD, endoscopic submucosal dissection; NOTES, natural orifice translumenal endoscopic surgery; OTSC, over the scope clip.

Very few complications related to POEM have been reported to date. Capnoperitoneum (8.3%)[18] and inadvertent mucosal perforation or mucosotomy (6.7%)[18] are minor technical adverse events that can be managed during the procedure. A Veress needle can be temporarily placed transabdominally to drain a capnoperitoneum. Mucosotomies can generally be managed endoscopically with clips or endoscopic suturing and seem to decrease in frequency with increase in operator's experience.[19–22] Serious adverse events (mediastinitis, abscess, leak, delayed bleeding[23]) are extremely rare (<0.1%)[24] with only 2 reports of esophageal perforation requiring surgical (laparoscopic and thoracoscopic) intervention.[25,26] Recently, Li and colleagues[23] reported on a total of 3 out of 428 patients (0.7%) who had postoperative delayed bleeding within the submucosal tunnel. Patients presented with severe retrosternal chest pain or hematemesis. The clips were removed and blood clots extracted from the tunnel, after which a bleeding vessel was identified and treated using hemostatic forceps in two-thirds of patients. In the third patient, a bleeding source could not be identified and a Sengstaken-Blakemore tube was immediately placed. The gastric balloon was immediately deflated and esophageal balloon deflated at 24 hours. All cases were managed endoscopically without need for surgical intervention or blood transfusion. Decompressing the tunnel prevented mucosal ischemia and necrosis, which could lead to full-thickness perforation. Intraprocedural bleeding is commonly encountered, although there are no reports of inability to complete POEM owing to massive bleeding.[27] Hemostatic techniques commonly used during POEM include use of coagraspers (Olympus, Center Valley, PA, USA; **Fig. 1**), water-jet–assisted knives (ERBE, Tübingen, Germany; **Fig. 2**), or mechanical tamponade using a blunt catheter or the distal cap.

Most operators perform POEM in the operating room.[18] However, we recently published efficacy and safety outcomes on 60 consecutive patients who underwent POEM in an endoscopy unit performed by an interventional gastroenterologist.[22] Mean procedure time was 99 minutes, and clinical success was achieved in 92.3% of patients. Only 10 adverse events occurred, and the majority were mild (n = 7) with no severe adverse events. Inadvertent mucosotomies occurred in 4 patients, all of which were controlled endoscopically (TTS clips, OTSC, and cyanoacrylate). Significant pneumoperitoneum occurred in 3 patients, which were successfully decompressed with a Veress needle (Genicon, Winter Park, FL, USA). One patient on chronic immunosuppression therapy (including steroids) experienced symptomatic intraprocedural pneumothorax, which was treated successfully with insertion of a chest tube within 10 minutes of diagnosis. There are many advantages to performing

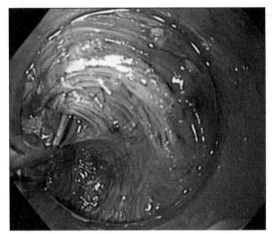

Fig. 1. Coagraspers (Olympus, Center Valley, PA, USA) are used to coagulate a vessel noted on the muscular side during peroral endosopic myotomy.

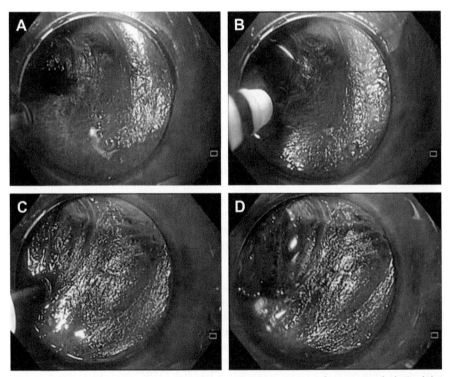

Fig. 2. A 54-year-old man underwent peroral endosopic myotomy for type 3 achalasia. (*A*) A bleeding vessel was noted on the mucosal side during submucosal tunneling. (*B*) The water-jet injection (ERBE hybrid knife; Tübingen, Germany) was used to inject underneath the vessel lift to lift it away from the mucosa. (*C*) The hybrid knife was used to coagulate the vessel. (*D*) Lifting the vessel away from the mucosa prevented transmission of coagulation current to the mucosal surface, which can lead to inadvertent mucosotomy.

POEM in the endoscopy unit. Gastroenterologists are adept at performing procedures in the endoscopy suite, which is usually set up in an ergonomic manner for various endoscopic procedures. Importantly, all necessary endoscopy equipment and accessories are available within short reach (particular for adverse event management). Furthermore, familiarity and comfort with the surrounding environment is important for both the endoscopist and the assisting team when performing challenging procedures such as POEM.

POEM is a successful and safe new NOTES procedure that has been adopted worldwide by both gastroenterologists and surgeons who have endoscopy and ESD experience and can be safely performed either in the operating room or endoscopy suite. Long-range NOTES or surgical experience does not seem to influence the operator's ability to safely and successfully perform POEM.

Peroral Endoscopic Pyloromyotomy

Gastric antral hypomotility and pyloric dysfunction have been demonstrated in patients with idiopathic or diabetic nausea and vomiting.[28] Hence, therapies eliminating the pyloric barrier may improve such symptoms in patients with gastroparesis. G-POEM is an incisionless, minimally invasive procedure analogous to POEM with proposed efficacy similar to surgical pyloroplasty. A mucosal incision is created 5 cm proximal to the pylorus either on the anterior or posterior wall. A submucosal tunnel is created to the level of the pyloric ring, which is then dissected. The mucosal incision is subsequently closed. Initial cases were performed by a surgical group in porcine models.[29] Subsequently, the first human case was reported by Khashab and colleagues[30] at Johns Hopkins Hospital. Another group of surgeons reported a series of 7 patients who had successful G-POEM; however, surgical laparoscopic guidance was also used in the majority (6/7) of patients, primarily because other laparoscopic interventions (cholecystectomy, fundoplication) were performed concomitantly. Overall clinical success rate approached 90%.[31] Only 1 complication related to G-POEM has been reported; a patient who failed to take proton pump inhibitor after G-POEM presented with a bleeding pyloric channel ulcer with visible vessel, which was treated endoscopically.[31] Chaves and colleagues[32] and Gonzalez and colleagues[33] have also reported successful G-POEM for refractory gastroparesis. Chung and colleagues[34] reported a case of G-POEM for management of gastric outlet obstruction after esophagectomy.

G-POEM can safely be performed as a pure endoscopic procedure, provided the operator is experienced with the same skillset required for POEM. The current G-POEM operators have endoscopic and ESD experience and are expert POEM operators.

Submucosal Tunneling and Endoscopic Resection

Once new NOTES endoscopists became comfortable in the third space, the natural progression was resection of tumors residing beneath the mucosa in the esophagus and stomach. After creation of a mucosal incision, a submucosal tunnel is created, followed by enucleation of the tumor using ESD techniques while preserving the integrity of the overlying mucosa. The tumor is extracted via the mucosal incision that is, subsequently closed (**Fig. 3**). Since 2012, more than 150 STER of medium sized lesions (19.5 mm) have been reported worldwide, contributed by both gastroenterologists and surgeons.[35–38] Technical success (complete resection rate) is reported at 100% in large series with no recurrence at follow-up (range, 3.9–12 months).[35–38] The most commonly reported adverse event was pneumothorax (26.6%), which was managed successfully with a chest drain. The modest rate of pneumothorax is likely

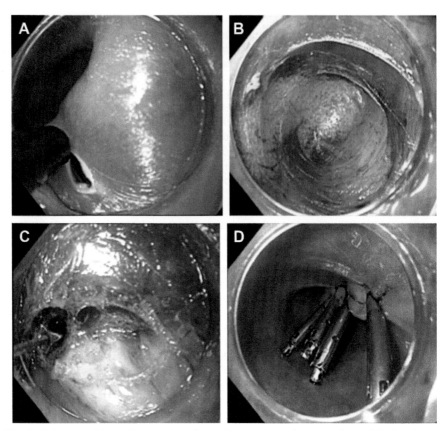

Fig. 3. Submucosal tunneling and endoscopic resection of an esophageal lesion is performed by creating a (A) mucosal bleb and incision 5 cm proximal to the subepithelial lesion. (B) The tunnel is created by dissecting the submucosal fibers using indigo carmine/saline solution and a triangle tip ESD knife (Olympus, Center Valley, PA, USA). (C) Once the gastrointestinal stromal tumor is identified, the submucosal fibers and muscle fibers are dissected away from the lesion. Once the tumor is free, it is removed from the tunnel. (D) The mucosal incision is closed with Endoclips.

related to (1) use of air insufflation rather than CO_2 in some early series and (2) requirement of full-thickness resection for tumors arising deep within the muscularis propria layer.

Both surgeons and gastroenterologists with extensive POEM experience are the current STER operators.

Endoscopic Full-Thickness Resection

Indications for full-thickness resection of GI lesions is evolving. Lesions arising from the submucosa can be resected by EMR or ESD techniques. However, lesions arising from the muscularis propria (GI stromal tumors, leiomyoma) require either STER or EFTR. Certain anatomic locations such as gastric fundus, body, and antrum may prove challenging for creation of a proximal tunnel to enable STER. Therefore, EFTR is required. Other indications include nonlifting adenomas and re-resection of T1 carcinomas. EFTR naturally results in a GI wall defect; hence, the mainstay of this technique is secure defect closure. There are 2 described approaches to EFTR: (1)

full-thickness resection followed by closure of the defect, or (2) securing GI wall closure (serosa-to-serosa) before resection.

EFTR followed by closure has been feasible and effective. After marking the perimeter of the lesion, the mucosa overlying the lesion is incised to reveal the tumor. Subsequently, the entire circumference is excavated deeply to the level of the muscularis propria. After the intraluminal aspect of the tumor is completely revealed, approximately 75% of the seromuscular layer of the tumor is incised. A double channel endoscope can then be used to (a) grasp the tumor and (b) resect the remainder of the tumor (with a snare or ESD knife). Grasping the tumor prevents it from accidentally falling into the peritoneal cavity while being resected.

There are many series reporting EFTR of gastric tumors. Overall, complete resection rates range from 98% to 100% among tumors sized 12 to 24 mm.[39–42] No recurrence is reported at 3 to 22 months of follow-up.

Closure of the defect is performed with clips. However, standard TTS clips may only have the capacity to grasp the superficial mucosa, which increases the risk of leakage. Furthermore, defects greater than 3 cm in size are difficult to close with TTS clips. Therefore, a clip plus endoloop method can be used. After passing an endoloop through the first channel, clips are advanced through the second channel to anchor the loop circumferentially around the edge of the defect. The endoloop is then tightened to obtain closure.[36] The OTSC is an innovation born out of the need for full-thickness closure devices during the advent of NOTES. Closure after EFTR is an ideal application for this device and has been used successfully.[39] Endoscopic suturing (overstitch device) is another feasible method for securing defect closure.

The manufacturer of the OTSC recently developed a full-thickness resection device (Ovesco, Tübingen, Germany) that is preloaded with a snare. The device can be mounted onto a gastroscope or colonoscope. However, the distal cap is much longer than the conventional OTSC (23 vs 6 mm) and may pose a challenge for intubation, visibility, and flexibility. After marking the lesion, the device is loaded onto the endoscope. The clip is first deployed over the lesion (grasper forceps may be used to assist) followed by immediate snare resection. At present, gastroenterologists have reported EFTR of upper GI and colonic lesions using the EFTR device.[43–45]

As is the case for other new NOTES procedures, endoscopists (gastroenterologists and surgeons) with ESD and POEM experience have placed EFTR into clinical practice. Proficiency with endoscopic closure and hemostatic techniques and devices remains essential for the success of such new NOTES procedures.

HOW DID WE TRAIN IN NEW NATURAL ORIFICE TRANSLUMENAL ENDOSCOPIC SURGERY?

In the past, many NOTES proponents have suggested that once the field has undergone significant developments, NOTES practitioners will likely need some form of fundamental surgical training, along with platform-specific and procedure-specific training.[46,47] It was widely recognized that NOTES training was unique in that it crosses specialty lines (surgery and gastroenterology) and most practitioners do not possess both the knowledge and skill to perform the traditional NOTES procedures.[48] Owing to the assumed requirements of both laparoscopic surgical and advanced endoscopic skills,[3,49] traditional NOTES training programs were lacking. Fellowships that combine extensive surgical training as well as advanced endoscopic training simply are not feasible.

The current worldwide clinical experience (and literature) suggests that dual surgical and endoscopic training is not essential for new NOTES operators. The new NOTES practitioner is an advanced GI endoscopist. The dexterity and skills for implementation of new NOTES are advanced endoscopy and submucosal endoscopy.

Because POEM seems to be a platform for most new NOTES procedures, the development of POEM programs and subsequent POEM training programs broadly illustrates the pathway of training required for new NOTES operators.[50] Currently, practicing and experienced advanced endoscopists initiate their self-directed POEM training with a combination of (i) observation of an expert performing clinical cases and (ii) hands-on training in an animal laboratory. Once proficiency is achieved within the laboratory setting, clinical cases are commenced, preferentially with direct proctorship of an expert operator.

The iPOEMs survey highlighted that the majority of POEM endoscopists have prior ESD experience.[18] Furthermore, POEM operators in 10 of 16 centers pursued preclinical training before human POEMs. Most centers used live animal training with a minority of centers using ex vivo models or cadavers. The extent of preclinical training varied widely (total hours spent on preclinical training ranged from 12 to 154 h). Nine of 16 centers reported having an expert proctor for the initial human POEM case or cases. The median number of proctored cases was 2 (range, 1–7).[18]

Once endoscopists become proficient in POEM, STER, EFTR, and G-POEM practice can be initiated. Discussing techniques to improve the technical and clinical aspects of the procedures with colleagues, peers, and mentors has been encouraged. The international POEM conference held at Digestive Diseases Week and United European Gastroenterology Week each year is an ideal forum for learning and sharing techniques. The forum also provides the opportunity for collaboration and research within the field of new NOTES.[51]

Therefore, the vast majority of the current generation of new NOTES operators are experienced advanced endoscopists and may have either a gastroenterology or surgical training background. The key element of all proceduralists is their broad endoscopy training.

TRAINING, LEARNING CURVE, AND PROGRAM DEVELOPMENT FOR THE NEXT GENERATION

As highlighted, the key elements required for the new NOTES operator are advanced and submucosal endoscopy training. Hence, the new NOTES operator needs proficiency in advanced endoscopic skills such as dexterity, submucosal dissection, use of various endoscopic equipment and accessories (OTSC, endoscopic suturing, and hemostatic devices), all of which assume basic skills in endoscopy (gastroscopy, colonoscopy) before embarking upon advanced endoscopy training. Thereafter (or concomitantly), training in submucosal endoscopy and POEM should be undertaken.

Two years ago, the iPOEM survey identified 25 centers across North America, Europe, and Asia performing POEM.[18] Many more centers have since emerged and now also span across Australia and South America. Ideally, a trainee would undertake their advanced endoscopy fellowship in a center where POEM is performed and as such would be incorporated into their training program. However, such training opportunities are still not widely available. Hence, postadvanced fellowship POEM training can be achieved by initially attending training courses that include hands-on sessions. The trainee should endeavor to obtain access to an animal laboratory for further training. Training on a nonsurvival model or on an explanted esophagus is initially advised until the procedure can be performed consistently without serious complications. Observing an expert POEM operator is then recommended, usually as part of a preceptorship program. In-depth familiarization with all the equipment is paramount (eg, electrosurgical generator settings, ESD knives, clips).[52] Subsequently, training in a live pig model should be performed. The pig is the most appropriate animal training model owing to the similarity of its anatomy to that of humans. Disadvantages of the pig model include the soft and less-vascular submucosal tissue in comparison with humans, rendering dissection less challenging and with much less bleeding risk. Limited bleeding is not uncommon during POEM in humans.[50]

Ascertaining the learning curve of this challenging procedure is an important aspect of developing a training program. Several POEM operators have attempted to define the learning curve for this intricate procedure. Procedure times have been used as a surrogate marker for performance. Kurian and colleagues[20] reported on their initial POEM experience in 40 cases. The senior surgeon was an experienced advanced endoscopist with EMR and ESD experience. The surgical trainees underwent intensive ESD, EMR, and endoscopic suturing and clipping training during their fellowship, followed by hands-on POEM training in porcine explants. A significant decrease in procedure time and inadvertent mucosotomies were noted with increasing experience and the learning curve seemed to plateau after 20 cases. Teitelbaum and colleagues[53] studied the learning curve of POEM when performed by 2 surgeons with prior experience in laparoscopic Heller myotomy and hybrid NOTES (transvaginal and transgastric cholecystectomy). The 2 operators performed 36 POEM procedures conjointly and did not find a significant decrease in procedure time with increasing experience. However, a learning rate of 8 procedures and plateau of 97 minutes were observed after excluding 2 outlier cases that required unusually prolonged times for mucosal entry closure. A recent large study reported on 93 consecutive cases performed by an interventional gastroenterologist with extensive prior ESD experience.[54] Efficiency was defined as the point in the learning curve in which the operator started engaging in performance refinements that lead to gradual decrease in procedure time. Mastery was defined as the point at which procedure time became consistent without further changes in mean procedure time.[55] Efficiency was obtained after 40 POEMs and mastery after 60 POEMs using cumulative sum analysis. However, clinical outcomes or rate of inadvertent mucosotomies did not correlate with increasing POEM experience. In another learning curve analysis of an interventional gastroenterologist, El Zein and colleagues[56] observed that the total procedure time decreased significantly with increasing experience and calculated a learning rate of 13 procedures and plateau of 102 minutes. In addition, the procedure was separated into its 4 steps and the learning curve was calculated for each step. The procedure time for performing mucosal entry, submucosal tunneling, and closure of mucosal entry decreased significantly with increasing experience, each at different learning rates. Learning plateau was attained at 16 cases for mucosal entry, 14 cases for submucosal tunneling, and 16 cases for mucosal closure. Myotomy time did not decrease with increasing operator experience. Using the mean time grouping method, a possible learning plateau was also observed around 15 cases. Overall, these results proposed that a gastroenterologist with expertise in therapeutic endoscopy and proper POEM training achieves proficiency in POEM at about 16 cases.

The reported learning curve rates in the literature vary greatly ranging from 8 to 40 cases. This may be owing to several reasons, including variable operator ability, previous experience, motivation, available technology, task complexity, case mix, operative findings, and institutional factors.[57,58] For instance, given the rarity of achalasia, a relatively short learning curve may be achievable in centers with large referral centers for motility disorders, whereas the converse may be true in centers with a low volume of referrals.

At our institution (Johns Hopkins Hospital), Khashab and colleagues developed a POEM program with the following steps: (1) in-depth review of available POEM literature and POEM videos performed by experts, (2), observation of 2 experts performing live POEM procedures with verbal instructions on the different steps and principles of the procedure, (3) performing nonsurvival POEM experiments in a porcine model, and (4) performing POEM in a survival porcine model. Finally, (5) a cohesive endoscopy team was formed composed of interventional endoscopists, interventional endoscopy nurses and technicians, anesthetists, and certified registered nurse anesthetists. The team practiced together and became knowledgeable about this novel procedure, including the steps, techniques, and potential complications before embarking upon clinical cases in patients. Most important, a multidisciplinary clinical team was formed composed of interventional endoscopists, motility gastroenterologists, and a laparoscopic surgeon. All patients who were potential POEM candidates were initially discussed in a multidisciplinary fashion.

Subsequently, the first trainee to graduate from the 2-year advanced endoscopy and POEM fellowship established a POEM program at her institution in Australia. Using the learned skills, Saxena prepared the endoscopy and clinical team. The team was already proficient in advanced endoscopy procedures (EMR, endoscopic retrograde cholangiopancreatography) but had no prior ESD experience. Didactic lectures and videos were used to educate the team about indications for POEM, equipment, and endoscopic accessories used for the novel procedure. In particular, she described the procedural principles, the various functions and features of ESD knives, cautery settings, and potential complications. Most important, various techniques for managing potential complications of the procedure (bleeding, mucosotomy, pneumoperitoneum, etc) were discussed and a "rescue kit" (see **Box 3**) was formed. The hospital's radiologists were also included in the team to increase understanding of the intricacies and difficulties of interpreting postprocedure imaging studies.[59] The POEM program was implemented successfully without any adverse events over the last 12 months. Proctoring other novice POEM operators has also been accomplished.

An adequate new NOTES training program for a trainee after completion of GI fellowship or surgical residency will likely span across another 1 to 2 years after basic endoscopic training, regardless of a surgical or gastroenterological training background. Furthermore, training may need to be carried across various centers and institutions to acquire the breadth of knowledge and endoscopic skill and experience required, not only with the endoscopic techniques, but also use of newer accessories and devices for the management of commonly encountered adverse events during new NOTES procedures. There may be a role for current working groups to help streamline the training process for the new generation of trainees.

WORKING GROUPS

The multidisciplinary effort to provide direction for NOTES has been worldwide. The skill set required to perform NOTES is reflected in the specialties represented by the societies that are contributing their efforts. The American societies, the American Society of Gastrointestinal Endoscopy and the Society of American Gastrointestinal Endoscopic Surgeons, combined to form the Natural Orifice Surgery Consortium for Assessment and Research in 2005. Similarly, the European Association for Endoscopic Surgery and the European Society of Gastrointestinal Endoscopy joined to form the Euro-NOTES Foundation.[60] In 2008, working groups in Germany known as Deustchland-NOTES, or D-NOTES were formed.[61] The working groups meet annually and the driving objectives of the working groups remain to ensure safe clinical application of NOTES and to provide an environment for gastroenterologists, GI surgeons and product design engineers, which is conducive to the development of solutions to existing challenges, particularly with regard to technological limitations for the progression of NOTES. Assessing yearly scientific progress and clinical outcomes has also been an integral component for Natural Orifice Surgery Consortium for Assessment and Research, Euro-NOTES, and D-NOTES, with publication of expert opinion guidelines based on existing data.

The annual program agenda and content of publications from these meetings has reflected the respectable progression of NOTES toward the "short-range" new NOTES procedures.

SUMMARY

Ten years later, NOTES represents one of the most intense areas of surgical and GI research, and is arguably the most significant endoscopic innovation of this decade. POEM was the first NOTES offshoot out of which was borne the novel collection of new NOTES. The training pathway for new NOTES is a relatively long journey encompassing advanced endoscopy training, mastery of endoscopic dexterity within the narrow submucosal or "third space" with an in-depth understanding of the tissue planes through training in submucosal endoscopy. Proficiency with new closure and hemostatic devices is also essential. There are few institutions worldwide that can provide all the cognitive and technical elements essential to train new NOTES trainees. Hence, many trainees may need to spend time across several institutions to ensure safe and effective practice of new NOTES.

REFERENCES

1. Kalloo AN, Singh VK, Jagannath SB, et al. Flexible transgastric peritoneoscopy: a novel approach to diagnostic and therapeutic interventions in the peritoneal cavity. Gastrointest Endosc 2004;60:114–7.
2. Rao GV, Reddy DN, Banerjee R. NOTES: human experience. Gastrointest Endosc Clin N Am 2008;18:361–70, x.
3. Rattner D, Kalloo A, Group ASW. ASGE/SAGES working group on natural orifice translumenal endoscopic surgery. October 2005. Surg Endosc 2006;20:329–33.
4. Marescaux J, Dallemagne B, Perretta S, et al. Surgery without scars: report of transluminal cholecystectomy in a human being. Arch Surg 2007;142:823–6 [discussion: 826–7].
5. Zorron R, Filgueiras M, Maggioni LC, et al. NOTES. Transvaginal cholecystectomy: report of the first case. Surg Innov 2007;14:279–83.
6. Branco AW, Branco Filho AJ, Kondo W, et al. Hybrid transvaginal nephrectomy. Eur Urol 2008;53:1290–4.
7. Dumont F, Goere D, Honore C, et al. Transanal endoscopic total mesorectal excision combined with single-port laparoscopy. Dis Colon Rectum 2012;55: 996–1001.
8. Fuchs KH. Comments on the current status and future development of natural orifice transluminal endoscopic surgery. ANZ J Surg 2015;85:201–2.
9. Khashab MA, Pasricha PJ. Conquering the third space: challenges and opportunities for diagnostic and therapeutic endoscopy. Gastrointest Endosc 2013;77: 146–8.
10. Rattner D. Introduction to NOTES white paper. Surg Endosc 2006;20:185.

11. Moss A, Williams SJ, Hourigan LF, et al. Long-term adenoma recurrence following wide-field endoscopic mucosal resection (WF-EMR) for advanced colonic mucosal neoplasia is infrequent: results and risk factors in 1000 cases from the Australian colonic EMR (ACE) study. Gut 2015;64:57–65.

12. Pimentel-Nunes P, Dinis-Ribeiro M, Ponchon T, et al. Endoscopic submucosal dissection: European society of gastrointestinal endoscopy (ESGE) guideline. Endoscopy 2015;47:829–54.

13. Pasricha PJ, Hawari R, Ahmed I, et al. Submucosal endoscopic esophageal myotomy: a novel experimental approach for the treatment of achalasia. Endoscopy 2007;39:761–4.

14. Inoue H, Kudo SE. Per-oral endoscopic myotomy (POEM) for 43 consecutive cases of esophageal achalasia. Nihon Rinsho 2010;68:1749–52 [in Japanese].

15. Inoue H, Minami H, Kobayashi Y, et al. Peroral endoscopic myotomy (POEM) for esophageal achalasia. Endoscopy 2010;42:265–71.

16. Khashab MA, Kumbhari V, Kalloo AN, et al. Peroral endoscopic myotomy: a 4-step approach to a challenging procedure. Gastrointest Endosc 2014;79:997–8.

17. Barbieri LA, Hassan C, Rosati R, et al. Systematic review and meta-analysis: efficacy and safety of POEM for achalasia. United European Gastroenterol J 2015;3:325–34.

18. Stavropoulos SN, Modayil RJ, Friedel D, et al. The international per oral endoscopic myotomy survey (IPOEMS): a snapshot of the global POEM experience. Surg Endosc 2013;27:3322–38.

19. Inoue H, Rubino F, Shimada Y, et al. Risk of gastric cancer after roux-en-Y gastric bypass. Arch Surg 2007;142:947–53.

20. Kurian AA, Dunst CM, Sharata A, et al. Peroral endoscopic esophageal myotomy: defining the learning curve. Gastrointest Endosc 2013;77:719–25.

21. Teitelbaum EN, Rajeswaran S, Zhang R, et al. Peroral esophageal myotomy (POEM) and laparoscopic Heller myotomy produce a similar short-term anatomic and functional effect. Surgery 2013;154:885–91 [discussion: 891–2].

22. Khashab MA, El Zein M, Kumbhari V, et al. Comprehensive analysis of efficacy and safety of peroral endoscopic myotomy performed by a gastroenterologist in the endoscopy unit: a single-center experience. Gastrointest Endosc 2015;83(1):117–25.

23. Li QL, Zhou PH, Yao LQ, et al. Early diagnosis and management of delayed bleeding in the submucosal tunnel after peroral endoscopic myotomy for achalasia (with video). Gastrointest Endosc 2013;78:370–4.

24. Committee NPWP, Stavropoulos SN, Desilets DJ, et al. Per-oral endoscopic myotomy white paper summary. Gastrointest Endosc 2014;80:1–15.

25. Hungness ES, Teitelbaum EN, Santos BF, et al. Comparison of perioperative outcomes between peroral esophageal myotomy (POEM) and laparoscopic Heller myotomy. J Gastrointest Surg 2013;17:228–35.

26. Ujiki MB, Yetasook AK, Zapf M, et al. Peroral endoscopic myotomy: a short-term comparison with the standard laparoscopic approach. Surgery 2013;154:893–7 [discussion: 897–900].

27. Bechara R, Ikeda H, Inoue H. Peroral endoscopic myotomy: an evolving treatment for achalasia. Nat Rev Gastroenterol Hepatol 2015;12:410–26.

28. Mearin F, Camilleri M, Malagelada JR. Pyloric dysfunction in diabetics with recurrent nausea and vomiting. Gastroenterology 1986;90:1919–25.

29. Kawai M, Peretta S, Burckhardt O, et al. Endoscopic pyloromyotomy: a new concept of minimally invasive surgery for pyloric stenosis. Endoscopy 2012;44: 169–73.
30. Khashab MA, Stein E, Clarke JO, et al. Gastric peroral endoscopic myotomy for refractory gastroparesis: first human endoscopic pyloromyotomy (with video). Gastrointest Endosc 2013;78:764–8.
31. Shlomovitz E, Pescarus R, Cassera MA, et al. Early human experience with per- oral endoscopic pyloromyotomy (POP). Surg Endosc 2015;29:543–51.
32. Chaves DM, de Moura EG, Mestieri LH, et al. Endoscopic pyloromyotomy via a gastric submucosal tunnel dissection for the treatment of gastroparesis after sur- gical vagal lesion. Gastrointest Endosc 2014;80:164.
33. Gonzalez JM, Vanbiervliet G, Vitton V, et al. First European human gastric peroral endoscopic myotomy, for treatment of refractory gastroparesis. Endoscopy 2015; 47(Suppl 1):E135–6.
34. Chung H, Dallemagne B, Perretta S, et al. Endoscopic pyloromyotomy for post- esophagectomy gastric outlet obstruction. Endoscopy 2014;46(Suppl 1):E345–6.
35. Wang XY, Xu MD, Yao LQ, et al. Submucosal tunneling endoscopic resection for submucosal tumors of the esophagogastric junction originating from the muscu- laris propria layer: a feasibility study (with videos). Surg Endosc 2014;28:1971–7.
36. Ye LP, Zhang Y, Mao XL, et al. Submucosal tunnelling endoscopic resection for the treatment of esophageal submucosal tumours originating from the muscularis propria layer: an analysis of 15 cases. Dig Liver Dis 2013;45:119–23.
37. Liu BR, Song JT, Kong LJ, et al. Tunneling endoscopic muscularis dissection for subepithelial tumors originating from the muscularis propria of the esophagus and gastric cardia. Surg Endosc 2013;27:4354–9.
38. Xu MD, Cai MY, Zhou PH, et al. Submucosal tunneling endoscopic resection: a new technique for treating upper GI submucosal tumors originating from the mus- cularis propria layer (with videos). Gastrointest Endosc 2012;75:195–9.
39. Guo J, Liu Z, Sun S, et al. Endoscopic full-thickness resection with defect closure using an over-the-scope clip for gastric subepithelial tumors originating from the muscularis propria. Surg Endosc 2015;29(11):3356–62.
40. Zhou PH, Yao LQ, Qin XY, et al. Endoscopic full-thickness resection without lapa- roscopic assistance for gastric submucosal tumors originated from the muscula- ris propria. Surg Endosc 2011;25:2926–31.
41. Ye LP, Yu Z, Mao XL, et al. Endoscopic full-thickness resection with defect closure using clips and an endoloop for gastric subepithelial tumors arising from the mus- cularis propria. Surg Endosc 2014;28:1978–83.
42. Schmidt A, Bauder M, Riecken B, et al. Endoscopic full-thickness resection of gastric subepithelial tumors: a single-center series. Endoscopy 2015;47:154–8.
43. Schmidt A, Meier B, Cahyadi O, et al. Duodenal endoscopic full-thickness resec- tion (with video). Gastrointest Endosc 2015;82:728–33.
44. Schmidt A, Bauerfeind P, Gubler C, et al. Endoscopic full-thickness resection in the colorectum with a novel over-the-scope device: first experience. Endoscopy 2015;47:719–25.
45. Snauwaert C, Jouret-Mourin A, Piessevaux H. Endoscopic full-thickness resec- tion of a nonlifting adenoma in an ileal pouch using an over-the-scope full-thick- ness resection device. Endoscopy 2015;47(Suppl 1):E344–5.
46. Santos BF, Hungness ES. Natural orifice translumenal endoscopic surgery: prog- ress in humans since white paper. World J Gastroenterol 2011;17:1655–65.
47. Mansard MJ, Reddy DN, Rao GV. NOTES: a review. Trop Gastroenterol 2009;30: 5–10.

48. Dunkin BJ. Natural orifice transluminal endoscopic surgery: educational challenge. World J Gastrointest Surg 2010;2:224–30.
49. Rattner DW, Hawes R, Schwaitzberg S, et al. The second SAGES/ASGE white paper on natural orifice transluminal endoscopic surgery: 5 years of progress. Surg Endosc 2011;25:2441–8.
50. Khashab MA. Thoughts on starting a peroral endoscopic myotomy program. Gastrointest Endosc 2013;77:109–10.
51. Available at: http://www.achalasia-poem.net. Accessed October 10, 2015.
52. Eleftheriadis N, Inoue H, Ikeda H, et al. Training in peroral endoscopic myotomy (POEM) for esophageal achalasia. Ther Clin Risk Manag 2012;8:329–42.
53. Teitelbaum EN, Soper NJ, Arafat FO, et al. Analysis of a learning curve and predictors of intraoperative difficulty for peroral esophageal myotomy (POEM). J Gastrointest Surg 2014;18:92–8 [discussion: 98–9].
54. Patel KS, Calixte R, Modayil RJ, et al. The light at the end of the tunnel: a single-operator learning curve analysis for per oral endoscopic myotomy. Gastrointest Endosc 2015;81:1181–7.
55. Li X, Wang J, Ferguson MK. Competence versus mastery: the time course for developing proficiency in video-assisted thoracoscopic lobectomy. J Thorac Cardiovasc Surg 2014;147:1150–4.
56. El Zein M, Kumbhari V, Saxena P, et al. Learning curve for peroral endoscopic myotomy deciphered: a comprehensive analysis using two different methodologies. Gastrointest Endosc 2015;81:AB167.
57. Sachdeva AK, Russell TR. Safe introduction of new procedures and emerging technologies in surgery: education, credentialing, and privileging. Surg Clin North Am 2007;87:853–66, vi–vii.
58. Cook JA, Ramsay CR, Fayers P. Statistical evaluation of learning curve effects in surgical trials. Clin Trials 2004;1:421–7.
59. Saxena P, Abdollahian D, Kompel A, et al. Radiologic imaging of over-the-scope-clips can be misunderstood: the "pooling sign". Endoscopy 2013;45(Suppl 2): E305–6.
60. Meining A, Spaun G, Fernandez-Esparrach G, et al. NOTES in Europe: summary of the working group reports of the 2012 EURO-NOTES meeting. Endoscopy 2013;45:214–7.
61. Fritscher-Ravens A, Feussner H, Kahler G, et al. State of NOTES development in Germany: status report of the D-NOTES-Congress 2011th. Z Gastroenterol 2012; 50:325–30 [in German].

Pre-clinical Training for New Notes Procedures
From Ex-vivo Models to Virtual Reality Simulators

Mark A. Gromski, MD[a],*, Woojin Ahn, PhD[b],
Kai Matthes, MD, PhD[c], Suvranu De, ScD[b]

KEYWORDS

- NOTES • New NOTES • Endoscopic surgery • Simulation • Training

KEY POINTS

- The field of natural orifice transluminal endoscopic surgery (NOTES) has evolved over the past decade.
- There is immense clinical and research interest in the current new NOTES procedures, and this version of NOTES is likely here to stay.
- With that comes the responsibility to inform health practitioners and effectively train those who may perform these procedures now and in the future.
- Given the complexity and distinct skills required of NOTES, simulation will continue to play a prominent role in the training paradigm for NOTES.
- It is likely that simulation will decrease the lengthy learning curves for these procedures. Simulation research will also continue to advance the developmental endoscopy field.

INTRODUCTION

Natural orifice transluminal endoscopic surgery (NOTES) is a relatively new field of advanced endoscopic surgery that has undergone dramatic development and evolution since its inception in 2004 with the seminal description of a transgastric peritoneal

Conflict of Interest Disclosure: Dr M.A. Gromski has served as a consultant for EndoSim, LLC. Dr K. Matthes is owner of EndoSim, LLC. No other authors reported a conflict of interest relevant to this study.
[a] Division of Gastroenterology/Hepatology, Indiana University School of Medicine, 702 Rotary Circle, Suite 225, Indianapolis, IN 46202, USA; [b] Department of Mechanical, Aerospace and Nuclear Engineering, Center for Modeling, Simulation and Imaging in Medicine, Rensselaer Polytechnic Institute, 110 8th St, Troy, NY 12180, USA; [c] Department of Anesthesiology, Perioperative and Pain Medicine, Children's Hospital Boston, Harvard Medical School, 300 Longwood Ave, Boston, MA 02115, USA
* Corresponding author.
E-mail address: mgromski@iupui.edu

Gastrointest Endoscopy Clin N Am 26 (2016) 401–412
http://dx.doi.org/10.1016/j.giec.2015.12.007
1052-5157/16/$ – see front matter © 2016 Elsevier Inc. All rights reserved.

access by Kalloo and colleagues.[1] The history of NOTES has been described elsewhere, and thus is not addressed within this paper.[2]

Early in the evolution of NOTES, there was a vigorous interest in NOTES approaches to standard and frequent laparoscopic operations, such as the cholecystectomy and appendectomy. Perhaps predictably, given the high standards for safety and efficacy of existing laparoscopic techniques for those common operations, many have not been convinced that moving to a NOTES approach can improve upon the current gold standard laparoscopic approaches. Those traditional procedures are referred to as "first-generation NOTES." The field in general has pivoted to concentrating research and clinical efforts on novel minimally invasive approaches to pathology within the luminal wall and adjacent to the luminal wall. Peroral endoscopic myotomy (POEM), submucosal endoscopy, full-thickness endoscopic resection (EFTR) of subepithelial tumors and peroral pyloromyotomy are examples of this new paradigm, which has been called new NOTES or "near NOTES."

As with any emerging technology, simulation provides a safe introduction of the technique to the clinic. This is important for new NOTES for several reasons. First, new NOTES procedures requires unique skills that are distinct from standard advanced endoscopic procedures, such as a requirement to have expertise of transluminal anatomy, and mastery in submucosal dissection and various novel endoscopic tools. Furthermore, there needs to be crisp and collegial communication and teamwork between endoscopic and surgical interplay (or backup) for such procedures. Some procedures treat relatively rare pathologic entities (such as achalasia for POEM). Other new NOTES procedures that require submucosal tunneling are born out of endoscopic submucosal dissection (ESD) techniques that were developed in Asia. The training ground is completely different there given the vastly higher number of superficial gastric malignancies that are treated endoscopically there. For these, simulation is critical to supplement low case volumes for new NOTES procedures.

In this review of simulation and training in NOTES, we discuss the importance of simulation in NOTES, describe available simulators and comment on the need for multimodal training. We emphasize developments in ex vivo simulation in new NOTES techniques and also development of virtual reality (VR) NOTES platforms, the 2 most dynamic aspects of NOTES simulation training currently.

OVERVIEW OF NATURAL ORIFICE TRANSLUMINAL ENDOSCOPIC SURGERY SIMULATION

NOTES procedures are universally complex and advanced. They have been developed and studied by world-renowned endoscopists and surgeons, and require exceptional endoscopic skill to be accomplished safely and effectively. Given that NOTES procedures are complex endoscopic tasks that require the development and modification of endoscopic skills that even general experienced endoscopists do not carry, simulation carries an important role in the training environment of NOTES.

Unlike using a novel endoscopic accessory such as a snare that requires little if any specific training before using in clinical practice, NOTES requires mastery of specific skills, such as detailed anatomic understanding, expertise in needle knives and electrosurgery, familiarity with novel endoscopic devices, comfort with closing full-thickness luminal defects and submucosal endoscopy, all of which require practice and dedicated study. The training environment requires repeated skills building with expert guidance, all of which lends well to simulation training.

Available simulation options for NOTES include mechanical simulators including part task trainers to fine tube basic endoscopic skills and full procedure NOTES simulators, ex vivo simulators to simulate entire specific NOTES procedures or components of NOTES procedures (such as full-thickness luminal closure, submucosal dissection), and VR simulators. With recent shifts in interest to new NOTES procedures such as POEM, EFTR, and submucosal endoscopy, the NOTES simulation arena is in a period of development and undergoing changes.

MECHANICAL SIMULATORS

Inanimate task trainers can be used by endoscopists to improve technical endoscopic skills used in day-to-day endoscopy. For endoscopists who wish to learn NOTES, it is absolutely essential to have mastery of standard endoscopy skills. Inanimate skills trainers can help test and improve those skills. The Thompson Endoscopic Skills Trainer was recently developed as a part task trainer for endoscopists interested in improving or maintaining endoscopic technical skill. The Thompson Endoscopic Skills Trainer is a plastic-based modular portable training center that allows for the endoscopist to perform 5 individual tasks (retroflexion, torque, knob control, polypectomy and navigation/loop reduction) that develop a particular skill used in endoscopy.[3] The appealing component of this simulator is that it can provide objective information for skills testing and tracking for trainees. Jirapinyo and colleagues[4] recently reported a study that confirmed validity of this skills simulator, confirming it can assess endoscopic skills objectively.[4] Next steps for the simulator included more widespread multicenter trials of trainees skills development and defining learning curves with the simulator.

Mechanical simulators specific to NOTES have been developed. These have been developed for the first-generation NOTES, such as NOTES appendectomy and cholecystectomy. These mechanical NOTES simulators have been reviewed in detail elsewhere.[5,6] Two of these simulators are the Endoscopic-Laparoscopic Interdisciplinary Training Entity (ELITE) trainer and the Natural Orifice Simulated Surgical Environment simulator. The ELITE is a plastic phantom developed in Germany, which has previously demonstrated construct validity.[7,8] There was recently a study reported that used the ELITE NOTES trainer to judge whether previous endoscopic versus surgical simulation training helped novices in performing a simulated NOTES procedures.[9] The study found that previous training in a simple endoscopy simulator was superior to a laparoscopy simulator to successfully complete a NOTES task in the ELITE simulator.[9] The Natural Orifice Simulated Surgical Environment is similar to a surgical laparoscopic box trainer and provides skills training for tasks particular to NOTES procedures.[10]

A recent study by Buscaglia and colleagues[11] used the ProMIS simulator (Haptica, Dublin, Ireland) to carry out simulated transanal NOTES sigmoidectomy procedures. This is a laparoscopic, inanimate surgical simulator that was modified. In this study, 4 participants performed 21 simulated resections, and it was found that the participants had nonsignificant improvements in total procedure time and in 8 individual steps of the operation.[11]

There has not yet been developed a validated and commercially available mechanical simulator for new NOTES procedures such as POEM or EFTR.

EX VIVO SIMULATORS

A mainstay of simulation in NOTES is the ex vivo simulator. The benefits of ex vivo simulation include the ability to simulate entire NOTES procedures or concentrate on individual tasks (eg, gastrotomy closure); ex vivo simulation is readily commercially available; realistic tissue manipulation is realized given the use of biological tissue, including electrocautery; and ex vivo simulators are relatively less expensive than mechanical simulators, VR simulators, or live animals. Drawbacks of ex vivo simulation include the inability to simulate certain components of a procedure, such as intraprocedural bleeding.

"First-generation" NOTES procedures including intraperitoneal tissue resection (eg, cholecystectomy, appendectomy) can be simulated using total organ porcine explant (**Fig. 1**) simulators outfitted in specialized simulation trays that simulate an abdominal cavity and allow for both laparoscopic and endoscopic access (EndoSim, LLC, Hudson, MA, USA; **Fig. 2**).

Furthermore, ex vivo simulators have been created for the simulation of various new NOTES procedures, including POEM, pyloromyotomy, submucosal endoscopy, and EFTR. Simulation sessions can be organized as single complete procedures to introduce the concept of the procedure to endoscopists or to referring physicians. Or, a series of simulation sessions can be arranged to build skills in a certain procedure for the endoscopist who is interested in potentially implementing a procedure into his practice in the future. Particularly helpful are workshops that concentrate on a certain task, such as submucosal tunneling or full-thickness closure (such as endoscopic suturing device or over-the-scope clip; **Fig. 3**). This allows the endoscopist to add a particular skill to their armamentarium like submucosal endoscopy and full-thickness closure, because these skills are transferrable to a variety of advanced endoscopic procedures.

The effectiveness of ex vivo simulation in advanced endoscopic procedures has been validated. In a group of endoscopists novice to ESD, in which each endoscopist performed 60 each gastric ESD procedures, it was found that there were significant improvements in the speed and quality of ESD resections after 30 cases.[12] Another prospective ex vivo study evaluated the performance of colorectal ESD in endoscopists experienced in gastric ESD yet novice to colorectal ESD.[13] Each endoscopist performed 30 complete resections. There was significant improvement of performance by each endoscopist in the study. When performance was evaluated with a composite performance score, including time of procedure and complications including perforation, the inflection point of the learning curve appeared after 9 procedures.[13] Given the complexity of ESD is similar to many new NOTES procedures, it is reasonable to

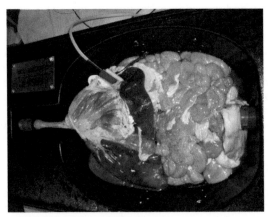

Fig. 1. Abdominopelvic porcine tissue explant arranged for first-generation natural orifice transluminal endoscopic surgery procedure.

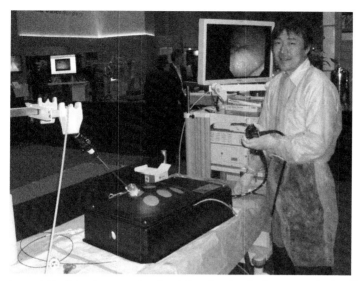

Fig. 2. Endoscopist training in an ex vivo simulator allowing for laparoscopic visualization of endoscopic procedure.

extrapolate that endoscopists would realize similar skills building with other specific NOTES ex vivo simulators. There are studies ongoing to answer this question.

Ex vivo simulators of NOTES procedures can be used to carry out research on clinical questions, as pilot studies before live porcine or human clinical studies. For instance, 1 ex vivo study investigated the maximal diameter of full-thickness gastric

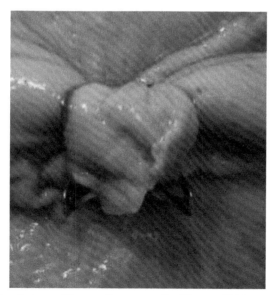

Fig. 3. Gastrotomy closure with over-the-scope clip (Ovesco, Tubingen, Germany) in an ex vivo model.

defect that could be closed with an over-the-scope clip (Ovesco, Tubingen, Germany).[14] Another study compared the efficacy of gastrotomy closure with different closure devices with either a submucosal tunnel access or transmural gastrotomy.[15] A submucosal tunnel closed with an over-the-scope clip was more secure than either a submucosal tunnel access closed with standard hemoclips or a transmural gastrotomy closed with an over-the-scope clip.[15] Another study used an adult and pediatric ex vivo model for endoscopic pyloromyotomy to investigate the optimal length of myotomy (**Fig. 4**).[16] In the ex vivo models, the optimal length of myotomy was 3 cm in the adult model and 2 cm in the pediatric model.[16]

VIRTUAL REALITY NATURAL ORIFICE TRANSLUMINAL ENDOSCOPIC SURGERY SIMULATORS

A VR-based NOTES simulator is a promising tool, both as a testbed for development of new procedures and instruments and as a training tool for acquiring well-established NOTES techniques and skills. As a testbed, unlike the current paradigm using porcine or cadaver models, a VR-NOTES simulator can provide a fully controllable operating room setting in a safe and risk-free environment without any ethical issues. A variety of scientific techniques used for modeling and simulation can be applied to resolve challenging issues in the field, such as evaluating safe closure techniques and the effects of pneumoperitoneum, before applying them to costly live animal studies or putting human patients at risk. As a training tool, the major benefits include quick and easy setup of various training scenarios, unlimited training materials, and automated, objective, quantitative analysis of surgical skills. Development of a VR-NOTES simulator, however, is a challenging task that requires innovative solutions to hardware and software design. A simulator is only useful if it is shown to be realistic and represent the procedure with sufficient fidelity. In particular, a rapidly developing field such as NOTES requires rapid prototyping technologies to quickly build new high-fidelity simulators for emerging NOTES procedures. To cope with this, our team is developing a VR-NOTES simulator called the Virtual Transluminal Endoscopic Surgical Trainer (VTEST) based on modularization of both software and hardware that facilitates the decomposition of the complex task of developing a

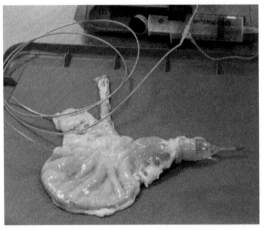

Fig. 4. Ex vivo simulation model for endoscopic pyloromyotomy, measuring the effectiveness of myotomy with EndoFlip (Crospon, Galway, Ireland).

new VR-NOTES system into a number of independent reusable and customizable modules.

Fig. 5 shows a schematic diagram of our VR-NOTES simulator that mainly consists of both interface and software components. This standard structure can be applied to build VR-NOTES simulators for the existing and future NOTES procedures in general. A user interacts with the virtual system via the interface that provides an immersive environment as the real operating room. The instruments used on actual NOTES procedures are inserted into the dummy patient that includes realistic natural orifice models, that is, a female reproductive organ model. The instruments are equipped with sensors to measure the motions and motors to provide force feedback to the user. The sensed signal is digitized and sent to the computer. The VR-NOTES software constructs and renders 3-dimensional organ models, and perform numerical computation for simulation of the interaction between the virtual instruments and organ models. The simulated scene is displayed to the user through high-definition display monitors. This is a VR-NOTES simulation cycle looping repeatedly a sequence of the user's hand motions, instrument interface, software computation, displaying the endoscopic view, and force feedback to the user. The system has to guarantee 30-Hz graphic and 1-kHz haptic refresh rates to provide high-fidelity combined sensory feedback. These real-time constraints become more challenging because a high level of visual and haptic realism requires more intensive computation. Thus, it is critical to build the simulation on a well-structured, high-performance software framework.

The VR-NOTES software is based on modular design. The idea is to decompose the complex VR-NOTES software into a number of independent modules. Ultimately, it facilitates rapid development of new simulation for future NOTES procedures by assembling the already developed modules and customizing them only for the specific requirements. For example, a graphic rendering module that visualizes the internal wall of the stomach and esophagus developed for simulation of transgastric appendectomy can be potentially reused for the development of new simulation for any transgastric NOTES procedures.

The hardware interface of a VR-NOTES simulator consists of modularized subsystems as the software does. The modularized hardware interface provides (1) an insufflated abdominal model with accessible ports (**Fig. 6**), (2) a rigid endoscope interface

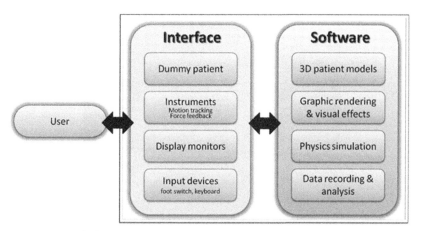

Fig. 5. Diagram of the virtual reality natural orifice transluminal endoscopic surgery simulator.

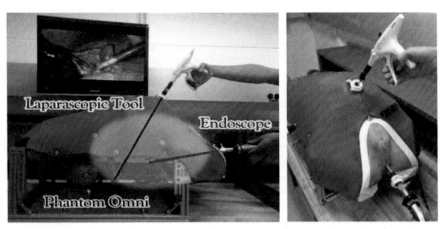

Fig. 6. A dummy patient for the virtual reality natural orifice transluminal endoscopic surgery simulator.

(**Fig. 7**), (3) a flexible endoscope interface (**Fig. 8**), (4) an interface for laparoscopic instruments, (5) modularized laparoscopic instrument handles, and (6) foot pedals. The hardware modules can be selected according to the requirements of a particular NOTES procedure, assembled with other modules, and integrated into the software module for controlling the hardware. For example, a simulator for pure transgastric NOTES cholecystectomy can be composed of the insufflated abdominal model and the flexible endoscope interface. The obvious benefit of this modular concept is to quickly build new hardware interfaces for new NOTES procedures by customizing the existing modules and assembling a set of the required modules.

The first version of the VTEST in **Fig. 9** is being developed based on the transvaginal NOTES hybrid (with laparoscopic assistance) cholecystectomy performed by Roberts and colleagues.[17] The decision to develop a VR-based NOTES training simulator for this procedure was based on a needs analysis at the 2011 Natural Orifice Consortium for Assessment and Research (NOSCAR) meeting.[18] The study found that NOTES

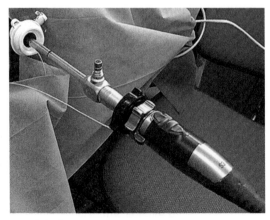

Fig. 7. Rigid endoscope interface.

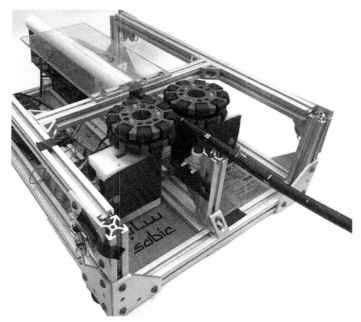

Fig. 8. Flexible endoscope interface.

cholecystectomy was the most widely performed NOTES procedure at the time and also the most preferred one to be simulated in a VR setting at the time. Also, the transvaginal route was preferred over the transgastric approach. The NOTES procedure has unique hand–eye coordination and does not allow bimanual cooperative operation

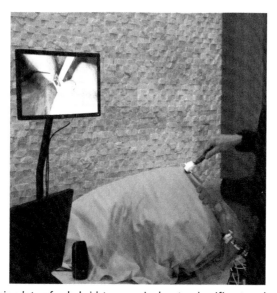

Fig. 9. A virtual simulator for hybrid transvaginal natural orifice transluminal endoscopic surgery cholecystectomy.

as in traditional laparoscopic surgery. The VTEST is designed to allow surgeons to adapt the new technique and instruments.

The hardware modules are assembled using the dummy patient, rigid endoscope, and laparoscopic interface modules, and integrated into novel software built with female 3-dimensional internal organ models. The transvaginal NOTES hybrid cholecystectomy procedure is divided into 7 sequential tasks based on our task analysis: stabilize gallbladder, identify cystic duct/artery, clip cystic duct/artery, cut cystic duct/artery, detach gallbladder, inspect the operation field, and remove gallbladder with endobag.[19] At the beginning of the simulation, the rigid endoscope is inserted and the tip is placed near the posterior vagina. The extracorporeal suture threads tightly retract the gallbladder for stabilization by assuming that the gallbladder is already stabilized. The trainee can start the simulation by navigating the abdomen cavity to reach the region of interest and performing the subsequent tasks. The simulation ends when the gallbladder is completely detached from the liver bed. **Fig. 10** shows simulation screen shots of the successive tasks.

The simulator has been displayed and we have elicited feedback at the NOSCAR meeting annually since 2013.[20] We are improving the simulator and planning to perform validation studies to determine the ability to differentiate the level of competence and the transferability of surgical skills from the simulator to the operating room. Although the VR-NOTES simulator under development is for the cholecystectomy procedure, the VTEST platform can be extended to the simulation of other procedures and techniques using the hardware and software modules. In particular, POEM is identified as a promising candidate for future simulator development from a series of our questionnaire studies at NOSCAR. Furthermore, we are developing automated scoring metrics that will allow real-time assessment of surgical competency. Once completed and validated, we anticipate that VTEST could be used as a training and assessment platform for safe and reliable surgical education.

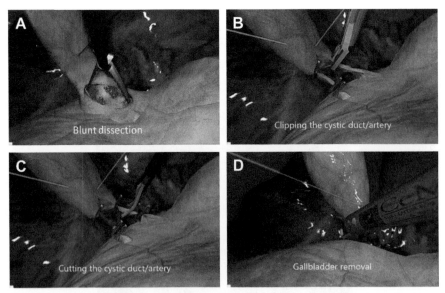

Fig. 10. Simulation scenes in virtual reality natural orifice transluminal endoscopic surgery cholecystectomy: (*A*) blunt dissection, (*B*) clipping of the cystic duct/artery, (*C*) cutting the cystic duct/artery, and (*D*) gallbladder removal.

MULTIMODAL TRAINING IN NATURAL ORIFICE TRANSLUMINAL ENDOSCOPIC SURGERY

The road to performing NOTES procedures in clinical practice at the moment is reserved for experts in advanced endoscopic and endoscopic surgical skills. Both first-generation NOTES and new NOTES procedures require distinct, technologically challenging skills that are often not used in the day-to-day practice of a general gastro-enterologist or surgeon. An inexperienced or poorly prepared endoscopist may have poor results with the adoption of NOTES into clinical practice. For this reason, it is important that those wishing to learning NOTES procedures undergo a multimodal training program to build the necessary skills to successfully perform the procedure of interest.[2,5] A prototypical training schedule may include initial exposure to the procedure or skills in question with a VR simulator or mechanical simulator. The next step would likely include skills building by performing multiple simulated procedures in an ex vivo model. Next, the training endoscopist should perform procedures in live animal models (most commonly porcine, less commonly canine or sheep), so as to be able to encounter aspects including intraprocedural bleeding and hemodynamic effects of the procedure that cannot otherwise be realistically simulated. At this stage of training, it is ideal to include the entire procedural team, including technician and nurse, so as to familiarize the team with the procedure and tools to be used. The final step of the training paradigm is to undergo proctored, gradual clinical experience with an established expert in the field that performs the procedure regularly.

SUMMARY

NOTES has evolved over the past decade. There is immense clinical and research interest in the current new NOTES procedures, and given the increasing adoption of these procedures here and abroad, this version of NOTES is likely here to stay. With that comes the responsibility to inform health practitioners and effectively train those who may perform these procedures now and in the future.

Given the complexity and distinct skills required of NOTES, simulation will continue to play a prominent role in the training paradigm for NOTES. It is likely that simulation will decrease the lengthy learning curves for these procedures. Simulation research will also continue to advance developmental endoscopy.

REFERENCES

1. Kalloo AN, Singh VK, Jagannath SB, et al. Flexible transgastric peritoneoscopy: a novel approach to diagnostic and therapeutic interventions in the peritoneal cavity. Gastrointest Endosc 2004;60:114–7.
2. Gromski M, Matthes K. Natural orifice translumenal endoscopic surgery (NOTES). In: Jones DB, Andrews R, Critchlow J, et al, editors. Minimally invasive surgery: laparoscopy, therapeutic endoscopy and NOTES. London: JP Medical Publishers; 2015. p. 199–207.
3. Thompson CC, Jirapinyo P, Kumar N, et al. Development and initial validation of an endoscopic part-task training box. Endoscopy 2014;46:735–44.
4. Jirapinyo P, Kumar N, Thompson CC. Validation of an endoscopic part-task training box as a skill assessment tool. Gastrointest Endosc 2015;81:967–73.
5. Matthes K, Gromski M, Hawes R. Training in natural orifice translumenal endoscopic surgery. In: Cohen J, editor. Successful training in gastrointestinal endoscopy. Wiley-Blackwell; 2011. p. 261–9.
6. Gromski M, Matthes K. Simulation in advanced endoscopy: state of the art and the next generation. Tech Gastrointest Endosc 2011;13:203–8.

7. Fiolka A, Gillen S, Meining A, et al. ELITE–the ex vivo training unit for NOTES: development and validation. Minim Invasive Ther Allied Technol 2010;19:281–6.

8. Gillen S, Wilhelm D, Meining A, et al. The "ELITE" model: construct validation of a new training system for natural orifice transluminal endoscopic surgery (NOTES). Endoscopy 2009;41:395–9.

9. Nehme J, Sodergren MH, Sugden C, et al. A randomized controlled trial evaluating endoscopic and laparoscopic training in skills transfer for novices performing a simulated NOTES task. Surg Innov 2013;20:631–8.

10. Clark J, Sodergren M, Noonan D, et al. The natural orifice simulated surgical environment (NOSsE): exploring the challenges of NOTES without the animal model. J Laparoendosc Adv Surg Tech A 2009;19:211–4.

11. Buscaglia JM, Karas J, Palladino N, et al. Simulated transanal NOTES sigmoidectomy training improves the responsiveness of surgical endoscopists. Gastrointest Endosc 2014;80:126–32.

12. Kato M, Gromski M, Jung Y, et al. The learning curve for endoscopic submucosal dissection in an established experimental setting. Surg Endosc 2013;27:154–61.

13. Gromski M, Saito K, Gonzalez JM, et al. Learning Colonic Endoscopic Submucosal Dissection (C-ESD): a prospective study assessing training using an ex-vivo simulator. Gastrointest Endosc 2014;79:AB270–1.

14. Matthes K, Jung Y, Kato M, et al. Efficacy of full-thickness GI perforation closure with a novel over-the-scope clip application device: an animal study. Gastrointest Endosc 2011;74:1369–75.

15. Gonzalez JM, Saito K, Kang C, et al. Prospective randomized comparison of gastrotomy closure associating tunnel access and over-the-scope clip (OTSC) with two other methods in an experimental ex vivo setting. Endosc Int Open 2015;3: E83–9.

16. Jung Y, Lee J, Gromski MA, et al. Assessment of the length of myotomy in peroral endoscopic pyloromyotomy (G-POEM) using a submucosal tunnel technique (video). Surg Endosc 2015;29:2377–84.

17. Roberts KE, Shetty S, Shariff AH, et al. Transvaginal NOTES hybrid cholecystectomy. Surg Innov 2012;19:230–5.

18. Sankaranarayanan G, Matthes K, Nemani A, et al. Needs analysis for developing a virtual-reality NOTES simulator. Surg Endosc 2013;27:1607–16.

19. Nemani A, Sankaranarayanan G, Roberts K, et al. Hierarchical task analysis of hybrid rigid scope Natural Orifice Translumenal Endoscopic Surgery (NOTES) cholecystectomy procedures. Stud Health Technol Inform 2013;184:293–7.

20. Ahn W, Dargar S, Halic T, et al. Preliminary face validation of a virtual translumenal endoscopic surgery trainer (VTEST). SAGES Annual Meeting. Salt Lake City (UT), April 2–5, 2014.

A Western Perspective on "New NOTES" from POEM to Full-thickness Resection and Beyond

Rani Modayil, MD[a], Stavros N. Stavropoulos, MD[b,c,d],*

KEYWORDS

- New NOTES • Peroral endoscopic myotomy (POEM) • Peroral pyloromyotomy (POP)
- GERD • Reflux esophagitis • Endoscopic full-thickness resection (EFTR)
- Submucosal tunnel endoscopic resection (STER) • Reimbursement

KEY POINTS

- There are East–West dichotomies in terms of operators and patients in new natural orifice translumenal endoscopic surgery (NOTES).
- A substantial proportion of peroral endoscopic myotomies (POEMs) are performed by gastroenterologists.
- The United States is leading the way in the important issue of post-POEM gastroesophageal reflux disease and in the development of peroral pyloromyotomy for gastroparesis.
- Endoscopic full-thickness resection and submucosal tunnel endoscopic resection are challenging new NOTES procedures that represent truly translumenal incursions into the thoracic or abdominal cavities.

INTRODUCTION

Because the cornerstone of new natural orifice translumenal endoscopic surgery (NOTES) procedures is endoscopic submucosal dissection (ESD), the parent procedure, so to speak, of all new NOTES interventions, Western endoscopists were at a distinct disadvantage compared with their Asian colleagues in the adoption and development of new NOTES procedures. ESD was invented in Japan for en bloc resection of early gastrointestinal (GI) neoplasms, mainly early gastric cancer (found in Asia at approximately 8 times the incidence in the United States), and was widely applied

Disclosures: No relevant disclosures.
[a] Winthrop University Hospital, 222 Station Plaza North Suite 429, Mineola, NY 11501, USA;
[b] Columbia University, 161 Fort Washington Ave., New York, NY 10032, USA; [c] Temple University, 3401 N Broad St., Philadelphia, PA 19140, USA; [d] Program in Advanced GI Endoscopy (P.A.G.E.), Winthrop University Hospital, 222 Station Plaza North Suite 429, Mineola, NY 11501, USA
* Corresponding author. Program in Advanced GI Endoscopy (P.A.G.E.), Winthrop University Hospital, 222 Station Plaza North Suite 429, Mineola, NY 11501.
E-mail addresses: sns10md@gmail.com; sstavropoulos@winthrop.org

giendo.theclinics.com

there starting in 2000. For more than a decade, ESD did not gain any significant adoption in the United States. This was in part owing to the scarcity in the West of easy ESD target lesions available in abundance in Asia (early gastric cancer and squamous carcinoma of the esophagus), and the perception of ESD as a time-consuming, technically demanding, difficult to learn, and risky technique without clearly proven benefits over endoscopic mucosal resection in the lesions most common in the West such as colorectal neoplasms.[1] Largely influenced by this negative climate, Olympus and ERBE did not pursue US Food and Drug Administration approval of ESD electrosurgical knives in the United States until 2010, after the advent of peroral endoscopic myotomy (POEM). Most knives became finally commercially available in the United States in 2011. At our center, early ESDs from 2005 to 2011 and POEMs from 2009 to 2011, were performed using a standard non-ESD needle knife resulting in a riskier and less efficient resection. Interestingly, the advent of POEM did, in 2 to 3 years more, to stimulate adoption of ESD in the United States than more than 10 years of favorable publications and demonstrations of ESD by Asian endoscopists. This is a paradoxical situation whereby an initially obscure offshoot of ESD to treat a rare and rather esoteric motility disorder is now driving adoption of the parent technique along with the entire field of "new NOTES" procedures. This has led to a pathway to new NOTES in the United States which, as we shall see, has unique features that distinguish it from that seen in Asia.

THE NEW NATURAL ORIFICE TRANSLUMENAL ENDOSCOPIC SURGERY PIONEERS, AN EAST–WEST DICHOTOMY

It is instructive to look at the background of POEM pioneers in North America in comparison with that of European and Asian pioneers based in part on data from our international POEM survey conducted in 2012 polling 16 of the 21 pioneering centers in the world at that time. These 16 centers included all high-volume POEM centers at that time (centers with $\geq$30 cases).[2] All Asian pioneers were surgeons (Inoue, Zhou, Shiwaku, Minami, Chiu) and all but one, Phillip Chiu, came to POEM exclusively from extensive ESD experience rather than NOTES experience. In Europe, early pioneers were almost exclusively gastroenterologists with advanced flexible endoscopy skills, including some ESD experience (Costamagna, Neuhaus, Seewald, Devierre, Fockens, Roesch; one, however, with surgical training as well, Guido Costamagna) with only 1 European POEM pioneer (Karl-Hermann Fuchs) being a surgeon coming to POEM from traditional NOTES experience. In the United States, in stark contradistinction with Asia and Europe, with the exception of our center (Winthrop, Mineola, NY), where the operator is a gastroenterologist with extensive prior ESD experience and no traditional NOTES experience, all other POEM pioneers were surgeons most of whom came to POEM mainly from "traditional NOTES" experience (Swanstrom, Hungness, Marks/Ponsky, Romanelli/Earle/Desilets, Horgan, Ujiki). **Table 1** illustrates the rapid growth of POEM in the United States from 1 center in 2009 to 38 centers by the end of 2014. In 27% of these 37 centers, POEM was performed by a gastroenterologist, in 35% by a team composed of a gastroenterologist and a surgeon, and in 38% by a surgeon alone. We venture to speculate that, if in 2009 our center was not the first center in the United States to perform POEM[3] (in fact, the first center to perform POEM outside of the first few cases in Yokohama by Haruhiro Inoue, a foregut surgeon) and do so safely and effectively, POEM and by extension the nascent new NOTES field may have rapidly become the exclusive territory of the surgeon. Based on multiple personal communications with interventional gastroenterologists around the country over the past 5 years, institutional review boards populated in part by traditional surgeons, particularly in

Table 1
POEM adoption in the United States, 2009–2014

Program	GI/Surgeon	First POEM	Volume
Winthrop, NY	G	10/2009	>150
University of California, San Diego, CA	G/S	02/2010	40s
Northwestern, IL	S	08/2010	70s
Oregon Clinic, OR	S	10/2010	>150
Baystate, MA	G/S	2011	~40s
Case Western, OH	S	05/2011	~50s
Northshore, IL	S	08/2011	~50s
McGill, Montreal	S	08/2011	20
Stanford, CA	S	2012	~60
Mayo Clinic, MN	G/S	04/2012	20s
Ohio State University	S	8/2012	40s
Johns Hopkins, MD	G	8/2012	60s
University of Southern California	S	10/2012	30s
Emory	G	2012	40s
University of Florida	G	2/2013	50s
West Penn Allegheny	G/S	3/2013	20s
Lenox Hill Hospital	G/S	3/2013	10
University of Colorado	G	5/2013	20s
Cornell	G/S	6/2013	30s
University of Michigan	G/S	2013	<10
University of Iowa	G/S	12/2013	<10
Hershey, PA	G	2014	~20
Albert Einstein, NY	S	2014	<10
GW University Hospital	G/S	2014	~15
University of Pennsylvania	G	2014	~10
Washington University, St Louis	G/S	2014	<10
Mass General	S	2014	<10
Swedish, Seattle	G/S	2014	<10
UC Irvine	G	2014	<10
NYU	S	2014	<10
Indiana University	G/S	2014	<10
Pittsburgh	S	2014	<10
Houston Methodist	S	2014	<10
USF, Tampa	S	2014	<10
Cleveland Clinic	G/S	2014	<10
Beth Israel Hospital, NY	G	2014	<10
UVA	G	2014	<10

Centers are listed in approximate chronologic order by date of first POEM. For each center we list the approximate date of first POEM, whether POEMs are performed by a gastroenterologist (G), a surgeon (S) or a team comprised by a gastroenterologist and a surgeon (G/S), and the approximate volume of POEMs by December 2014.
Abbreviation: POEM, per oral endoscopic myotomy.

major academic centers, regarded the performance of what is essentially minimally invasive thoracic surgery by gastroenterologists with great trepidation. We believe that our early foray into POEM and the excellent initial results supporting the feasibility, efficacy, and safety of POEM performed by a gastroenterologist, as well as our active involvement in proctoring, training, and counseling of both gastroenterologists and surgeons in other institutions (eg, Hopkins, Cornell, Temple, Geisinger, University of California at Irvine, University of Southern California), helped to pave the way for a more equitable participation of gastroenterologists in new NOTES than was the case with traditional NOTES. In this respect, it also helped that as early as March 2011 we were able to demonstrate POEMs performed by a gastroenterologist under the scrutiny of live transmission at our live therapeutic endoscopy course (Long Island Live) followed in subsequent years (2012–2015) by multiple simultaneous live POEMs and live new NOTES subepithelial tumor resections performed in a US endoscopy unit by a gastroenterologist (Stavropoulos) alongside accomplished surgeons (Inoue, Zhou) with comparable procedural facility and outcomes (archived live case videos at www.winthropendoscopy.org). Another important point that can be easily deduced from **Table 1** is that as late as the end of 2014 (>6 years after the first human POEM in Yokohama Japan and >5 years after the first POEM in the United States), only 2 centers had performed more than 150 cases and 10 centers had performed 40 to 80 cases, with the remaining 25 centers at 0 to 30 cases. Thus, based on published data from our group on the learning curve of POEM indicating that competence occurs at 40 procedures and mastery at 60 procedures,[4] most centers were still very early in the learning curve.

FROM ENDOSCOPIC SUBMUCOSAL DISSECTION TO NEW NATURAL ORIFICE TRANSLUMENAL ENDOSCOPIC SURGERY: A WESTERN EXPERIENCE

Apart from leading the way in POEM adoption in the United States and continuing to possess the highest operator volume for POEMs in the United States, our center is also leading the way in NOTES full-thickness resection of GI tumors with the first endoscopic full-thickness resection (EFTR) and submucosal tunnel endoscopic resection (STER) human cases in the United States performed at our center in 2012 initiating what is still the only reported large Western series of such resections.[5,6] Our center is also now engaged in developing peroral pyloromyotomy (POP) via a unique interinstitutional collaboration. As such, we briefly review our center's experience as emblematic of new NOTES development in the United States.

Per Oral Endoscopic Myotomy

POEM represents an aggressive paradigm shift in surgery. Introducing such a procedure in the highly regulated, high medicolegal risk health care environment of the United States and even more egregiously having a gastroenterologist do so in 2009, when the grand total of worldwide publications on POEM consisted of a Digestive Diseases Week video forum abstract from Haruhiro Inoue, required a perfect storm of favorable factors that included (1) extensive prior operator experience in ESD before this became fashionable in the United States, (2) open-minded surgical leadership that provided critical support and advice; (3) an institutional review board that could provide outstanding patient protection while allowing innovation, and (4) stalwart institutional support, including provision of top-notch anesthesia and endoscopy staff, endoscopic equipment, and other resources and research infrastructure, financial support for animal laboratory facilities and live endoscopy activities with Asian NOTES masters, and expert assistance with billing coding and reimbursement issues and negotiations with payers. **Fig. 1** demonstrates our gradual methodical progression

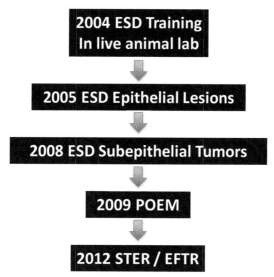

Fig. 1. Progression from endoscopic submucosal dissection (ESD) to new natural orifice translumenal endoscopic surgery (NOTES) at Winthrop University Hospital. EFTR, endoscopic full-thickness resection; STER, submucosal tunnel endoscopic resection.

from ESD to new NOTES procedures of increasing risk and technical complexity. In 2012, we presented data on 89 human ESD cases accumulated between 2008 and 2012[7] and a study completed in 2011 and 2012 involving 63 ESDs in an acute live animal model in a randomized comparison of 3 knives.[8] The vast majority of POEM operators in the United States after the initial wave of pioneers proceeded to POEM with relatively limited or no ESD experience and no NOTES experience. They sought to develop both POEM and ESD in parallel. This may result in more modest POEM outcomes compared with those of the pioneer group. Of particular concern, however, is the potential increase in severe or life-threatening adverse events, many of which may remain unreported. Recent such events (based on personal communications) that may present the tip of the proverbial iceberg have included septic shock owing to delayed esophagopericardial fistula, empyema, and several cases of severe intratunnel bleeds. Another important finding from our POEM series, which is also seen to a somewhat lesser degree in other US series but does not seem to be shared by most Asian series, is the higher complexity and surgical risk of the cases (**Table 2**). In our series of 248 patients, 122 patients (49%) were treated previously and in particular 53 (21%) had prior Botox (including patients with up to 18 and 30 Botox treatments), 39 (16%) had prior surgical Heller myotomy (including 3 patients with 2 prior Heller myotomy surgeries each). In addition, 45 of our patients (18%) had endstage, sigmoid esophagus; 60 (24%) had severe comorbidities and 25 (10%) were older than 80 years old (mean age for the series 54; range, 10–93). These are categories of patients in whom POEM is technically challenging and/or carries a higher surgical risk. In contrast, in the recent publication by Inoue of his series of 500 patients, patients are overall significantly younger by more than a decade (mean age, 43 years old) with very few patients having had prior treatment (Botox 6 patients, 1%; Heller 10 patients, 2%) and a lower proportion of advanced achalasia patients (21 patients [4%] >6 mm diameter and 29 patients [6%] with severe sigmoidization [S2]).[9] These differences result from a number of factors. First, in the United States there was

Table 2 Winthrop POEM series baseline patient characteristics	
Variable	**Value**
No. of patients	248
Male	141
Female	107
Age (y), mean	54 (10–93); [a]23 patients >80 y old, 2 patients ≥90 y old
Prior achalasia treatment	122 (49%) previously treated[a]
Pneumatic balloon dilation	33
Suboptimal balloon dilation	57
Botox	53[a] (1 treated 18 times, 1 treated 30 times)
Heller myotomy	39[a] (3 patients had Heller myotomy 2 times)
POEM	3[a]
Esophageal diameter, mean (range)	4.9 cm (2.0–16.9)
Sigmoid esophagus	203 nonsigmoid, 45 sigmoid[a]
Achalasia stage	
I (<3 cm)	34 (14%)
II (3–6 cm)	146 (59%)
III (6–8 cm)	22 (9%)[a]
IV (>8 cm/sigmoid)	46 (18%; 45/46 all sigmoid, diameter 4–16.9 cm)[a]
ASA classification	
1	18 (7%)
2	170 (69%)
3	60 (24%)[a]

Abbreviations: ASA, American Society of Anesthesiologists; POEM, per oral endoscopic myotomy.
[a] High surgical risk and/or high technical challenge categories of patients.

substantial initial resistance to POEM by most gastroenterologists and surgeons, which likely resulted in a referral bias whereby only patients that were poor candidates for Heller myotomy (older, comorbid patients with advanced achalasia, and/or extensive prior therapies including prior Heller) were referred for POEM. During the first years of POEM many of the low-risk/low challenge ideal candidates for POEM who came to our center seeking POEM had discovered POEM on their own through achalasia support groups and then, ignoring the usual advice from their physicians to undergo laparoscopic Heller or other "standard treatments," would travel great distances to expert POEM centers to have a POEM. For example, at our center, 90 of 248 of our patients (36%) to date traveled to Winthrop from 23 different states and 4 foreign countries (**Fig. 2**). Second, in contravention to all published guidelines recommending that Botox be reserved for the frail elderly, in the United States, Botox remains unfortunately the most commonly used first-line treatment,[10] despite making subsequent POEM (or Heller myotomy) potentially more complicated. Third, in the United States with its highly distributed decentralized system of health care delivery, many patients with achalasia are being treated in community centers rather than centers of excellence. Given the rarity of achalasia, this results in inexpert management that includes, in addition to inappropriate use of Botox, Heller myotomies performed by surgeons with very limited experience and thus more modest outcomes than those published by centers of excellence. This situation, unfortunately, will also increasingly

Winthrop Out-of-Area POEM patients
90/248 (36%) (23 states, 4 foreign countries)

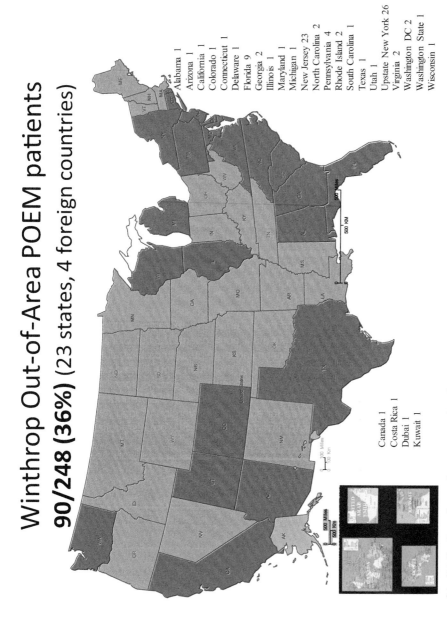

Alabama 1
Arizona 1
California 1
Colorado 1
Connecticut 1
Delaware 1
Florida 9
Georgia 2
Illinois 1
Maryland 1
Michigan 1
New Jersey 23
North Carolina 2
Pennsylvania 4
Rhode Island 2
South Carolina 1
Texas 1
Utah 1
Upstate New York 26
Virginia 2
Washington DC 2
Washington State 1
Wisconsin 1

Canada 1
Costa Rica 1
Dubai 1
Kuwait 1

Fig. 2. Geographic distribution of out-of-area per oral endoscopic myotomy (POEM) patients seeking POEM at Winthrop University Hospital in Mineola, New York.

be the case with POEM as we move from pioneers and early adopters to wider adoption. With the number of POEM centers in the United States now estimated at 60 and increasing rapidly, and the number of achalasia patients who are candidates for POEM by some estimates at only 3000 annually, for many US centers, attaining adequate procedural volumes may be challenging and will get increasingly more so in the future. The outcomes in centers with high-volume operators are similar to the outcomes in our series with success rates remaining greater than 90% beyond 1 year (**Table 3**) despite the inclusion of many patients who generally respond poorly to any treatment, including POEM, such as sigmoid and severely dilated patients (>6 cm esophageal diameter; accounting for 27% in our series). However, with the inevitable spread of POEM to low-volume centers, outcomes may be more modest, and adverse events, as alluded to previously, may be more severe than the mild, manageable adverse events that have been reported so far by most pioneering US centers including ours (**Table 4**).

ENDOSCOPIC FULL-THICKNESS RESECTION/SUBMUCOSAL TUNNEL ENDOSCOPIC RESECTION

After 3 years of POEM at our center from 2009 to 2012, as the first reports of EFTR[11] and STER[12,13] appeared in 2011 and 2012 from the 2 groups with the highest POEM volumes in the world in Yokohama and Shanghai, we were able to follow suit with the first cases of EFTR and STER in the United States in 2012. From April 2012 to November 2015, we have performed 62 EFTR/STER cases (**Table 5**), the only large series of such resections in the West. These are true NOTES procedures that are substantially riskier than POEM, which, strictly speaking, is not truly transluminal because the endoscope stays within the safe confines of the outer muscularis propria or adventitia. EFTR and STER involve a much deeper dissection that follows the tumor contour through the muscle and beyond in the peritoneal or thoracic cavity, because these tumors often have a significant extraluminal component. The risk of injury to surrounding structures including adjacent organs and large paratumoral extraluminal vessels is substantial and this risk is compounded by the much more limited devices to effect hemostasis than are available to the laparoscopic surgeon. As seen in **Table 5**, there are more adverse events than in POEM but they are still mild or moderate events that are manageable without any need for surgical intervention or long-term sequelae in our series. The operator needs to have mastery of ESD, but also collaborate closely

Table 3 Winthrop POEM efficacy outcomes				
	Baseline	**After POEM**	**P Value**	**Efficacy[a]**
Eckardt score	7.8 (4–12)	0.8 (0–3) 3-mo assessment	<.0001	≥3 mo: 224/236 (95%) ≥6 mo: 199/211 (94%) ≥12 mo: 174/183 (95%)
LES pressure (mm Hg) at 3 mo[b]	43.3 (5.4–114)	18.5 (0–50)	<.0001	—
Timed barium esophagram at 6 mo (% emptying at 5 min)	—	>50% emptying >80% emptying 100% emptying	—	81/81 (100%) 74/81 (91%) 46/81 (57%)

Abbreviations: LES, lower esophageal sphincter; POEM, per oral endoscopic myotomy.
  [a] Defined as post-POEM Eckardt score of ≤3.
  [b] Post-POEM manometry results available on 101 patients.

Table 4
Winthrop POEM series, length of stay, adverse events, and readmissions

Variable	Value
Mean length of hospital stay (d)	1.9 (1–30)
Major adverse events/mortality	0
Aborted POEM/surgical intervention/conversion	0
Minor/moderate adverse events	9/248 (4%)
$\leq$24-h ICU stay for extubation (obesity, sleep apnea, difficult intubation)	3
Transient atrial fibrillation in 2 elderly patients >80 y old with CAD	2
RML atelectasis in patient with emphysema resolved in hours without tx	1
Moderate right pleural effusion, conservative tx, no drain	1
SBO requiring LOA	1
Anemia requiring 1 U of blood transfusion in elderly patient	1
Pain requiring narcotics once on hospital floor (no patient discharged home on narcotics)	107/248 (43%)
Readmissions within 30 d related to POEM	3/248 (1%)
Bipolar patient on steroids for polymyalgia rheumatica: eloped ×36 h on POD 1, small tunnel dehiscence, no leak; 19 d stay for observation, antibiotics (no drain or other intervention)	1
Low-grade fever; EGD, deep ulcer at GEJ; NPO ×48 h, PPI, discharge on PPI, antibiotics	1
Bleeding from suture puncture site treated with endoscopic clip 5 d LOS	1
Readmissions within 30 owing to other causes	8/248 (3%)
PPM malfunction owing to defective lead in 89-y-old woman, LOS 2 d	1
Anxiety/subjective fevers in 35-y-old man, LOS 2 d	1
Episodes of SVT in patient with known SVT, LOS 2 d	1
Generalized weakness/dehydration, LOS 2 d	3
Clostridium difficile infection, LOS 18 d	1
Peripheral small PE 2 wk after POEM, LOS 5 d (anticoagulation)	1

Abbreviations: CAD, coronary artery disease; EGD, esophagogastroduodenoscopy; GEJ, gastroesophageal junction; ICU, intensive care unit; LOA, lysis of adhesions; NPO, nil per os; POD, postoperative day; POEM, per oral endoscopic myotomy; PPI, proton pump inhibitor; PPM, permanent pacemaker; RML, right middle lobe; SBO, small bowel obstruction; SVT, supraventricular tachycardia; tx, treatment.

with a minimally invasive foregut surgeon. Although most of our full-thickness resection procedures are performed in the endoscopy unit, in cases where the tumor is located mostly or completely extraluminally, particularly if it is in proximity to large extraluminal vessels, we schedule the procedure in the operating room with surgical backup. However, in only 4 of 62 cases (6%) did we require surgical assistance. In 1 patient, owing to severe tumor vascularity, we asked our collaborating surgeon to provide laparoscopic overview of our procedure; however, no surgical manipulation or intervention was required. In 2 cases of larger 3- to 4-cm SETs, we could not extract the resected tumor through the patient's small caliber esophagus. Therefore, after using endoscopic suturing to securely close the resection defect on the posterior gastric wall, we asked our collaborating surgery to perform a minimal laparoscopic intervention to extract the specimen intact within a specimen bag through a small anterior gastrotomy and an 11-mm umbilical port. Finally, in 1 case, during seromuscular dissection we noted that the extraluminal portion of the tumor was abutting the main trunk of the left gastric artery. At this point, we felt that continuing with EFTR

Table 5
Winthrop EFTR/STER series April 2012 to November 2015

Variable	Value
Age (y)	58 (18–86)
Gender (M: F)	21:41
ASA classification	
I	6 (10%)
II	46 (73%)
III	10 (17%)
Location in GI tract	
Esophagus	13 (21%)
Stomach	36 (57%)
Duodenum	1 (2%)
Colon	12 (20%)
Technique	
EFTR	48 (77%)
STER	14 (23%)
Anesthesia	
General	39 (62%)
Propofol sedation	23 (38%)
Procedure time (min)	87 (21–400)
Gross pathology size (cm)	2.3 (1–5.5)
Closure technique	
Endoscopic suture	37 (58%)
Endoscopic clips	17 (28%)
Both sutures and clips	7 (12%)
Complete en bloc resection	57 (92%)
Piecemeal resection	4 (6%)
Conversion to surgical resection	1 (2%)
Histopathology	
SETs with malignant potential	77%
GIST	27 (43%)
Leiomyoma	13 (21%)
Leiomyosarcoma	1 (1.6%)
Schwannoma	1 (1.6%)
Carcinoid	3 (4.9%)
Granular cell tumor	2 (3.3%)
Glomus tumor	1 (1.6%)
Plexiform angiomyxoid myofibroblastic tumor	1 (1.6%)
Calcified hyalinized neoplasm	1 (1.6%)
Pancreatic hamartoma	1 (1.6%)
Low grade adenocarcinoma in transmural scar	1 (1.6%)
Adenoma in deep transmural scar	1 (1.6%)
Benign (Pancreatic rest, pneumatosis, lipoma, etc)	9 (15%)

(continued on next page)

Table 5 *(continued)*	
Variable	Value
Length of stay (d)	2.4 (1–35)
Adverse/Unanticipated events	
12–24 h ICU observation	5 (8%)
Prolonged hospitalization (>5 d)	1 (1.6%)
Chest tube for pleural effusion	1 (1.6%)
Prolonged intraprocedural hemostasis	3 (5%)
Blood transfusion (for marginal Hct)	2 (3%)
Laparoscopic overview of EFTR	1 (5%)
Laparoscopic specimen extraction	2 (3%)
Laparoscopic conversion	1 (1.6%)
Needle venting of capnoperitoneum	4 (7%)
Clostridium difficile infection	1 (1.6%)
Dilation of postresection stricture	1 (1.6%)

Abbreviations: ASA, American Society of Anesthesiologists; EFTR, endoscopic full-thickness resection; GI, gastrointestinal; GIST, gastrointestinal stromal tumor; Hct, hematocrit; ICU, intensive care unit; SET, subepithelial tumor; STER, submucosal tunnel endoscopic resection.

would carry a high risk for injury to this artery and potential catastrophic bleeding and asked our collaborating surgeon to perform laparoscopic resection. Clearly, these cases illustrate the importance of close collaboration with surgical colleagues for this type of complex new NOTES procedures at the frontiers of what current endoscopic instrumentation permits.

We have found that close collaboration with a dedicated pathologist is also essential. The proper assessment of margins in these minimally invasive full-thickness endoscopic resections of SETs is poorly understood. The resection specimens of these relatively small, often benign tumors, usually gastrointestinal stromal tumors or leiomyomas, reveal no true capsule under microscopic examination and have 3 quite different anatomic borders: (1) normal GI wall at their "equator" where the tumor was circumferentially excised from the GI wall; (2) mucosa and submucosa (that may or may not be intact or present depending on the resection technique) on the luminal "pole" of the tumor; and (3) tumor surface (grossly seen as a smooth "pseudocapsule") on the extraluminal pole of the tumor. Clearly, because EFTR and STER "hug" the pseudocapsule of these tumors during the resection and because these tumors have a free surface on their extraluminal side, the traditional negative pathologic margin consisting of normal tissue extending beyond the border of the tumor is neither achievable nor relevant on the extraluminal surface of the tumor. Therefore, proper assessment of complete resection involves a collaboration between the endoscopist and the pathologist, as well as an understanding of the complex 3-dimensional geometry of these specimens. In our discussion of a US perspective on EFTR and STER, we would be remiss if we did not emphasize the importance of a critical enabling device for new NOTES resection procedures in the United States, the Overstitch endoscopic suturing system (Apollo Endosurgery, Austin, Texas, USA).[14] The improved current version of this device was released in the United States in October 2011 revolutionizing the endoscopist's ability to securely close full-thickness defects in the GI tract just as the first EFTR procedures were being reported from China. Interestingly, this device is still not available in China, where nearly all EFTR procedures are currently performed and therefore closure there is performed with less secure clip-and-endoloop techniques.[15] In Europe, the device is prohibitively expensive at more than $2000 compared with only $800 to $900 in the United States. The cost effectiveness of this device in the United States is further amplified by the lack of availability of inexpensive endoscopic through-the-scope clips (EZ-clip, Olympus Medical, Tokyo, Japan), which are widely available in Asia and Europe and, at approximately $15 per clip, cost one-tenth of the endoscopic clips available in the United States. We recently compared standard endoscopic clips with endoscopic suturing for POEM tunnel closure.[14] The opening of the POEM tunnel provides an excellent "standardized" defect with unvarying location and size that represents an excellent target for comparing closure techniques. We have consistently used the suturing device for POEM closure starting in 2012 and in our analysis (**Table 6**) we found it to be equivalent to endoscopic clips (used earlier in our POEM series) in terms of time needed for closure and cost. Interestingly, a recent retrospective study comparing only 5 POEM closures with each of this devices by the surgical group in Portland found a very long closure duration with Overstitch of 33 minutes (much longer than our group's 8 minutes), which resulted in a greater cost in the Overstitch closures owing to the cost of operating room time (despite similar equipment cost). These findings may be related to learning curve issues for this device or other factors such as the use of an overtube, which, although recommended by the manufacturer, our group has not found necessary and has never used in now more than 300 Overstitch cases.

With a large variety of ESD knives and a robust suturing device now available in the United States, the "NOTES toolkit" is richer than ever before. However, an important additional ingredient required for NOTES interventions beyond the confines of the GI wall is operator mastery of ESD skills and techniques. With the massive increase in

Table 6
Comparison of endoscopic clips versus endoscopic suturing for POEM tunnel closure

Variable	Endoclip	Suturing	P
n	73	142	—
Efficacy (%)	100	98.6	NS
AEs	No leaks Increased LOS (4 d) in one patient with thick mucosal edges approximated with clips and endoloop	No leaks One partial dehiscence One suture puncture site bleed One aborted closure owing to a mucosal tear in the hypopharynx during Overstitch insertion; mild sore throat for 4 d	NS
Cost/procedure duration comparison of 35 consecutive closures for each technique after excluding the initial 30 cases with each technique (to eliminate any learning curve effect)			
Time†	8 (4–30)	8.5 (3–28)	NS
Cost†	$960 (455–2215)	$818	NS
LOS†	2 (1–5)	1 (1–5)	.013

Abbreviations: †, mean; AEs, adverse events; LOS, length of stay; NS, not significant; POEM, per oral endoscopic myotomy.

Adapted from Stavropoulos SN, Modayil R, Friedel D. Current applications of endoscopic suturing. World J Gastrointest Endosc 2015;7(8):783; with permission.

ESD training and adoption in the United States stimulated by POEM, it should only be a matter of time before true transluminal NOTES as exemplified by full-thickness resection of SETs gains traction and hopefully stimulates further device development, such as better energy devices for cutting/hemostasis and endoscopic staplers.

PER ORAL PYLOROMYOTOMY

Haruhiro Inoue performed the first human peroral pyloromyotomy worldwide in April 2013 in the United States on a patient with gastroparesis. This author was present along with Mouen Khashab in this landmark procedure, later published as a case report,[16] and the technical similarities to POEM were striking. However, this is where the similarity ends. Gastroparesis is a much more heterogeneous and ill-defined motility disorder than achalasia and, unlike myotomy for achalasia, pyloromyotomy may only be effective in certain subsets of gastroparesis patients in whom pyloric dysfunction may significantly contribute to symptoms. Furthermore, the posterior gastroduodenal junction is a much riskier area than the GE junction, because the dissection needs to avoid the delicate duodenal mucosa and muscularis as well as large vessels while operating with a "floppier" endoscope than is the case in POEM, without good "one-to-one" motion of the tip of the scope owing to endo-scope "looping" in the stomach. Thus, optimal application of this technique requires the combination of, on the one hand, extensive experience in gastroparesis assess-ment and management to ensure proper patient selection for POP and sophisticated postprocedural evaluation and management, and, on the other hand, advanced NOTES surgical skills to ensure maximum POP safety and efficacy. Such multidisci-plinary breadth of expertise may not exist in the same center, even among centers of excellence, and particularly for uncommon diseases such as gastroparesis and a very novel and technically challenging procedure such as POP. In an effort to provide just such a multidisciplinary top-notch team, our center in New York with its exten-sive expertise in new NOTES procedures forged a unique collaboration with Temple University in Philadelphia, an internationally recognized referral center for gastropa-resis. This unique arrangement may serve as a model for multidisciplinary "teams of excellence" that cross institutional and even geographic borders; it allows POPs at both Winthrop and Temple to be performed by the same operator with extensive prior experience in new NOTES and POEM while the patients also benefit from comprehensive preoperative and postoperative assessment by a team of motility experts with unparalleled experience in the assessment and management of gastro-paresis. Data from this Winthrop-Temple series are forthcoming; **Fig. 3** illustrates our current technique. Preliminary data on 7 POP procedures have been published by Lee Swanstrom and colleagues from Portland, representing the only published series to date (albeit one where in most patients laparoscopic surgery was performed at the same time as endoscopic pyloromyotomy raising some methodological concerns). POP appears to be the only New NOTES procedure where the US is leading the way and is reviewed in detail (See Swanstrom LL: Per-oral pyloromyotomy, in this issue).

GASTROESOPHAGEAL REFLUX DISEASE AFTER PER ORAL ENDOSCOPIC MYOTOMY, WEST VERSUS EAST OR INITIAL OPTIMISM DISPELLED BY OBJECTIVE DATA?

Early POEM series particularly from Asia but also some from Europe[17–19] reported little or no gastroesophageal reflux disease (GERD) after POEM ($\leq$10%). In retrospect, it seems that these extremely favorable findings were likely owing to dependence mostly on symptom scores or unstructured clinical interviews. In 2012, the Portland

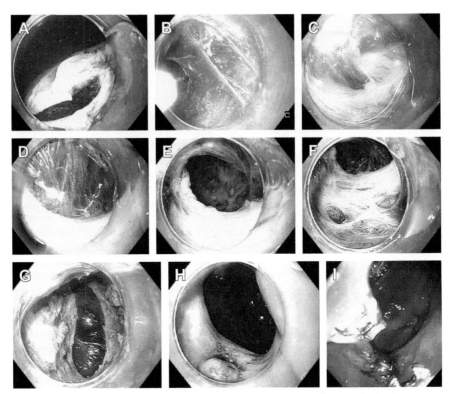

Fig. 3. Peroral pyloromyotomy. (*A*) Mucosal incision at the tunnel entry site in the antrum. (*B*) Dissection of the submucosal tunnel. (*C*) Penetrating vessels requiring careful hemostasis. (*D*) Pyloric muscle fibers at 6 o'clock. Duodenal submucosa and mucosa at 12 o'clock. (*E*) Tunnel completion. Dissection has been extended to the duodenal submucosa isolating the pyloric ring. (*F*) More detailed view of the pyloric muscle fibers. (*G*) Full-thickness pyloromyotomy to the level of the serosa. (*H*) Patulous pyloric orifice seen after completion of the pyloromyotomy. Note mild blanching of the mucosa overlying the tunnel as a result of the tunnel dissection. (*I*) Sutured closure of the tunnel entry site using the overstitch endoscopic suturing system.

group published data on objective assessment of reflux by pH study in 13 POEM patients.[20] Somewhat alarmingly, abnormal acid exposure was found in 46% of patients. Follow-up reports from Asia looking at objective measures of GERD found erosive esophagitis in 18 of 105 (17%) by Inoue[21] and in 11 of 28 (39%) by Minami in Nagasaki,[22] and positive pH studies in 3 of 15 (20%) by Chiu in Hong Kong.[23] Interestingly, in a now familiar upward drift on the GERD incidence data, in the most recent report by Inoue reflux esophagitis was seen at 1 year in 113 of 191 (59%), whereas reflux symptoms were present in 56 of 289 (19.4%).[9] No pH data were available in this series, as is usually the case in studies from Asia. These results, however, seem to dispel the idea that there may be an East–West dichotomy with more GERD reported in US studies owing to higher body mass index and other factors particular to US/Western patients. To date, only 4 centers, all from the West (3 from the United States and 1 from Europe), have presented substantial data on GERD assessment by all 3 methodologies (symptom assessment, endoscopic evaluation, and ambulatory pH studies).[24–27] The most recent data from each of these centers are presented in **Table 7**.

Table 7
Series with comprehensive objective assessment of GERD after POEM

Center	Year	GERD Symptoms, n/N (%)	Erosive Esophagitis, n/N (%)	+pH Study, n/N (%)
Chicago, IL[24]	2014	15/41 (15)	13/22 (59)	4/13 (31)
Portland, OR[25]	2015	12/100 (15)	20/73 (27)	26/68 (38)
Mineola, NY[26]	2015	40/174 (23)	29/86 (34)	29/84 (36)
Rome, Italy[27]	2015	19/103 (18)	21/103 (20)	52/103 (51)

Abbreviations: GERD, gastroesophageal reflux disease; POEM, per oral endoscopic myotomy.

Based on these data, 20% to 59% of patients have endoscopic signs of GERD after POEM (mainly LA class A or B esophagitis), 31% to 51% have positive pH studies and 15% to 23% have frequent GERD symptoms. The vast majority of patients with GERD were effectively treated with proton pump inhibitors. The Rome group introduced the concept of "clinically relevant GERD," defined as abnormal acid exposure PLUS heartburn and/or esophagitis, in what seems to be an effort to discount positive pH studies in patients without corroborating endoscopic findings or symptoms of GERD. In achalasia patients, such abnormal pH studies can occur owing to stasis and fermentation.[28] Distinguishing these patients from patients with abnormal acid exposure owing to true GERD may require expert analysis of pH data by various methodologies.[29] Our center is studying this issue at present. Of 117 patients with Bravo studies performed after POEM, 91 had their studies performed at our center, allowing detailed analysis of the raw data and tracings (data to be presented at Digestive Diseases Week 2016). Of the 91 patients, 50 (55%), a rate similar to the most recent reports from the Costamagna group,[27] had a positive Bravo study by standard Bravo analysis at pH less than 4. However, only 30 of the 91 patients (33%) had a positive Bravo study when analyzed using a pH of less than 3 ($P<.01$) methodology as suggested by Crookes and colleagues.[29] Twenty of the 50 patients (40%) with a positive study at a pH of less than 4 became negative when analyzed at a pH of less than 3. Of 50 patients who had a positive BRAVO study as assessed by pH less than 4 methodology, 27 (54%) had reflux erosions whereas 22 of 30 patients (73%) who were positive at a pH of less than 3 had reflux erosions. In a 3-center (Portland, Rome, Hamburg) multicenter study[30] that focused on longer term data from patients who had completed 2-year follow-up, 37% had erosive esophagitis and 37% were on proton pump inhibitor at 2 or more years of follow-up (mean, 29 months; range 24–41). No pH data were provided. Interestingly in that study, the strongest predictor of dysphagia relief after POEM seemed to be the presence of GERD (odds ratio, 6.7), which lends support to the widely held belief that the more effective the lower esophageal sphincter disruption, the more effective the relief of dysphagia, but at the expense of a greater risk for GERD. It is important to emphasize that up to 50% of GERD may be asymptomatic and diligent post-POEM follow-up is required with at least 1 pH study postoperatively and endoscopic surveillance at 1- to 2-year intervals to detect patients with GERD early and to treat them so as to forestall long-standing reflux complications, such as Barrett's esophagus and peptic strictures. Such reflux related complications were the most common cause of late failure after laparoscopic Heller myotomy (LHM) with Dor fundoplication.[31] It should also be noted here that high-quality studies from expert LHM centers in the United States have shown abnormal acid exposure rates in 18% to 42% of patients after LHM with fundoplication,[32–34] rates not too dissimilar to those after POEM. This may be owing to the fact that, unlike standard LHM technique, POEM preserves the "suspensory ligaments" of the esophagus, most notably the phrenoesophageal membrane, thought to have an important antireflux function separate from the esophageal "sphincter" itself. Two recent Western studies lend support to this hypothesis by demonstrating that a modified LHM technique with very limited dissection of the hiatus and without fundoplication results in much lower rates of GERD (9% and 31%, respectively)[35,36] than the rates seen in traditional LHM without fundoplication, which often exceed 80%.

THE PLIGHT OF CODING AND REIMBURSEMENT IN THE UNITED STATES

This discussion will focus on POEM as the prototypical and best established New NOTES procedure with extensive published data supporting its utility that suggest equivalence or superiority to Heller myotomy in most outcome measures (See Bechara R, Inoue H: POEM, the prototypical "new NOTES" procedure and first successful NOTES procedure, in this issue). Unlike health care coverage in most other countries, in the United States a large proportion of health care is paid for by private payers rather than some form of national health service or government-funded universal health coverage. In such a decentralized setting, with a large number of private payers with different policies regarding new procedures, it is difficult for thought leaders in the physician community to advocate effectively for valuable new procedures and technologies. An effort in that direction was the Preservation and Incorporation of Valuable Innovation (PIVI) initiative by the American Society for Gastrointestinal Endoscopy (ASGE) designed to provide unbiased reviews of valuable endoscopic technologies that can inform reimbursement policy decisions and minimize the risk of stifling innovation owing to lack of coverage by payers. Such a PIVI document was actually produced for POEM and recently published.[37] Certain procedures that use new and expensive devices, for example, antireflux procedures such as transoral incisionless fundoplication with the Esophyx device[38] or endoscopic anterior fundoplication with the MUSE device[39] can benefit from "industry champions" whose business viability depends on coverage of these procedures and who have more financial and other resources than physicians to navigate the byzantine and often irrational seeming process of obtaining a Current Procedural Terminology (CPT) code (one of the most important steps in securing payer coverage of a new procedure). POEM and the other "new NOTES" procedures use a few inexpensive devices (most often just an electrosurgical ESD knife, a plastic distal cap attachment, and a coagulation forceps) and thus cannot depend on much help from "industry champions." Paradoxically, then, their low-cost equipment is a handicap in the pathway to reimbursement.

Currently, there is no CPT code for POEM. Among participants in the international POEMS survey essentially all high-volume pioneering US centers in 2012 reported using, as is appropriate, an "unlisted esophageal surgery" code (CPT code 43499) billed at the relative value units of a thoracoscopic Heller myotomy, LHM, or an average of the 2 procedures.[2] Some centers have used a LHM code for POEM in an effort to bypass the difficulties in obtaining POEM authorization and reimbursement when the unlisted procedure code is used. This is not in compliance with current billing and coding rules and may result in penalties for fraudulent billing, including at a minimum return of monies paid for POEMs billed in such a manner and exclusion of the physician from health plans. This is also the case when "undercoding" is employed using codes such as those for esophagogastroduodenoscopy with endoscopic submucosal injection and tissue ablation to bill for POEM. Some centers have performed POEM in conjunction with laparoscopic Dor fundoplication and billed this hybrid procedure under a LHM code. Even though such a procedure allows the patient to benefit from some of the aspects of POEM that make it potentially superior to Heller myotomy (better identification of the lower esophageal sphincter, easier extension of the myotomy into the chest in patients who need longer myotomy such as spastic patients, lower blood loss, etc), the minimal invasiveness of true natural orifice surgery is lost. Furthermore, with this hybrid procedure, even if one uses the highest published estimates for GERD after POEM of 45% to 50% (see section on GERD), at least one-half of the patients undergo an unnecessary Dor fundoplication that may in fact put them at risk for lesser relief of dysphagia in addition to its invasiveness, whereas the other half could have easily been managed with proton pump inhibitors or, if they so desire, pursue a Dor fundoplication electively at a later time.

Finally, some centers in competitive markets have decided to "absorb the cost" of POEMs that are not reimbursed in an effort to remain at the forefront of this exciting nascent field of new NOTES procedures until such time as a CPT code is obtained. At our center, one of the highest volume centers in the United States with POEM volumes of 90 to 100 cases per year, we authorize and bill the procedure under the unlisted procedure code. We only perform POEM if authorization is obtained. In approximately 10% of cases, we encounter denials that are vigorously appealed (at great expenditure in time and effort) through peer review, internal review, external review, and often, if allowed, independent review at state board level. This process, which often takes 1 to 2 months, is a source of great frustration for both patient and physician and, unfortunately, is the norm in cases of payers that have formulated written policies denying coverage for POEM (**Fig. 4**). These policies, interestingly,

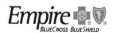 **Medical Policy**

Subject:	Transendoscopic Therapy for Gastroesophageal Reflux Disease and Dysphagia
Policy #:	SURG.00047
Status:	Reviewed

Current Effective Date: 10/06/2015
Last Review Date: 08/06/2015

Description/Scope

This document addresses selected transendoscopic therapies for the treatment of gastroesophageal reflux disease (GERD) and dysphagia. This document does not address procedures which approach the esophagus through abdominal laparoscopic or open surgical approaches.

Note: For additional information please see:

- SURG.00106 Ablative Techniques as a Treatment for Barrett's Esophagus
- SURG.00131 Lower Esophageal Sphincter Augmentation Devices for the Treatment of Gastroesophageal Reflux Disease (GERD)

Position Statement

Investigational and Not Medically Necessary:

The following transendoscopic treatments for gastroesophageal reflux disease (GERD) and dysphagia are considered **investigational and not medically necessary** in all cases:

1. Endoluminal gastric plication (ELGP); or
2. Transendoscopic gastroplasty; or
3. Transoral incisionless fundoplication (TIF); or
4. Endoscopic submucosal injection of bulking agents, beads or other substances; or
5. Transesophageal radiofrequency therapy (note: this does NOT include treatment of Barrett's Esophagus with radiofrequency energy); or
6. Per-oral endoscopic myotomy (POEM).

Fig. 4. Typical coverage policy determination for US private insurance plans that deny POEM coverage.

invariably mention prominently and with great reverence 2 older practice guidelines by the Society of American Gastrointestinal and Endoscopic Surgeons and the American College of Gastroenterology[40,41] drafted in 2011 to 2012, while ignoring or dismissing subsequent comprehensive documents on POEM such as the Natural Orifice Consortium for Assessment and Research POEM White Paper[42] produced jointly by the Society of American Gastrointestinal and Endoscopic Surgeons and the ASGE with approval from the governing boards of both societies and the PIVI document[37] on POEM from the ASGE systematically reviewing POEM outcomes against standard therapies. It is also particularly vexing that the POEM policy seems to have been addended to a previous policy on GERD by adding the word dysphagia after "reflux" and tacking POEM to the end of a list of GERD-related procedures, including endoscopic antireflux procedures (see **Fig. 4**) that, unlike POEM, are substantially less effective than standard surgical therapy (Nissen fundoplication) with their minimal invasiveness being their main advantage over surgery. What is even more startling is that these endoscopic fundoplication procedures such as those performed with the Esophyx and MUSE devices will have a category I CPT code starting in 2016, whereas no such code is expected for POEM. This recent development probably attests to the importance of industry support in the complex process of applying for a CPT code. Nevertheless, with evidence rapidly accumulating in favor of POEM and POEM continuously gaining ground at the expense of LHM as a first-line therapy for achalasia, obtaining a CPT code is a matter of time. A collaborative initiative by the ASGE and the Society of American Gastrointestinal and Endoscopic Surgeons would be important in accelerating this process.

REFERENCES

1. Chandrasekhara V, Ginsberg GG. ESD for colorectal neoplasms: dissecting value from virtue. Gastrointest Endosc 2011;74(5):1084–6.
2. Stavropoulos SN, Modayil RJ, Friedel D, et al. The international per oral endoscopic myotomy survey (IPOEMS): a snapshot of the global POEM experience. Surg Endosc 2013;27:3322–38.
3. Stavropoulos SN, Harris MD, Hida S, et al. Endoscopic submucosal myotomy for the treatment of achalasia (with video). Gastrointest Endosc 2010;72:1309–11.
4. Patel KS, Calixte R, Modayil RJ, et al. The light at the end of the tunnel: a single-operator learning curve analysis for per oral endoscopic myotomy. Gastrointest Endosc 2015;81(5):1181–7.
5. Stavropoulos SN, Modayil RJ, Friedel D, et al. Natural orifice endoscopic surgery (NOTES) techniques for full thickness R0 endoscopic resection of deep seated subepithelial tumors (SETs): a single center experience. Gastrointest Endosc 2015;81(5):AB249–50.
6. Stavropoulos SN, Modayil RJ, Friedel D, et al. Endoscopic full-thickness resection for GI stromal tumors. Gastrointest Endosc 2014;80(2):334–5.
7. Stavropoulos SN, Widmer J, Kevin K, et al. Early experience with endoscopic submucosal dissection (ESD) for early mucosal neoplasms (EMNs) and subepithelial tumors (SETs) at a U.S. center. Am J Gastroenterol 2012;107(Suppl 1s):S781.
8. Stavropoulos SN, Ghevariya V, DeJesus D, et al. Prospective, randomized comparison of three endoscopic submucosal dissection (ESD) knives in an acute porcine model: results from a U.S. Center. Am J Gastroenterol 2012;107(Suppl 1s):S781.

9. Inoue H, Sato H, Ikeda H, et al. Per-oral endoscopic myotomy: a series of 500 patients. J Am Coll Surg 2015;221(2):256–64.

10. Enestvedt BK, Williams JL, Sonnenberg A. Epidemiology and practice patterns of achalasia in a large multi-centre database. Aliment Pharmacol Ther 2011;33(11): 1209–14.

11. Zhou PH, Yao LQ, Qin XY, et al. Endoscopic full-thickness resection without laparoscopic assistance for gastric submucosal tumors originated from the muscularis propria. Surg Endosc 2011;25(9):2926–31.

12. Inoue H, Ikeda H, Hosoya T, et al. Submucosal endoscopic tumor resection for subepithelial tumors in the esophagus and cardia. Endoscopy 2012;44(3): 225–30.

13. Xu MD, Cai MY, Zhou PH, et al. Submucosal tunneling endoscopic resection: a new technique for treating upper GI submucosal tumors originating from the muscularis propria layer (with videos). Gastrointest Endosc 2012;75(1):195–9.

14. Stavropoulos SN, Modayil R, Friedel D. Current applications of endoscopic suturing. World J Gastrointest Endosc 2015;7(8):777–89.

15. Ye LP, Yu Z, Mao XL, et al. Endoscopic full-thickness resection with defect closure using clips and an endoloop for gastric subepithelial tumors arising from the muscularis propria. Surg Endosc 2014;28(6):1978–83.

16. Khashab MA, Stein E, Clarke JO, et al. Gastric peroral endoscopic myotomy for refractory gastroparesis: first human endoscopic pyloromyotomy (with video). Gastrointest Endosc 2013;78(5):764–8.

17. Inoue H, Minami H, Kobayashi Y, et al. Peroral endoscopic myotomy (POEM) for esophageal achalasia. Endoscopy 2010;42:265–71.

18. von Renteln D, Inoue H, Minami H, et al. Peroral endoscopic myotomy for the treatment of achalasia: a prospective single center study. Am J Gastroenterol 2012;107(3):411–7.

19. Costamagna G, Marchese M, Familiari P, et al. Peroral endoscopic myotomy (POEM) for oesophageal achalasia: preliminary results in humans. Dig Liver Dis 2012;44(10):827–32.

20. Swanstrom LL, Kurian A, Dunst CM, et al. Long-term outcomes of an endoscopic myotomy for achalasia: the POEM procedure. Ann Surg 2012;256(4):659–67.

21. Inoue H, Tianle KM, Ikeda H, et al. Peroral endoscopic myotomy for esophageal achalasia: technique, indication, and outcomes. Thorac Surg Clin 2011;21(4): 519–25.

22. Minami H, Isomoto H, Yamaguchi N, et al. Peroral endoscopic myotomy for esophageal achalasia: clinical impact of 28 cases. Dig Endosc 2014;26(1): 43–51.

23. Chiu PW, Wu JC, Teoh AY, et al. Peroral endoscopic myotomy for treatment of achalasia: from bench to bedside (with video). Gastrointest Endosc 2013;77(1): 29–38.

24. Teitelbaum EN, Soper NJ, Santos BF, et al. Symptomatic and physiologic outcomes one year after peroral esophageal myotomy (POEM) for treatment of achalasia. Surg Endosc 2014;28(12):3359–65.

25. Sharata AM, Dunst CM, Pescarus R, et al. Peroral endoscopic myotomy (POEM) for esophageal primary motility disorders: analysis of 100 consecutive patients. J Gastrointest Surg 2015;19(1):161–70 [discussion: 170].

26. Stavropoulos SN, Modayil RJ, Brathwaite CE, et al. Outcomes of a 5-year, large prospective series of per oral endoscopic myotomy (POEM). Emphasis on objective assessment for GERD and luminal patency. Gastrointest Endosc 2015; 81(5S):AB118–9.

27. Familiari P, Greco S, Gigante G, et al. Gastroesophageal reflux disease after peroral endoscopic myotomy: analysis of clinical, procedural and functional factors, associated with gastroesophageal reflux disease and esophagitis. Dig Endosc 2015. http://dx.doi.org/10.1111/den.12511.

28. Novais PA, Lemme EM. 24-h pH monitoring patterns and clinical response after achalasia treatment with pneumatic dilation or laparoscopic Heller myotomy. Aliment Pharmacol Ther 2010;32(10):1257–65.

29. PF Crookes, Corkill S, DeMeester TR. Gastroesophageal reflux in achalasia. When is reflux really reflux? Dig Dis Sci 1997;42(7):1354–61.

30. Werner YB, Costamagna G, Swanström LL, et al. Clinical response to peroral endoscopic myotomy in patients with idiopathic achalasia at a minimum follow-up of 2 years. Gut 2015. http://dx.doi.org/10.1136/gutjnl-2014-308649.

31. Csendes A, Braghetto I, Burdiles P, et al. Very late results of esophagomyotomy for patients with achalasia: clinical, endoscopic, histologic, manometric, and acid reflux studies in 67 patients for a mean follow-up of 190 months. Ann Surg 2006; 243(2):196–203.

32. Kumagai K, Kjellin A, Tsai JA, et al. Toupet versus Dor as a procedure to prevent reflux after cardiomyotomy for achalasia: results of a randomised clinical trial. Int J Surg 2014;12(7):673–80.

33. Khajanchee YS, Kanneganti S, Leatherwood AE, et al. Laparoscopic Heller myotomy with Toupet fundoplication: outcomes predictors in 121 consecutive patients. Arch Surg 2005;140:827–33.

34. Rawlings A, Soper NJ, Oelschlager B, et al. Laparoscopic Dor versus Toupet fundoplication following Heller myotomy for achalasia: results of a multicenter, prospective, randomized-controlled trial. Surg Endosc 2012;26:18–26.

35. Simić AP, Radovanović NS, Skrobić OM, et al. Significance of limited hiatal dissection in surgery for achalasia. J Gastrointest Surg 2010;14(4):587–93.

36. Zurita Macías Valadez LC, Pescarus R, Hsieh T, et al. Laparoscopic limited Heller myotomy without anti-reflux procedure does not induce significant long-term gastroesophageal reflux. Surg Endosc 2015;29(6):1462–8.

37. ASGE PIVI Committee, Chandrasekhara V, Desilets D, et al. The American Society for Gastrointestinal Endoscopy PIVI (Preservation and Incorporation of Valuable Endoscopic Innovations) on peroral endoscopic myotomy. Gastrointest Endosc 2015;81(5):1087–100.e1.

38. Håkansson B, Montgomery M, Cadiere GB, et al. Randomised clinical trial: transoral incisionless fundoplication vs. sham intervention to control chronic GERD. Aliment Pharmacol Ther 2015;42(11–12):1261–70.

39. Kim HJ, Kwon CI, Kessler WR, et al. Long-term follow-up results of endoscopic treatment of gastroesophageal reflux disease with the MUSE™ endoscopic stapling device. Surg Endosc 2015. [Epub ahead of print].

40. Society of American Gastrointestinal and Endoscopic Surgeons, Stefanidis D, Richardson W, et al. SAGES guidelines for the surgical treatment of esophageal achalasia. Surg Endosc 2012;26(2):296–311.

41. Vaezi MF, Pandolfino JE, Vela MF. ACG clinical guideline: diagnosis and management of achalasia. Am J Gastroenterol 2013;108(8):1238–49 [quiz: 1250].

42. NOSCAR POEM White Paper Committee, Stavropoulos SN, Desilets DJ, et al. Per-oral endoscopic myotomy white paper summary. Gastrointest Endosc 2014;80(1):1–15.

Moving?

Make sure your subscription moves with you!

To notify us of your new address, find your **Clinics Account Number** (located on your mailing label above your name), and contact customer service at:

Email: journalscustomerservice-usa@elsevier.com

800-654-2452 (subscribers in the U.S. & Canada)
314-447-8871 (subscribers outside of the U.S. & Canada)

Fax number: 314-447-8029

Elsevier Health Sciences Division
Subscription Customer Service
3251 Riverport Lane
Maryland Heights, MO 63043

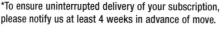

ELSEVIER

Printed and bound by CPI Group (UK) Ltd, Croydon, CR0 4YY

14/05/2025

01870847-0002